Make-up

artistry

for professional qualifications

Julia Conway

D0452396

www.heinemann.co.uk
✓ Free online support
✓ Useful weblinks
✓ 24 hour online ordering

01865 888058

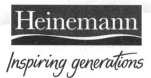

Heinemann

Inspiring generations

Heinemann Educational Publishers
Halley Court, Jordan Hill, Oxford OX2 8EJ
Part of Harcourt Education

Heinemann is the registered trademark of
Harcourt Education Limited

Text © Julia Conway, 2004

First published 2004

10 09 08 07 06 05 04
10 9 8 7 6 5 4 3 2 1

British Library Cataloguing in Publication Data is
available from the British Library on request.

ISBN 0 435 45330 0

Designed by Hardlines Ltd

Cover design by The Wooden Ark Studios

Printed in Spain by Edelvives

Cover photo: © Mark Tasker

Acknowledgments
Every effort has been made to contact copyright
holders of material reproduced in this book. Any
omissions will be rectified in subsequent printings if
notice is given to the publishers.

Unless otherwise stated, original illustrations
© Harcourt Education Limited, 2004

Artwork acknowledgments
The publisher would like to thank the following people
for contributing their artwork to this book:
Mark Barrett: page 83
Julia Conway: pages 78, 79, 85, 86, 180, 182, 215,
250, 254, 322, 335, 338, 344, 346, 348
Paul Conway: page 83
Amanda Duxbury: page 84
Louisa Morgan: pages 174, 339
Fern Raymond: pages 337, 352
Kristen Tunley: pages 84, 342, 349, 351

The publisher would also like to thank Elsevier for
providing permission to use images on pages 302,
303, 305, 306, 307, 328 and 333. These are
reprinted from *Wigs and Make-Up* by
Patsy Baker (1993).

Websites
There are links to relevant websites in this book. In
order to ensure that the links work, and that the sites
are not inadvertently linked to sites that could be
considered offensive, we have made the links
available on the Heinemann website at
www.heinemann.co.uk/hotlinks. When you access the
site, the express code is 3300P. Additional material is
also available on the Make-Up Artistry web pages.
Follow the links from
www.heinemann.co.uk/vocational.

Contents

Radbrook LRC

Foreword

The study of make-up is not simply a matter of knowing how to use cosmetics. Candidates study fashion and photographic make-up, cosmetic camouflage, body art, special effects, hairdressing and wig making and creation and design of prosthetics. These skills are built on a foundation of anatomy and physiology, basic design techniques and health and safety. Qualifications with make-up pathways include HABIA Level 3 Make-Up route, HABIA Advanced Practice Units, ITEC Fashion and Theatrical Make-up Diploma, VTCT Level 2 Certificate in Cosmetic Make-Up and Beauty Consultancy, VTCT Level 3 Diploma in Theatrical and Media Make-Up, Skill Set National Occupational Standards Hair and Make-Up, and BTEC National Certificate in Performing Arts. This book is designed to provide you with a realistic and comprehensive guide to accompany any training and study within the field of make-up artistry. It will provide you with a comprehensive, theoretical and practical reference guide, to help in you in your goal of becoming a professional make-up artist.

Features of the book

Information in this book is presented in a number of ways.

Remember boxes offer a guide to good practice, helping you to anticipate any problems that may arise. They cover health and safety matters as well as good professional working practice.

Key Notes highlight specific areas you need to pay attention to. These may be definitions of particular terms, or important facts you'll need to remember when working.

Step-by-Step guidelines break techniques down into manageable sections, giving you the opportunity to try out techniques for yourself.

Hands On activities let you start to become an artist. No two make-up artists work in the same way and these tasks will allow you to explore your own creativity and develop your individual style.

Knowledge Check questions at the end of each chapter let you test yourself on what you've learnt.

You can find additional resources on Heinemann's Make-Up Artistry website, by going to www.heinemann.co.uk/vocational and following the links.

A final word

The author has contributed her expertise and extensive knowledge in order to support you in your chosen studies and to help you to develop your interest in make-up artistry and its application in the fashion and media industries.

We hope that it will also be a reference book that you will find useful to dip into long after you have finished your qualification. Good luck!

Acknowledgements

I would like to thank everyone who has contributed to the production of this book, including a big thanks to:

* The team at Heinemann for their unstinting hard work and professionalism, with special thanks to Julia and Pen for their expertise and support always given with kindness – I have really enjoyed working with you both.

* To Jane, my photo researcher, for all her efforts and to Gareth and Tony for making the step-by-step photo shoot such good fun – the pics look great (and Tony, I think you should give serious consideration to growing a real one!)

* To Pilar and Alesha for their professionalism, enthusiasm and patience during the photoshoot – good luck in your careers.

* To Joanne Price for her contribution and assistance – you are a great make-up artist.

* To all the make-up artists and students who have contributed to the visual content of the book – you are all very talented.

* To all the photographers who have graciously allowed me to use their images. Mark Tasker – you are a star and possibly one of the nicest people I know! AJ – thank you for everything you have taught me about photography.

* To Angela (ADF Management, Manchester) for allowing me to use images of your beautiful models. Thanks for always thinking of me when opportunities arise.

* To South Trafford College for the wonderful training opportunities offered to me over the years.

* To Carolyn Cowan and Kathy Ducker for their inspirational contributions.

* To Shu Uemura for allowing me to use images of their products.

* To my family for their unquestioning support and love.

* To my friends for their support and enthusiasm.

* And finally to Paul, my husband and best friend – thank you for everything. And to Daisy, my daughter, who spent nine months in my belly with a laptop resting on her head. The pair of you make me very happy and I love you both very much.

Introduction

Chapter 1 Careers and opportunities in make-up artistry

Careers and opportunities in make-up artistry

A career in make-up artistry is based around the design and application of cosmetics, where cosmetics is taken in its broadest sense and may include many different types of materials applied to the body and hair.

The term 'cosmetics' or 'cosmetology' arises from the Greek word *kosmeetin*, which means to decorate. The use of cosmetics has always been part of human life: humans in primitive societies used natural pigments from the earth to create 'cosmetics' that were applied to the body as a form of decoration and were often used as part of rituals and ceremonies. This link between cosmetics and ceremony or performance has developed through history and has resulted in a career pathway for the media make-up artist.

Make-up artists usually work in one or more of the following main areas.

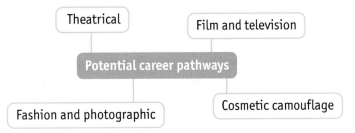

These main pathways can offer a number of specific routes:

* wigmaking and wigdressing
* theatre
* body art
* films
* television
* commercials
* music videos
* special effects
* animatronics
* editorial
* catwalk / runway
* bridal
* retail and demonstration work
* mortuaries
* model making, painting mannequins, Madame Tussauds
* teaching.

Working in theatre

Performers have always understood the use of make-up in transforming their appearance to portray different characters to the audience, and ensuring they are seen in large auditoriums. Ancient civilisations (Greek and Roman) used to perform in massive amphitheatres and used masks to help identify characters to the audience. Eastern theatre uses highly stylised make-up designs for the same purpose.

In Elizabethan England, a period when theatre reached new heights in popularity, actors often used crude forms of cosmetics from unusual sources, such as soot that was applied to define the eyes. But as stage lighting improved, a more subtle application of make-up was required, resulting in the invention of greasepaint in the 1860s, a form of which is still used in theatre today.

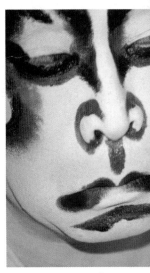

A Japanese actor in traditional Kabuki make-up

The role and responsibilities of the theatrical make-up artist

Make-up artists employed in the theatre must enjoy working with hair and postiche (wigs and facial hair) as this will make up a large proportion of their workload. Indeed, they are often referred to as **wig masters** or **wig mistresses**, heading a team of **wig dressers**, and are responsible for the postiche in a production and assisting the actors with applying their make-up. However, the actual responsibilities of the wig / make-up department will vary according to the size of production and production company. Nowadays, it is only the larger production companies that employ a wig master or mistress on a permanent basis; the rest of the team are hired freelancers who are usually employed on a casual or short-term contract basis.

For large productions, such as those found in London's West End theatres and in national opera houses, a make-up / wig designer will often work in collaboration with the director, costume designer and set designer. The wig master or mistress is then responsible for designing the make-up and wigs for the cast and implementing the designs. He or she will teach the cast members how to apply the make-up on themselves, leaving the wig / make-up team

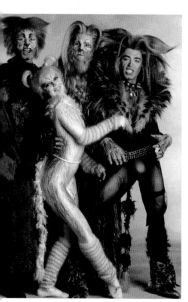

Some effects are applied by the actors themselves

free to care for and apply the postiche or hairstyles. However, exceptions may occur when special effect make-up techniques are required. In this case, a member of the team is designated this responsibility for the run of the production.

The roles and responsibilities of a theatrical make-up artist will vary according to their position within the department. A wide range of knowledge and skills are required if you wish to pursue a career in this area. For smaller productions, wig and make-up departments may combine these roles, for example the designer may also take on the role of wig master or mistress. You may start your career as an assistant wig dresser / make-up artist, which is the same as an apprentice. Please refer to the Make-Up Artistry website for an interview with the make-up artist Jo Price. You'll also find a detailed breakdown of different job roles and responsibilities for make-up artists.

Career considerations for theatre work

Working in theatre can be a thoroughly rewarding career choice for the make-up artist, but as in all careers there are certain aspects of the job to consider before deciding whether it may be right for you.

* You will probably be working irregular and unsocial hours. Most production runs will consist of evening and occasional matinee performances. As a wig dresser you will be required to arrive in plenty of time to prepare postiche and undertake any other duties delegated to you by the wig master or mistress prior to the start of the performance. You may also be the last to leave after the performance has finished, as postiche will need re-dressing and cleaning.

* Work can be irregular (unless you are lucky enough to gain employment on a long-running production) and you will probably find yourself working to short-term contracts.

* Unless you live near a big city (or near a large established theatre), you may have to travel to find regular work. In addition, sometimes you may find yourself working for companies that go on tour with productions – this is great if you like to travel, but if you have a family or other commitments this may be unsuitable for your lifestyle.

* Theatre work tends to be less well paid than the film and television or fashion industries.

However, work conditions tend to be better and more regulated as there is a stronger union influence in the theatrical world.

* Because each performance is 'live' there tends to be an exciting buzz behind the scenes. You will often be working under pressure: applying make-up and postiche on cast members when they turn up late for their calls, undertaking quick changes in the stage wings, ensuring the hairstyles and wigs are secure and remain intact throughout the live performance – responsibilities not for the faint hearted.

Working in film and television

When film technology was first introduced, the images were in black and white, the lighting crude and the moving images lacked the definition found on the big screen of today. This resulted in the faces and features of actors tending to look 'flat' on screen. The make-up artists of this time relied heavily on the principles of light and shade to counteract this effect, and literally used strong highlighting and shading techniques to sculpt the performers' faces.

It was the dramatic use of make-up on the early screen sirens, such as Theda Bara, that influenced the average woman to experiment with cosmetics. Bara's make-up artists created heavily darkened eyes, a pale complexion and a deeply stained mouth. It was a make-up designed to create drama and impact on the big screen, but it was soon imitated by fashionable women all over America. Around this time, a new type of semi-liquid make-up was created, especially for film, by a young make-up artist called Max Factor.

The importance of make-up within the film industry was suddenly taken far more seriously. The 1920s saw the emergence of the 'it' girls: Clara Bow and Louise Brooks became firm favourites with the public, who followed their lead by rimming their eyes with kohl, thinning their eyebrows and making small cupid bow shaped

mouths. Max Factor, along with many other make-up artists, continued to develop new cosmetics in response to demands from both actresses and the general public, and in the 1920s introduced the hugely popular 'Cake Make-up'. The world of the big screen had become irrevocably entwined with the world of cosmetics.

Improvements in cinematic technology continued: television was introduced, and cameras were able to pick up fine detail in close-up, so the techniques of make-up artists had to change to move with the times. But perhaps the biggest changes came with the invention of colour film. Make-up artists now had to deal with the problem of colour balance and correction as well as light and shade. Today's make-up artists face their own challenges, most recently the introduction of digital technology.

Roles and responsibilities of the film and television make-up artist

Today, make-up artists who work in film and television are required to master a wide variety of skills and undertake tasks that include designing and applying make-ups that change the appearance of actors so they look beautiful, ugly, old, inhuman, injured, etc. – the list goes on and on. Whilst completing these characterisations, the make-up artist is expected to work safely; exhibit excellent communication skills; be able to restore the skin to the condition prior to the application of cosmetics; and recreate the make-up to look exactly the same, day after day (continuity). In addition, with the exception of big budget productions, make-up artists are expected to be equally competent in hairstyling and wig dressing skills as in make-up application.

The roles and responsibilities of a film and television make-up artist will vary according to their position within the department. A wide variety of knowledge and skills are required if you wish to pursue a career in this area. Please refer to the Make-Up Artistry website for more information.

In addition, a hair or make-up department working on a production with large wig content may employ the services of a **wig specialist**. The sole responsibility of the wig specialist would be to maintain, dress and fit the wigs. A production with a need for complicated special effects may also hire a **prosthetic** or **special effect make-up artist** to make and fit prosthetic pieces.

On any production, there will usually be a regular team of people contracted to work within the hair and make-up department. For days with heavy schedules, additional assistants – referred to as 'daily' make-up artists – will be brought in on a casual basis.

Career considerations for film and television work

* In the UK, most television companies have significantly reduced the size and structure of their hair and make-up departments, preferring to employ make-up artists on a casual basis rather than offering them permanent contracts. The result of this move is that most make-up artists in film and television are freelancers. This makes their income unpredictable, but allows them the freedom to work for different production companies and undertake film work if desired. The film industry tends to offer work lasting several months at a time, involving incredibly long hours in a day and often six days a week.

* Working in film and television can be exciting and very rewarding – there is nothing quite as thrilling (or nerve-racking) as seeing your work projected onto a large screen. You will almost certainly get to travel and meet interesting people, and there is usually a strong team spirit amongst the crew on a production. You may even get to attend a few glamorous after-show parties!

* However, do not be fooled into thinking that being a make-up artist will lead to a life of glamour. Twelve-hour days (or more), six-day weeks, very early starts and working into the night are all quite normal. Travelling can sound appealing but the reality is often very different – you may be required to go to cold, unappealing places as well as hot, exotic locations. You may also be away from home for many weeks at a time, which will not suit everyone's lifestyle. In addition, you must be fit and healthy – working on an external shoot at 5am on a winter's morning is not unusual.

* The range of work in television and film is very varied: one day you may be applying conventional make-up and hairstyling to a newsreader, the next you may be required to age an artiste, recreate a period make-up, apply horrific casualty effects, create a tattoo or design an alien.

* Once established, pay for make-up artists working in film and television is generally good. Below are the guidelines as recommended by BECTU (Broadcasting, Entertainment, Cinematography and Theatre Union).

Please refer to the Make-Up Artistry website for an interview with the film make-up artist, Kathy Ducker.

Position	Rate of pay per day (8 hours)	Rate of pay per day (12 hours)
Junior make-up / hair assistant	£99	£173
Make-up / hair assistant	£113	£197
Make-up / hair artist	£130	£228
Animatronics technician	£139	£243
Make-up designer prosthetics	£149	£262
Chief make-up / hair designer	£169	£296

BECTU recommended minimum rates of pay 2003, based on a basic 40-hour week

Working in the fashion industry

During the 1920s, in response to consumer demands brought about by the development of motion pictures and the illustrated press, there emerged a new genre of photography, centred on images of fashion and glamour. This new genre brought together the interests of commercialism and art and gave photographers a chance to show their work to a more widespread audience. Early fashion photographers included Cheney Johnston, Platt-Lynes, Madam d'Ora and Cecil Beaton. Heavily influenced by art movements of this time, such as Art Deco and Surrealism, they transformed fashion into a world of theatrical showcases.

By the 1930s, the world of haute couture had reached new heights, increasing the popularity of the fashion magazine and giving status to the art of high fashion photography. By the 1950s, developments in printing technology had increased the circulation of fashion magazines, bringing fashion photography to all the social classes. Most fashion photographers were still creating images of austere models in luxurious settings, but there were two exceptions – Richard Avedon and Irving Penn, who developed a completely individual style of their own. Penn rejected luxurious settings for neutral backgrounds and Avedon's approach was based on the bizarre and unexpected.

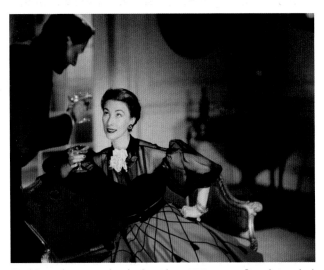

Fashion photography during the 1950s was often intended to be aspirational

The 1960s saw a social and cultural revolution, and fashion photography was not left out. Photographers such as David Bailey began to create images with a new, exciting vibe, often displaying sexual overtones, reflecting a new sense of freedom that emerged during this time. The 1960s also witnessed the emergence of the super model phenomenon – Twiggy became an iconic figure of this decade. Suddenly, the fashion industry was taking over from the movie industry and producing glamorous personalities that influenced and captured the imagination of the public.

The fashion image of the 1970s was heavily influenced by forms of sexual expression, sometimes producing shocking images that seemed to say less about clothes and more about a story or mystery behind the photograph. Helmut Newton was famous for his provocative images, often showing women as sexual aggressors. The 1980s saw an eclectic mix of styles, with designers such as Vivienne Westwood promoting a return to theatrical drama for the printed image and catwalk runways. The 1990s saw a return to the more natural image, with photographers such as Corinne Day taking fashion to a particularly unglamorous state. This continued with stylists, make-up artists and designers creating the much criticised 'heroin chic' style.

Today, the fashion image has been heavily influenced by the development of digital technology, taking visual imagery to a whole new level.

Roles and responsibilities of the fashion and photographic make-up artist

The fashion and photographic make-up artist is working in an ever changing and fairly aggressive industry and must therefore be ready to meet the challenges this presents. In addition to excellent application skills, they must not only be up to date with the latest fashion trends, but must be ahead of them. This means carrying out lots of research – reading cutting-edge fashion magazines, watching fashion shows and looking at the work of make-up artists at the top of their profession. They must also familiarise themselves with other design trends in areas such as interior design and art, as these will heavily influence ideas in contemporary fashion. The innovative and successful make-up artist will always need to keep an open mind and be ready to adapt and work with new ideas.

On a photographic shoot, the make-up artist will be required to work with some or all of the following people:

* photographer
* stylist
* models
* client, editor, designer or advertising agency
* art director
* hairdresser (on large budget shoots).

The client determines a brief and the creative parties – the photographer, stylist, hairdresser, make-up artist and sometimes the art director – discuss ideas and concepts. The storyboard, location, clothes, props and models are chosen and it is the role of the make-up artist to translate the original concept onto the face (and sometimes body) of the models.

HANDS ON

Start collecting images from 'underground' magazines. They may be a little more difficult to source (particularly if you do not live near a big city), but most newsagents will be able to order you copies and the visual imagery you will discover will be worth the extra effort. Magazines to look out for include: *The Face*, *i-D*, *Arena*, *Self Service*, *Spoon*, *Dutch* and *Tank*.

You may find yourself working in one of the following areas:

* editorial (shoots carried out for magazines)
* advertising (shoots carried out to promote a company image or product)
* fashion shows (also known as catwalk or runways – the show is in front of a live audience, and therefore has an element of theatre)
* catalogue (shoots to promote clothing ranges to a mass market)
* portrait (shoots photographing people, usually celebrities, for newspapers or magazines)
* glamour (shoots photographing models in the nude or wearing lingerie for the glamour industry).

A make-up artist wishing to work in fashion will sometimes begin his or her career assisting an established make-up artist, as this is a great way to develop skills and learn about the industry. Alternatively, you could start out working with other potential talent, building up a portfolio of images on test shoots. Tests are usually unpaid, but they are a great way of gaining experience and getting photographs of your work.

Career considerations for fashion and photographic work

* It may take up to two years to build your portfolio to a standard that will be acceptable by professional photographers and agencies. During these initial years, you will be working on test shoots for little or no money, therefore you will need to supplement your income. Many make-up artists starting out will also gain employment in retail and demonstration work – this enables them to build up their kit at reduced cost, and gives them lots of practice at making up lots of different faces.

* Most make-up artists will eventually work through agencies. With the right agent, this will open up possibilities of working with big commercial clients, but the agency will keep part of your fee as commission (20 per cent as a rough estimate).

* Even established make-up artists will spend a proportion of their week 'cold calling' or attending interviews. This involves visiting photographers and potential clients with their

portfolio, with the aim of securing jobs. When approaching these interviews the right attitude is vital – you may get knock-back after knock-back and it is important to remain enthusiastic and confident.

* Not all photographic shoots take place in the studio; many will take place on location, which may involve some travelling. When working on the major fashion shows, you may work in Paris, Milan, Madrid, London and New York.

* Personal presentation is vitally important when working in the fashion industry. Your choice of clothes and hairstyle will be noticed by others and will be taken as a reflection of your personal sense of style. There is also more awareness and 'snobbery' about brands of products you keep in your kit.

Working in retail

Retailing involves selling products and services to customers. It is a people-oriented business and it would be hard to find a profession that places a bigger emphasis on enthusiasm and communication skills. People with good attitudes and a willingness to be flexible and resourceful succeed in retail. Unless you are a buyer or promoter, you will not normally be required to travel. This means you'll have a good chance of being able to spend more time in your home environment than would be possible if you were working in the media. Retail also allows you to perfect your skills on people with different features, skin types and tones on a daily basis.

The daily activities of a retailer are more structured than those of make-up artists in other working environments. However, retailers often work long, irregular hours and since retail stores are usually open nights and weekends, some work schedules may be erratic. Starting salaries tend to be on the low side, but pay can increase as the individual moves into management.

Cosmetic houses such as Nars, Stila, Bobbi Brown, Benefit and MAC are great to work for because they are make-up rather than skin-care orientated. Because make-up artists founded them, they have a particularly creative approach. This kind of company prefers to employ staff that have had make-up rather than sales training, and show personality and creativity.

Many make-up artists begin their careers in retail on the shop floor. If you can work for a company that encourages career progression, from here you could progress to account manager and trainer. You may eventually end up working as a demonstrator, senior trainer or as a senior artist working on fashion shows and shoots as part of their creative development team and choosing next season's colours.

Other career options

Not everyone will be suited to life as a high profile make-up artist, travelling the world and spending days or weeks at a time away from home. Remember, you can create your own personal success in an environment that suits you. There are many career options that you could pursue following training as a make-up artist.

* retail and demonstration work
* mortuaries
* teaching
* cosmetic camouflage
* model making, painting mannequins, Madame Tussauds.

Qualities required of a make-up artist

In order to fulfil the role and responsibilities of a make-up artist successfully, you will need to possess the following personal qualities.

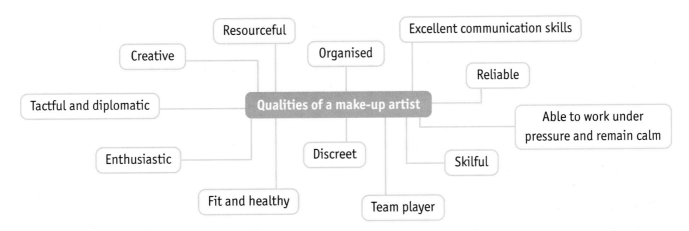

In addition to these personal qualities, you must also acquire a breadth of knowledge that extends past the obvious requirements of excellent application skills in hair and make-up, to include:

* lighting
* colour theory
* production and photographic processes
* contemporary and period imagery and styling
* theatre, film, photographic and art genres
* script analysis and breakdown
* research techniques
* health and safety
* budgeting and scheduling techniques.

Even with all the right personal qualities and acquired knowledge, there is no guarantee you will become a successful make-up artist. However, it will give you the best chance possible in a hugely competitive industry. What is also required, which no textbook or training programme can provide, is the right attitude for success: determination, perseverance and a passion for creating visual imagery with make-up and hair.

Routes into make-up artistry

You may already have a preference as to which area you think you may like to work in, for example fashion, but it is best not to narrow your options at this early stage. The field of make-up artistry is competitive and hard to break into (as are many rewarding careers), so the more skills you

acquire, the more jobs you will be able to accept with confidence. During the early stages of your career, you should be grabbing every opportunity with both hands. Even the most uninspiring jobs will lead to new contacts, and new contacts may eventually lead to that dream job. If you are offered work experience whilst training, make sure you take this valuable opportunity to practise your skills; whilst many colleges offer excellent training and facilities nowadays, nothing can compare with the experience of working in industry.

Suggested GCSEs and AS / A level subjects

Even if you are sure you would like to pursue a career in make-up artistry, it is important to keep your options as open as possible and study a range of subjects. The list below is not definitive and is in no particular order, but it may help with these important decisions:

* art
* history of art
* design-based subjects (for example photography)
* media / communication studies
* English literature
* history
* science (biology or chemistry when specialising at A level)
* a European language, for example French or Italian.

Studying an art or design-based subject is strongly advised. Most training organisations require a portfolio of artwork demonstrating creativity and artistic skills at interview.

Further education options

After GCSEs you can progress onto AS / A level study or you may prefer to pursue a technical qualification, provided by many local colleges. Suggested AS / A level subjects are listed above, and suggested technical programmes below. When non-art based subjects are studied, in addition to the academic qualification, a portfolio of artwork demonstrating a creative flair is usually required at interview in order to progress onto higher education. Technical programmes include the following:

* Art & Design Foundation Programme
* Advanced GNVQ in art and design subjects
* BTEC National Diplomas in related subjects (art, design, fashion or media studies)
* NVQ level 2 or 3 in related subjects (the above subjects or hairdressing or combined hair and beauty qualification)
* AVCE single or double award in a related subject.

Alternatively, there are a number of level 2 and 3 qualifications specialising in make-up design and application. Check with individual colleges for entry criteria. Awarding bodies offering these qualifications include:

* VTCT
* ITEC
* City and Guilds
* BTEC (EDEXCEL)
* SKILL SET (industry based).

Higher education options

Various options are available at higher education level. These courses, in make-up application and design, are available for prospective students aged 18 +. Check with educational establishments for entry criteria. Courses include:

* Foundation Degrees (Higher National Diplomas are currently being phased out and replaced by Foundation Degrees)
* BA (Hons)
* NVQ level 4.

Private and independent colleges

A number of independent, fee-paying colleges offer courses in make-up design. You will normally leave with a college certificate, the value of which will depend on the reputation of the college in question. If you decide this may be the route for you, make sure you research the college thoroughly before committing yourself.

Researching the right college

Before deciding on a college to study at, whether it is private or government funded, it is important to carry out some research.

* Check out the facilities, and attend an open day if possible.
* Check out the lecturers – what experience do they have?
* Check out what their past students are doing now.
* Do they offer work experience opportunities?
* Do they enter students into national competitions and if so, have they had any success?
* What qualifications will you achieve on successfully completing the course?

Apprenticeships

Specialised training and experience in industry is available, though positions are hard to secure. There are many more applicants than places for each intake so organisations can afford to be very choosy. Accepted starting points are candidates with academic qualifications to HND or degree level in art and design or related subjects (fashion studies, make-up design, beauty therapy, hairdressing, theatre craft). In addition to an academic qualification, a strong portfolio of work demonstrating art and design skills is usually required.

Mature students

The industry looks favourably on mature individuals, and most colleges will accept candidates with relevant experience who can demonstrate a strong creative flair and passion for visual imagery. Some colleges also offer access courses that prepare the student for entry into further and higher education programmes.

Useful addresses and contacts

UCAS (Universities and Colleges Admissions Service)
Rosehill
New Barn Lane
Prestbury
Cheltenham
GL52 3LZ

Skill Set
Prospect House
80–110 New Oxford Street
London
WC1A 1HB

FT2 – Film and Television Freelance Training
4th Floor, Warwick House
9 Warwick Street
London
W1R 5RA

BECTU (Broadcasting, Entertainment, Cinematography and Theatre Union)
111 Wardour Street
London
W1V 4AY

Follow the links from www.heinemann.co.uk/hotlinks to go to the websites of these organisations.

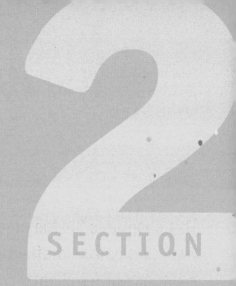

Building Blocks

Health and safety –
Reducing risks in the workplace

This chapter is fundamental to your training as a make-up artist. It will encourage you to work in a safe and effective manner and ensure the workplace is a secure and healthy environment for clients, colleagues and yourself.

Aim and objectives

Aim of this chapter: to provide you with the knowledge and understanding to ensure your own actions do not create health and safety risks and to enable you to identify hazards within the workplace, reducing risks with appropriate action.

You should achieve the following **objectives**:

* Discuss health and safety requirements, including relevant legislation and policies within the workplace
* Check your own working practices and work area for any risk to others and yourself
* Identify risks arising from hazards in your workplace
* Take appropriate action to reduce risks, i.e. safely deal with them yourself or report them to a 'responsible person'
* Follow appropriate steps and procedures when reducing health and safety risks yourself
* Carry out tasks safely and in accordance with legislation and workplace requirements
* Follow suppliers' and manufacturers' instructions for the safe use of equipment, materials and products

* Discuss the importance of personal presentation and conduct for maintaining standards of hygiene and safety in the workplace
* Follow recommended sterilising and hygienic procedures
* List statutory and other insurance considerations
* Maintain a make-up kit safely, securely and hygienically
* Follow basic first aid procedures
* Record accidents appropriately, and in line with current legislation
* Dispose of waste appropriately
* Discuss the importance of record cards and allergy tests
* Demonstrate a thorough awareness of contra-indications and contra-actions and appropriate action should they occur.

Hazard and risk

The Health and Safety Executive (HSE) is the body appointed by the government to enforce health and safety legislation. In reviewing this law, reference is frequently made to two terms: hazard and risk. It is important that you have a comprehensive understanding of what they mean.

Hazard	A hazard is something with potential to cause harm
Exposure	How many times a person (or persons) is exposed to the hazard
Risk	A risk is the likelihood, high or low, of someone being harmed by the hazard

Therefore,

hazard X exposure = risk

For example, a trailing lead from the plug of a piece of electrical equipment is a hazard. If the lead were trailing along the edge of a room, there would be less likelihood of someone tripping and falling than if it were placed across a doorway. Therefore the trailing lead across a doorway presents a high risk.

The main causes of accidents can be classified as:

Human – carelessness; improper behaviour; lack of training; poor supervision; tiredness

Environmental – faulty equipment; unattended equipment; inadequate ventilation; obstructions; overcrowded areas

Health and safety legislation

Health and safety laws aim to:

* protect a person's health, safety and welfare at work
* ensure an employer protects the health and safety of his or her employees, as far as is 'reasonably practicable'
* ensure employees look after themselves and others

* ensure any problems with regard to health and safety are discussed between employees and employers or safety representatives.

> **KEY NOTE**
>
> Acting as far as is 'reasonably practicable' means the employer has to balance the cost against the risk. However, HSE guidelines and legislation must be followed.

Health and Safety at Work Act 1974

This Act of Parliament is the main piece of legislation that most of the other regulations fall under. It affects employers, employees, the self-employed and anyone on work premises. Listed below are the key points of the Act.

In general the employer has a legal duty to:

* have a 'written safety policy statement' that includes the **organisation** of people and responsibilities and **arrangements** of systems and procedures for carrying it out if there are five or more employees; it is also the employer's responsibility to bring the policy to the attention of the employees, usually by displaying it in a prominent position
* ensure the workplace is safe and free from risks to health
* ensure work equipment is suitable, safe and properly maintained for use and that systems of work, as laid down in the policy statement, are followed
* ensure articles and substances are moved, stored, used and disposed of safely
* provide adequate welfare and first aid facilities
* provide adequate training, information and supervision to ensure the health and safety of employees and others.

Employees have a legal duty to:

* take reasonable care of their own health and safety, and that of others who may be affected by what they do, or do not do

Health and safety policy statement

Health and Safety at Work etc Act 1974

This is the Health And Safety Policy Statement of

(name of company)

Our statement of general policy is:

- to provide adequate control of the health and safety risks arising from our work activities;
- to consult with our employees on matters affecting their health and safety;
- to provide and maintain safe plant and equipment;
- to ensure safe handling and use of substances;
- to provide information, instruction and

- supervision for employees
- to ensure all employees are competent to do their tasks, and to give them adequate training;
- to prevent accidents and cases of work-related ill health;
- to maintain safe and healthy working conditions; and
- to revise this policy as necessary at regular intervals

Signed

(Employer)

Date   Review date

Infoline **08701 545500**   HSE website **www.hse.gov.uk**   HSE direct **www.hsedirect.com**

An example of a health and safety policy statement

* co-operate with supervisors and employers on health and safety issues

* correctly use equipment and items provided by the employer, in accordance with training and instructions

* not interfere with, or misuse anything provided for their health, safety and welfare

* report all health and safety concerns to an 'appropriate person'.

If you think there is a health and safety problem in your workplace you should first discuss it with an 'appropriate person' – this is usually your employer or manager. If there is a safety representative, you

may also wish to discuss it with him or her. If the employer then makes no attempt to reduce the risk and you feel they are not carrying out their legal duty, you could contact the enforcing authority, who may send health and safety inspectors with the power to enforce the law.

Health and Safety inspectors can enter any the premises without warning

Powers of Inspectors

They have the right to demand access to the entire premises

They can remove equipment or items for further examination

If an employer or employee has been found to put others in danger, he or she may face prosecution, even if it was not done on purpose. This may lead to unlimited fines or imprisonment.

Workplace (Health, Safety and Welfare) Regulations 1992

Employers must ensure that the workplace complies with the requirements set out in these regulations which cover:

* ventilation
* temperature
* lighting
* cleanliness
* waste materials
* room dimensions
* workstations and seating
* condition of the floor
* falls or falling objects
* transparent surfaces
* windows and sky lights
* doors and gates
* sanitary conveniences and washing facilities
* drinking water
* rest and changing facilities.

By law, the minimum temperature in the workplace should be 16°C (61°F). Although it is obvious that the workplace should not be too hot, there is currently no upper limit on temperature.

The following areas of the Act are particularly relevant to the make-up artist.

Spillages

Precautions should be taken to avoid spillages in the first place, but if they do occur, the following procedure is recommended.

Mark off the area with warning signs or cones to prevent an increased risk of slipping

⬇

Assess the spillage and take adequate measures to protect yourself, e.g. wearing gloves

⬇

If the spill is of hazardous material, follow COSHH or the manufacturer's instructions – if in doubt seek assistance

⬇

Clean the spillage as quickly as possible

⬇

Dispose of appropriately

⬇

Only remove cones or warning signs if the area is dry and does not pose a risk

The procedure for dealing with spillages

Waste disposal

Ordinary waste products, for example cotton wool, should be disposed of in a lined, covered bin, which is emptied regularly.

Hazardous waste, for example flammable chemicals and special effect products, should be disposed of according to COSHH guidelines and manufacturers' instructions. Do not empty waste down the sink until you have checked it is safe to do so.

Sharp waste, for example needles and broken glass, should be disposed of in a specially sealed, yellow 'sharps bin'.

Ventilation

Workplaces should be adequately ventilated so that hot or humid, stale air is replaced at a reasonable rate by fresh or purified air, and unpleasant smells are reduced. Windows or other openings usually provide sufficient ventilation. However, air exchange and movement may need to be increased during some procedures carried out by the make-up artist, particularly when using chemicals that create noxious fumes, such as making bald caps or airbrushing. It is well known that chemicals such as Acetone, Glatzan and cold and hot foams, which make-up artists cannot avoid coming into contact with, are harmful to health. Manufacturers recommend that make-up artists should only work with such substances in well-ventilated rooms. This may rely on additional mechanical (extractor fans) or air-conditioned (involving filters) ventilation, or exhaust systems being in place.

Short-term effects from noxious fumes can include: headaches, dizziness, palpitations, breathing difficulties, nausea, fainting or tiredness. Long-term effects may lead to more serious, chronic conditions.

Electricity at Work Regulations 1989

Electric shocks can cause severe injuries, even fatal ones. Faulty electrical equipment or misuse of equipment can lead to fires that may also cause damage and injury or death. The Electricity at Work Regulations are concerned with the safe use of electricity in the workplace. They require employers to:

* organise the inspection by a '*competent* person' of all electrical equipment, called PAT testing, on a regular basis (at least once a year)

* ensure that equipment is in safe working order

* keep a record of tests for inspection purposes to include dates, repairs, serial numbers, name and signature of competent person.

It is the responsibility of all employees to co-operate with their employer in complying with the regulations.

> **KEY NOTE**
>
> A 'competent person' does not necessarily refer to a qualified electrician, although this is generally the preferred option, but the person must be capable of performing basic safety checks.

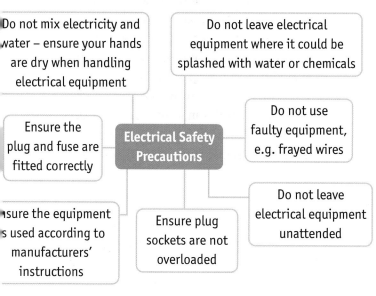

Do not mix electricity and water – ensure your hands are dry when handling electrical equipment

Do not leave electrical equipment where it could be splashed with water or chemicals

Electrical Safety Precautions

Ensure the plug and fuse are fitted correctly

Do not use faulty equipment, e.g. frayed wires

Ensure the equipment is used according to manufacturers' instructions

Ensure plug sockets are not overloaded

Do not leave electrical equipment unattended

Manual Handling Operations Regulations 1992

Manual handling is the moving or carrying of loads by hand or using bodily force. Many people injure themselves by lifting everyday loads; indeed, one of the main reasons for absences from work is back problems. Problems may arise for the make-up artist when moving or lifting equipment and stock.

Repetitive strain injuries are upper limb disorders caused by repetitive movements carried out in awkward postures over a length of time. These injuries can cause muscular aches and pains, which if not properly managed may lead to more serious, chronic conditions.

Most injuries associated with manual handling can be avoided with adequate training and the provision of suitable lifting equipment. These regulations require employers to:

* take appropriate steps to reduce the risk of injury that could be caused to employees by the manual handling of loads

* inform employees of any risks when handling loads and how best to avoid such risks.

Control of Substances Hazardous to Health Regulations 2002 (COSHH)

Many people are exposed to hazardous substances at work. Make-up artists will come across many chemicals and substances that, if used incorrectly, could be hazardous. Hazardous substances may

> **KEY NOTE**
>
> More than one-third of all injuries requiring the person to be absent from work for three days or more that are reported each year to the HSE and local authorities are the result of manual handling.

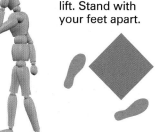

1 Think about the lift. Where is the load to be placed? Do you need help? Are handling aids available?

2 Get ready to lift. Stand with your feet apart.

3 Bend the knees. Keep the back straight. Tuck in your chin. Lean slightly forward over the load to get a good grip.

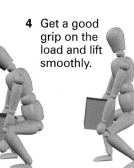

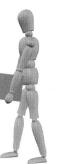

4 Get a good grip on the load and lift smoothly.

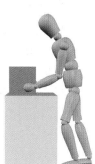

Manual handling techniques

come in the form of dust, fumes, chemicals and bacteria. They can be a hazard to health by:

* inhalation (breathing them in)
* direct contact (with skin or eyes)
* ingestion (swallowing them).

Illness or death may occur if exposure is not prevented or managed appropriately: cancer, asthma, infection and dermatitis can all be caused by contact with hazardous substances. To prevent illness of employees and clients, the law requires employers to control exposure to these substances in the workplace by ensuring that a systematic approach is taken to identify precautions that can be taken to control the risks. The HSE recommends the following eight steps:

STEP 1: Assess the risks

STEP 2: Decide what precautions are needed

STEP 3: Prevent or adequately control exposure

STEP 4: Ensure that control measures are used and maintained

STEP 5: Monitor the exposure

STEP 6: Carry out appropriate health surveillance

STEP 7: Prepare plans and procedures to deal with accidents, incidents and emergencies

STEP 8: Ensure employees are properly informed, trained and supervised

Eight steps of controlling risk

Safety warning symbols

Under the **Chemicals (Hazard Information and Packaging for Supply) Regulations (CHIP)**, substances or mixtures of substances classified as dangerous to health must have warning symbols on their containers, indicating COSHH is relevant when used in the workplace. Where no symbol is present, COSHH will not apply to its use. Suppliers

of substances affected by COSHH must provide a safety data sheet for the substances.

Chemicals used by a make-up artist

Make-up artists use a number of chemicals that should be safe if used correctly. The following safety guidelines should help to prevent accidents.

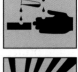 (a) Corrosive

 (b) Explosive

 (c) Harmful

 (d) Highly flamm...

 (e) Irritant

 (f) Oxidizing

 (g) Toxic

* Follow the manufacturers' instructions exactly.
* Wear protective garments and gloves where indicated.
* Maintain a high standard of hygiene in the workplace.
* Never mix products unless the manufacturer recommends this.
* Check that containers not in use are properly sealed.
* Make sure unused mixtures and empty containers are disposed of carefully.
* Make sure all stock is properly rotated and never allowed to deteriorate.

COSHH symbols

* Only store chemicals in labelled, appropriate containers.
* Keep aerosols away from naked flames or sources of heat.
* If there are any signs of abrasion or soreness on a client, do not use any product on that area.
* Keep all products out of reach of children.

Personal Protective Equipment at Work Regulations 1992

Prevention or control of the use of hazardous substances is always preferable. However, it may not always be possible to deal with these risks without the use of personal protective equipment (PPE). It may sometimes be necessary to protect employees' health by issuing protective clothing such as overalls, aprons, masks, eye goggles, gloves or footwear. Examples of when this may be necessary for a make-up artist include:

* when making prosthetics
* when carrying out procedures using hazardous chemicals
* when prolonged and frequent use of non-hazardous products can cause irritation.

Reporting of Injuries, Diseases and Dangerous Occurrences Regulations (RIDDOR) 1995

Reporting accidents and work-related ill health is a legal requirement. These regulations cover employees and clients who suffer injury or illness at the workplace, including freelance and mobile work situations. They state that the enforcing authority (the local authority or HSE) should be contacted immediately and a written report sent within ten days.

The HSE also considers it good practice for businesses to keep an 'accident book'. This is especially important in cases where the parties involved may consider suing. The accident book should contain the following information:

* date, time and place of the incident
* name and job of the injured person
* details of the illness or injury and what first aid was given
* whether the person then continued work, was taken to hospital and so on.

These details, signed and dated by the appointed person or first-aider, should be kept for three years.

ACCIDENT REPORT FORM

SECTION 1 PERSONAL DETAILS

Full name of first aider/staff member: _____

Position held in salon: _____

Date: _____

Accident (injury) ☐ Incident (illness) ☐

Time and date of accident/incident: _____

Full name of injured/ill person: _____

Staff member ☐ Client ☐ Other ☐

Address: _____

Tel. no: _____

SECTION 2 ACCIDENT/INCIDENT DETAILS

Describe what happened. In the case of an accident, state clearly what the injured person was doing. _____
_____

Name and address/tel. no. of witness(es), if any: _____
_____

Action taken

Ambulance called ☐   Taken to hospital ☐   Sent to hospital ☐   First aid given ☐

Taken home ☐   Sent home ☐   Returned to work ☐

SECTION 3 PREVENTATIVE ACTION

Preventative action implemented ☐

Describe action taken: _____
_____

Date implemented: _____

Signature of first aider/staff member: _____

Signature salon manager/owner: _____

Date: _____

An accident report form

Health and Safety (First Aid) Regulations 1981

This legislation sets out essential first aid requirements for the workplace and ensures injured parties receive immediate attention and that an ambulance is called in serious cases. It requires that adequate equipment and facilities are available for first aid to be given. Specific requirements will vary according to individual circumstances, but the minimum requirements for any workplace are:

* a suitably stocked first aid box
* an 'appointed person' to take charge of first aid arrangements.

KEY NOTE

An appointed person is someone who can take charge of an emergency situation should the need arise. An appointed person is ideal for small businesses or as a back up for more qualified first aiders. An appointed person should not attempt to carry out any first aid procedures he or she has not been trained in.

Contents of a first aid box in a workplace with five employees

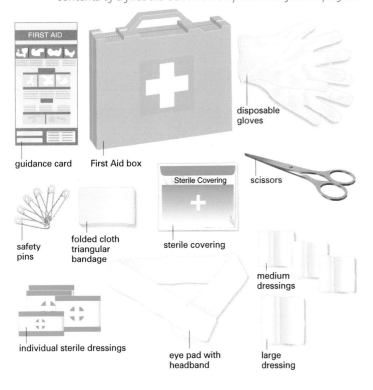

guidance card   First Aid box

FIRST AID

disposable gloves

safety pins

folded cloth triangular bandage

Sterile Covering

sterile covering

scissors

individual sterile dressings

eye pad with headband

medium dressings

large dressing

A first aid kit must be provided in the workplace but there is no standard list of items that it should contain. Requirements will depend on the assessment of the workplace needs. The box should be easily recognisable and should be green with a white cross. It should be kept in an accessible place, preferably near to hand-washing facilities. All employees should be aware of where the first aid box is kept so they can easily locate it in an emergency.

There should be no drugs or medicines in the first aid kit.

First aid procedures

There are no legal requirements with regard to the number of first aiders or appointed persons in the workplace but it is important that employees are aware of who the nominated persons are and how they can be contacted. The responsibilities of a first aid representative will depend on their level training.

Training for 'appointed person' HSE approved certificates includes:	Training for 'first aider at work' HSE approved certificates includes:
Accident prevention	Accident prevention
Initial assessment	Management of incidents
Wounds	Resuscitation
Identification of conditions	Treatment of shock
Priorities of first aid	Treatment of heart attack
Emergency procedures	Dressings
	Burns
	Priorities of first aid
	Control of bleeding
	Fractures
	Record keeping

Only trained personnel, who have an up-to-date first aid at work certificate approved by the HSE, should carry out first aid. Certificates are currently valid for three years at a time.

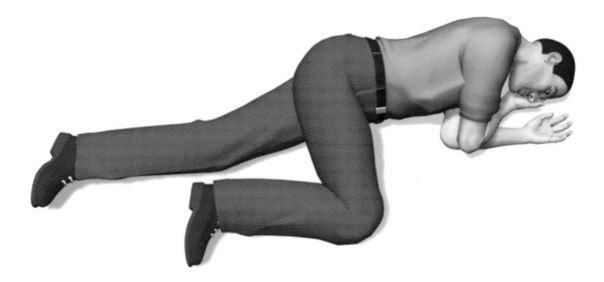

The recovery position

The Fire Precautions (Workplace) Regulations 1997

With the introduction of the Fire Precautions (Workplace) Regulations, which came into force on 1 December 1997, the employer is required to assess:

* what the fire safety risks are
* how serious the risk of fire is
* what, if anything, needs to be done.

The employer should establish a written programme to address fire hazards and preparation for emergencies, ensuring that all employees understand basic emergency action plans including alarms, emergency shutdown, evacuation routes and assembly areas. As a minimum, annual emergency drills should be carried out to test the effectiveness of the emergency action plan. Emergency alarms, exit doors, emergency lighting and other equipment must be inspected on a regular basis. Exits must be clearly illuminated, identified and accessible at all times and every employee must have access to two or more exits. All exits should give onto a clear and unobstructed pathway, and barriers should not obstruct persons from exiting the building.

Basic fire prevention

Fire relies on the following:

$$\text{oxygen} \times \text{fuel} + \text{ignition} = \text{fire}$$

Fuel is anything that burns: paper, wood, chemicals, etc. Ignition may occur from electrical sparks, chemical reactions or excessive heat sources. Removing one of the above elements from the equation will prevent fires from occurring. Following sensible fire precautions will reduce the risk of fire.

* COSHH guidelines should be followed and control measures should be put in place.
* Waste should be disposed of appropriately and regularly.
* Electrical equipment must be in good working condition and checked regularly.
* Electrical equipment should not be left on unattended.
* Plug sockets should not be overloaded.
* Electric fans and heaters should be placed in safe positions.
* Smoking should only be permitted in designated safe areas.

✳ Flammable products should be stored according to COSHH and local regulations. This usually involves a lockable, metal cabinet, labelled with safety symbols.

Use of extinguishers

When there is no immediate danger, as in the case of a very small fire, fire extinguishers may be used to put the fire out. At least two persons should be present and their safety must not be endangered. Remember even small fires spread rapidly and may produce smoke and fumes that can quickly overcome individuals. It is important that the correct extinguisher is used for the type of fire that has broken out. All fire extinguishers are red, but a coloured band near to the top indicates their contents and use. They should be maintained regularly and located at appropriate points.

Content	Coloured band	Used on
Dry powder	Blue	Wood, paper, textiles, fabrics, burning liquid, electrical fires and flammable liquids
Carbon dioxide (CO$_2$)	Black	Burning liquid, electrical fires and flammable liquids
Water	Red	Wood, paper, textiles, fabrics
Foam	Cream or yellow	Burning liquid

Other ways of extinguishing fire

Fire blankets can be wrapped around a person whose clothes are on fire. Care must be taken not to 'flap' the blanket as this will flare the flames. Sand can be used to soak up flammable spillages. Remember, if in doubt, evacuate the area and call 999.

Fire evacuation procedures

Raise the alarm.

↓

Call 999 and request the fire brigade.

↓

Close the windows, switch off equipment and lights, close the door behind you.

↓

Evacuate the building by the nearest exit as quickly as possible. Do not use the lifts.

↓

Assemble at the designated meeting point.

↓

Inform the fire brigade if anyone is trapped in the building.

↓

Do not re-enter the building until you have been told it is safe.

What to do if you discover a fire

Cosmetic Products (Safety Regulations) 1996

These regulations are part of the consumer protection legislation that sets strict guidelines affecting the packaging and composition of

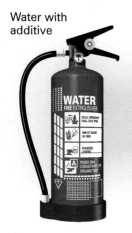

Water with additive

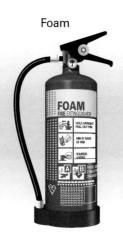

Foam

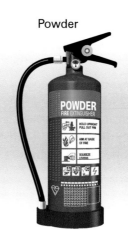

Powder

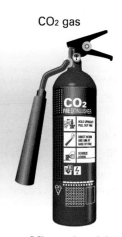

CO$_2$ gas

Types of fire extinguisher

cosmetic products. The following information should be marked on the container or packaging and sometimes both:

* name and address of manufacturer
* best before date (where necessary)
* product's function (where necessary)
* specific information and precautions
* ingredients, listed in descending order of quantity
* batch identification.

Where this is impractical, a leaflet should be enclosed or attached to the product, and the consumer informed of its presence on the container or packaging.

> **KEY NOTE**
>
> Further information regarding health and safety legislation can be found by following the links to the HSE website from www.heinemann.co.uk/hotlinks.

Workplace policies

In addition to statutory legislation, there may also be procedures and rules to follow that are laid down by individual work establishments. These often share the industry's suggested code of conduct guidelines and ensure a consistent, effective approach to health and safety throughout the department. Workplace policies will often relate to:

* sterilisation and hygiene
* preparation of the model or client
* record cards
* maintenance of stocks
* disposal of waste
* safety procedures.

Sterilisation and hygiene

Terminology

Healthy and hygienic working conditions are very important and should always be of the highest standard to ensure a safe environment for everyone involved.

Below are some terms you may come across when considering sterilisation and hygiene.

Sterilise	To make free from all living micro-organisms, to make sterile. It is an absolute term – an object is either sterile or not.
Sanitise	To inhibit growth of micro-organisms, to maintain or improve conditions with regard to dirt and infection.
Septic	Contaminated by bacteria and other micro-organisms.
Aseptic	Free from bacteria and other micro-organisms.
Disinfectant	A chemical agent capable of destroying most micro-organisms to a level where they are not harmful to health.
Antiseptic	A chemical agent that inhibits growth and multiplication of micro-organisms.
Bactericide, fungicide, virucide	A chemical agent that kills specific types of infection, i.e. bactericide kills bacteria, fungicide kills fungi and virucide kills viruses.
Cross-contamination	The spread of infectious or non-infectious organic matter from one person to another, a person to an object or vice-versa.
Cross-infection	The spread of infectious organic matter as above.

Basic bacteriology

Lack of cleanliness can lead to the spread of:

Bacterial infections	Minute, single-celled organisms found nearly everywhere. There are two general types of bacteria: non-pathogenic, which are harmless to humans, and pathogenic, which are harmful and cause disease such as respiratory diseases and skin infections like impetigo.
Virus infections	Organisms smaller than bacteria. Viruses can only live and reproduce

	within living cells. They are able to cause disease, e.g. hepatitis, influenza, herpes simplex (cold sores).
Fungal infections	Spongy, yeast growth, very contagious, e.g. tinea (ringworm).
Insect infestations	Head lice is the most common, also scabies, caused by female itch mite burrowing under the epidermis and laying her eggs.

Bacteria and viruses enter the body in the following ways:

* by inhalation (airborne)
* by ingestion (via the mouth)
* by direct contact (via cross-contamination, from another person or object)
* in the blood stream (via contaminated sharps material).

In the make-up studio, infection may occur when dirty equipment is used or a make-up artist works unhygienically.

Avoiding cross-infection

When discussing acceptable methods for effectively cleaning equipment used by make-up artists, it is important to recall the definitions of the terms sterile, sanitise and disinfect. It is very difficult to sterilise much of the equipment used in this industry, as professional sterilising equipment requires heating items to over 120°C. However, sterilisation is essential when equipment is contaminated with blood or bodily fluids, as may happen with tweezers. It is generally accepted that where sterilisation is not possible, make-up artists should follow aseptic procedures by cleaning and disinfecting equipment to reduce the risk of cross-infection to a minimal level.

There are a number of different ways to clean make-up equipment to avoid cross-infection. The method you choose will depend on the piece of equipment in question.

Methods of sterilisation, sanitation and disinfection

Whatever method of sterilisation, disinfection or sanitation is being used, it is important to physically clean contaminated equipment first to remove any residual material that may prevent the penetration of steam or chemicals to the contaminated surface.

Steam or wet heat (autoclave)

This method uses steam or wet heat to sterilise. It requires temperatures of between 121 and 134°C. A container known as an autoclave sterilises using this method. It is particularly suitable for small pieces of metal equipment such as tweezers and scissors.

Chemicals and alcohols

Many products are available, with various trade names, to disinfect equipment and surfaces. Many of these products are based on two alcohols – ethyl and isopropyl, which are diluted to varying strengths. Surgical spirit is the most common form of ethyl alcohol. These products have bactericidal properties but their virucidal effect is limited and variable. However, HIV is likely to be destroyed. According to their dilution, they can be used to sanitise the skin prior to treatment and to wipe non-sterilisable plastics such as make-up chairs. Hibitane (a form of chlorhexidine) is a product that has good anti-bacterial properties and some virucidal effects. It is available in a form called 'Hibiscrub' that can be used to sanitise the hands. Barbicide is a registered hospital disinfectant that is bactericidal, fungicidal and virucidal, and kills HIV, herpes, tinea and numerous other pathogenic organisms. Metals can be immersed without fear of rusting. It is also biodegradable.

Ultraviolet (UV) radiation

UV radiation is classed as a sanitiser, as it is only effective against a limited range of organisms. Objects must be turned to ensure UV rays penetrate the entire surface. Even then effectiveness may be limited by dust on the surface. However, UV cabinets are useful for storing sterilised equipment prior to use.

Brush cleaners

Brush cleaners remove cosmetic residue, grease and oil from brushes. Many products will also disinfect at the same time, whilst conditioning the brush hairs to keep them supple.

Methods for cleaning specific tools

Method 1: Wash in warm soapy water, rinse and immerse in barbicide solution for recommended time. Rinse well. Place in UV cabinet until ready for use.
Suitable for: sectioning clips, combs

Method 2: Wash out with barbicide solution. Rinse well.
Suitable for: water sprays

Method 3: Wipe clean with alcohol or a sterile wipe. Sterilise in autoclave. Place in UV cabinet until ready for use.
Suitable for: scissors, tweezers

Method 4: If unsuitable for cleaning, dispose of item.
Suitable for: sponges, heavily soiled powder puffs

Method 5: Wash in washing machine at 60°C. Tumble dry on hot cycle.
Suitable for: lightly soiled powder puffs, towels, head bands, make-up gowns

Method 6: Remove excess cosmetics on a tissue. Use a professional brush-cleaning product, which cleans and disinfects.
Suitable for: make-up brushes

Necessary hygienic and safety precautions for the make-up artist

The working environment

* The make-up room should be well lit and at a comfortable working temperature.
* The floor should be easily washable and have a non-slip surface.

* Worktops, trolleys and chairs should be wiped down frequently with a disinfecting fluid such as surgical spirit.
* Mirrors should be clean. Wipe them over with a suitable glass cleaner.
* A bin should be placed by the sink area and preferably at each workstation. The bins should be lined, have a lid and be emptied regularly. They should never be allowed to overflow.
* The make-up room should be a non-smoking zone.
* The room should have plenty of electrical plug sockets, but located away from water supplies and chemical storage.
* Products and equipment should preferably be stored in cupboards rather than on shelves. This will protect them against dust and light. Heavy or frequently used objects should be placed at a low level and be easily accessible.
* The make-up chair should be comfortable and provide good support for the client. Ideally it should possess the following qualities: adjustable height, reclining back, adjustable headrest, footrest.

Personal hygiene and conduct

* Hair should be clean. Long hair should be worn off the face so it does not dangle in the client's face.
* Clean clothes should be worn.
* Strong perfumes or aftershave should be avoided.
* Nails should be short and clean. Polish should not be worn, as some clients may be sensitive to it.
* Jewellery, particularly rings and bracelets, should not be worn as they may scratch or irritate the client.
* The make-up artist's hands should be cleansed before each client with a suitable hand wash, for example Hibiscrub.

* Wounds and open sores on the make-up artist's hands should be covered with a suitable waterproof dressing.

* Good oral hygiene is important, particularly if you are a smoker or have eaten strongly flavoured food the night before.

* Chewing gum whilst working should be avoided.

* Low or flat heels should be worn for safety and to encourage good posture.

* Always follow legislative and workplace rules and regulations.

Preparing the model or artiste

* Check the client is comfortable, and the client's neck, back and feet are supported.

* Continue to check that they remain comfortable throughout the procedure. If they are required to be in make-up for a long period of time, ensure they have frequent short breaks and have access to refreshments.

* Ask the client to remove any jewellery, contact lenses or eyeglasses as appropriate. The client should look after these items. Do not put them in your own pockets, as this could lead to a difficult situation if they are forgotten.

* Gowns should be used to protect the client against accidental spillages and make-up products soiling their clothes. Clean towels or gowns must be used for each client. Disposable gowns are useful when making up large numbers of extras. Costume lines around the neck can be given extra protection by placing tissues around this area.

* Ensure the client's hair is protected. If you use a headband, ensure it is clean, and do not make it too tight as it may mark the client's skin. It may also cover the skin around the hairline, so make sure you do not forget to blend any bases up to the hairline if it is hidden. It is important to dress the hair flat, otherwise the front hairline will stand on end once the band is removed. Often the preferable option is to use

clips to secure hair away from the face. The clips may be wrapped with tissue to prevent marking the hair.

Posture and client positioning

The make-up artist will spend a large proportion of the day on his or her feet and therefore consideration should be given to correct posture. Poor positioning of either the client or the operator could result in tense muscles, stiff joints, trapped nerves and back problems. Most make-up artists prefer to work from the same side of the client as their working hand. It is useful to become accustomed to working from one side of the client for most make-up procedures, particularly when working in a confined area. However, it is important not to stretch or lean across the client and the make-up artist's weight should always remain evenly distributed between both feet. This may mean temporarily turning the make-up chair to face the operator during application. To avoid bending unnecessarily, the make-up chair should be adjusted to a suitable height for the make-up artist. Finally, **never** lean on the client's head – if you need to steady yourself, use the headrest.

Working procedures

* Worktops should be disinfected and covered with paper roll. Products and equipment, such as sponges and powder puffs, should be placed on the paper in a logical working order. Try to ensure you have everything you require for the entire procedure.

* Equipment should be sterilised or disinfected as appropriate before use and between clients.

* Products should never be placed towards the front of the worktop as they may be accidentally knocked over and may spill over the client, equipment or the floor.

* Waste must be disposed of appropriately and not be left lying around on the worktop.

* Lids should be kept on jars and bottles to prevent spillage and contamination.

* Spatulas must be used to remove creams from containers – never dip fingers into containers. Make-up can then be transferred from the applicator to the client's skin and back to the palette without risking cross-contaminating the product in the container.

* Loose powders should be shaken onto a tissue – never dip a brush directly into the container.

* Eye and lip pencils should be sharpened before and after use with a metal sharpener that can be easily sterilised.

* Mascara should be applied with disposable mascara wands, unless it is being used exclusively on one client, in which case, the brush it comes with can be used.

* Brushes should be disinfected between clients. Where large numbers of artistes are being made up, disposable brushes are invaluable.

* Extra care should be taken with clients wearing contact lenses, particularly when applying powder products around the eyes.

* Apply barrier cream when using known irritants such as skin adhesives and latex.

* Keep your work area clean and tidy as you are working. Do not spread your equipment on to the workstation next to you; this will make you unpopular with neighbouring colleagues.

Maintenance of your kit

Most make-up artists work from a make-up kit; if it is disorganised, dirty and poorly maintained this will be seen as a reflection of their professionalism. It is important to keep the kit clean, both internally and externally; products and equipment should be cleaned and disinfected before being placed in the kit. In addition to hygiene, make-up artists should also give consideration to the weight and bulkiness of the kit, which they will have to transport around. There are many make-up boxes available to purchase, some of them very expensive and heavy. However, a lightweight toolbox from a DIY store

offers an excellent, affordable alternative. Unless you are intending to fly abroad with your kit, a heavy metal case is usually unnecessary. Always pick up and examine a box before purchasing it. If it feels heavy and bulky now, consider how heavy it will be when filled with products.

Thought should also be given to the containers in which products are stored: larger bottles of products such as cleaners, moisturisers and surgical spirit can be dispensed into smaller containers so they are easier to carry. It is essential to label them appropriately, including safety symbols if applicable. Also ensure you use the correct type of containers; some chemicals will 'melt' plastics and in these cases glass bottles should be used. Many make-up artists also choose to transfer products such as lipsticks into more practical containers. You can purchase empty paint palettes from art shops; lipsticks can then be crushed into the palettes, allowing easy access and viewing of the colours. It is also advisable to have a kit that is lockable for security.

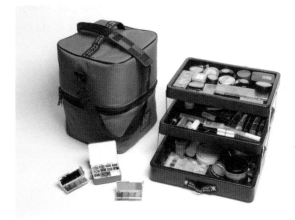

A make-up kit and practical lipstick container

Most cosmetics have a long shelf life. However, if used unhygienically there is a risk of contamination from bacteria, which will reduce the lifespan of even the most stable of products. Stable products are 'dry' cosmetics such as pressed powders; products most susceptible to contamination are those using cream formulations, such as lipsticks and cleansers. When a product starts to separate or discolour, lose its fragrance, or harden, it has probably outlived its shelf life. The following guidelines will ensure products are kept in optimum condition.

* Keep products in a cool, dry environment out of direct sunlight, and ensure that containers are airtight. Heat, light and moisture all have a damaging effect on cosmetics, and all cosmetics are subject to oxidisation (contamination from oxygen in the air).

* Lids should always be replaced directly after use to prevent contamination.

* Always dispense and apply products in a hygienic manner.

* Throw out anything from your kit that is past its shelf life. If products are out of date, they are more likely to cause reactions on clients.

Security in the workplace

It is wise to take precautions against theft within the make-up studio. Make-up kits and studio stock are particularly vulnerable when working in busy environments or on location. Follow the guidelines outlined below to avoid becoming a victim of crime.

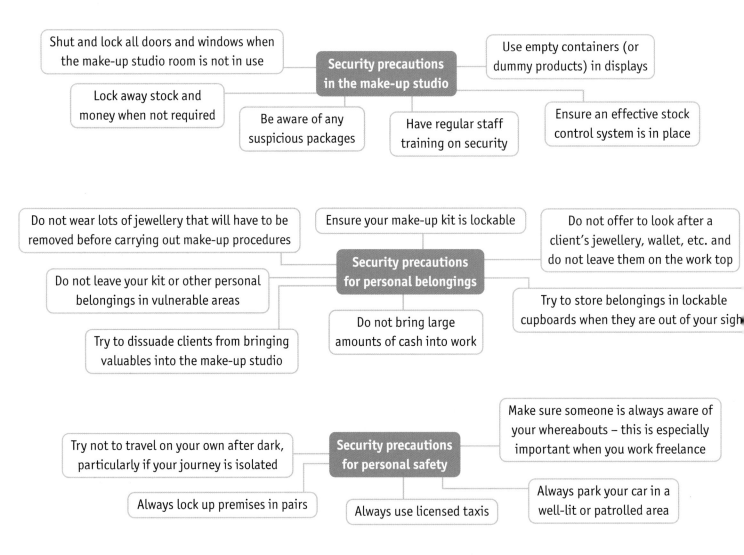

Shut and lock all doors and windows when the make-up studio room is not in use

Lock away stock and money when not required

Be aware of any suspicious packages

Security precautions in the make-up studio

Have regular staff training on security

Use empty containers (or dummy products) in displays

Ensure an effective stock control system is in place

Do not wear lots of jewellery that will have to be removed before carrying out make-up procedures

Do not leave your kit or other personal belongings in vulnerable areas

Try to dissuade clients from bringing valuables into the make-up studio

Ensure your make-up kit is lockable

Security precautions for personal belongings

Do not bring large amounts of cash into work

Do not offer to look after a client's jewellery, wallet, etc. and do not leave them on the work top

Try to store belongings in lockable cupboards when they are out of your sight

Try not to travel on your own after dark, particularly if your journey is isolated

Always lock up premises in pairs

Security precautions for personal safety

Always use licensed taxis

Make sure someone is always aware of your whereabouts – this is especially important when you work freelance

Always park your car in a well-lit or patrolled area

Contra-indications and contra-actions

A **contra-indication** refers to a condition that is present on a client that will prevent or restrict make-up procedures being carried out or will require medical approval before procedures can go ahead. Contra-indications may include external conditions such as contagious skin diseases, or internal medical conditions that become apparent during the consultation (though this is unusual in make-up procedures). Performing procedures on clients that exhibit contra-indications will:

* put the client at risk – make-up application may make the condition worse

* put other clients and the make-up artist at risk from cross-infection

* lead to insurance claims and the make-up artist being sued.

There are potentially many contra-indications to make-up procedures. It is important that you are able to recognise them and take appropriate action. Refer to page 58 for definitions and information regarding skin diseases and disorders. Below is a table of the most common contra-indications to make-up procedures and the action required.

With the exception of moles, for which medical referral should be sought, disorders of pigmentation do not contra-indicate make-up procedures.

If a contra-indication is present, it is important to handle the situation discreetly and with tact. The make-up artist must not alarm the client and under no circumstances should he or she attempt to diagnose the condition. The client should be informed, preferably in private, and should not be made to feel embarrassed or uncomfortable. Excellent communication skills are required for this

Contra-indication	Prevents treatment?	Medical approval?	Restricts treatment?
Contagious bacterial skin diseases – impetigo, folliculitis	Yes		
Non-contagious bacterial skin disorders – acne vulgaris, acne rosacea, boils	If infection present	If severe	If infected
Contagious viral skin disease – herpes simplex (cold sores), warts			Avoid area or use disposable applicators and follow strict hygiene precautions
Contagious eye disorder – conjunctivitis	Yes		
Non-contagious eye disorders – styes			Avoid area; use separate applicators on each eye
Insect infestations – lice, scabies	Yes		
Any long-term congenital skin disorder – psoriasis, eczema, dermatitis		Preferable	Avoid area if severe and infected
Fungal infection – tinea (ringworm)	Yes		
Cuts and abrasions			Avoid area; make-up artist may wish to wear protective gloves
Recent scar tissue (under six months old)		Yes	
Bruising or swelling		Yes – if post operative	If painful to touch or swelling is present
Skin cancers	Yes		

kind of situation (further information can be found in Chapter 3, page 35).

A **contra-action** is an undesirable reaction that occurs during or after a make-up procedure, requiring the procedure to be stopped mid-way or preventing it from being repeated in the future. Possible contra-actions to a make-up procedure include the following.

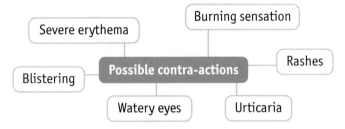

If a client is allergic or hypersensitive to the make-up products this could certainly cause most of the contra-actions mentioned above. There are certain ingredients in some products that some people are likely to have allergic reactions to.

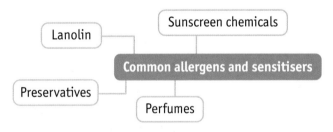

KEY NOTE

Erythema is one of the more common skin reactions. This occurs when the blood capillaries just below the epidermis dilate and a reddening appears on the skin's surface.

Urticaria is an acute allergic reaction causing red wheals of varying size on the surface of the skin. The attack may be localised or widespread and lesions can subside after several hours.

Anaphylactic shock is an extreme but rare reaction that may cause loss of consciousness and death. Check for known allergies during the consultation.

Hypo-allergenic cosmetics

The 'hypo' in hypo-allergenic means 'less' not 'none'. However, if a client does have a sensitive skin, a hypo-allergenic range can be useful in reducing the risk of contra-actions occurring. Products usually exclude known sensitisers.

If a contra-action occurs during a treatment, the following procedure should be followed.

> The product should be removed immediately
>
> ⬇
>
> A cool, soothing lotion (such as witch hazel) should be applied to the area
>
> ⬇
>
> The reaction should be noted on the client's record card
>
> ⬇
>
> If the adverse reaction persists, medical attention should be sought

The risk of contra-actions taking place can be reduced by performing allergy patch tests when using known irritants such as skin adhesives, latex, etc. Barrier cream can also be applied to the skin prior to the application of these products.

Allergy tests and record cards

A record card should be completed for each client and information given should be treated in strictest confidence. You should ensure that the record card is complete, accurate and legible because it has the following important functions.

* It will record a client's relevant personal details. This means the make-up artist will be able to contact the client if necessary.

* It will record necessary medical information, such as known allergies or conditions, enabling the make-up artist to treat the client safely.

* It will record make-up procedures, indicating the best way results can be achieved effectively and quickly.

* It will record any contra-actions, to avoid a repeat of adverse skin reactions in the future.

T RECORD CARD

/ Artiste's Name:			
of production:			
ct Telephone Number:	Day:		Eve:
r's Name and Tel. Number	Name:		Tel. No.
al History:	Asthma	Diabetes	Epilepsy
e indicate if applicable)	Known Allergies:		
a-indications Noted:	Details		Action
a-actions	Details		Action
al Requests:			

s of Procedures Undertaken

	Procedures and notes	Make-up artist

specific procedures, for example, postiche fittings, make-up design sheets should be attached to this card

An example of a record card

* It is important for continuity, and makes it possible for a new make-up artist to take over in a fully professional and competent manner.

* It will protect the make-up artist against insurance claims for damage or negligence.

Records should be kept in a system that is easily accessible to the make-up artist but is secure from prying eyes. This may be computer (data) or paper based. Record keeping is legislated by the following Act of Parliament.

Data Protection Act 1998

This Act enforces the following principles of good practice for anyone dealing with personal data.

Data must:

* be fairly and lawfully processed
* be processed for limited purposes
* be adequate, relevant and not excessive
* be accurate
* be kept no longer than necessary
* be processed in accordance with the data subject's rights
* be secure
* not be transferred to countries without adequate protection.

Further information can be found by following the links at www.heinemann.co.uk/hotlinks.

Insurance requirements

Insurance is important to protect make-up artists against legal claims, loss or damage. There are several types of insurance that are highly recommended.

Professional indemnity insurance

Make-up artists have a responsibility to their clients and any breach of that responsibility could lead to a claim against you. Professional indemnity insurance will protect against having to pay damages and legal costs should a claim be made against you. Every make-up artist should have this insurance regardless of how many make-up procedures they perform. It will protect against:

* breach of professional duty
* breach of confidentiality
* libel and slander
* loss of documents.

Public liability insurance

This is a general term applied to forms of third party liability insurance with respect to both bodily injury and property damage liability. It protects the insured against legal claims brought by clients and members of the public.

Theft, loss or damage of make-up kit and equipment

It is strongly advised that make-up artists insure their kits. Annual premiums may seem an unnecessary expense when you start out, but remember that without your kit and equipment you will not be able to work. Without insurance the contents of your kit, which you have probably built up over a period of time, may be irreplaceable because of cost.

KEY NOTE

Insurance policies may be null and void if legislation and good working practices are not followed.

Employer's Liability (Compulsory Insurance) Act 1969 and Employer's Liability (Compulsory Insurance) Regulations 1998

The Act requires *employers* to insure against their liability for personal injury to their employees. It protects them against compensation and legal costs arising from accidental death, injury, illness and disease. The regulations state that the amount of cover should not be less than £5m for each employee. All employers are required to display a certificate of insurance.

Knowledge Check

1. What is meant be the terms hazard and risk?
2. Discuss the responsibilities of employees under the Health and Safety Act 1974.
3. How should hazardous waste be disposed of?
4. List four electrical safety precautions.
5. What does COSHH stand for?
6. List three details that should appear in the accident record book.
7. Under the first aid regulations, what is meant by 'an appointed person'?
8. What is the priority of a first aider when dealing with an epileptic fit?
9. What does a fire extinguisher with a blue band contain and what type of fire could you use it on?
10. Suggest a safe procedure for evacuation in the workplace in the case of a fire breaking out.
11. What is meant by workplace policies?
12. What is meant by cross-infection?
13. Describe fungal infections and give an example.
14. What is the best method for sterilising tweezers?
15. How do you avoid cross-infection from used sponges?
16. Suggest four precautions for personal hygiene.
17. List four procedures when preparing the client for a make-up treatment.
18. List three guidelines for ensuring products are kept in optimum condition.
19. Discuss how you could reduce the risk of crime in the make-up studio.
20. What is meant by a contra-indication?
21. What is meant by a contra-action and what would you expect to occur?
22. Describe erythema.
23. Why is it important to keep accurate and complete record cards?
24. What implications does the Data Protection Act have for the make-up artist?
25. List three types of insurance that are highly advisable for the make-up artist.

Establishing positive relationships in the workplace

This chapter is about building positive relationships with other people in the workplace. It begins by looking at the make-up artist's relationship with clients, discussing how best to support their needs throughout the make-up procedure. It also looks at developing good working relationships with colleagues, which is important for establishing a harmonious and pleasant atmosphere in the make-up studio for all concerned.

Aim and objectives

Aim of this chapter: to provide you with the knowledge and understanding to establish positive working relationships with clients and colleagues.

You should achieve the following **objectives**:

* Discuss professionalism and professional ethics and how these affect behaviour in the workplace
* Provide a high standard of service
* Establish excellent care and support for the client
* Enable clients to discuss their expectations, concerns and needs
* Review options and decide on a course of action
* Identify client rights
* Discuss the importance of updating skills by researching the latest make-up techniques and products
* Establish excellent communication in the workplace
* Discuss effective teamwork
* Define equal opportunities and discrimination.

Professionalism and ethics

The make-up artist must act in a professional manner towards clients, colleagues, suppliers and other contacts.

What do we mean by 'professionalism'?

Professionalism is a standard of behaviour and implies responsibility and commitment that reflects the high standards of a professional occupation. It means providing an excellent service through an awareness of role, image, skills and knowledge.

What do we mean by 'professional ethics'?

Ethics can be defined as 'moral principles' or as 'rules of conduct', i.e. whether or not an action or conduct is correct or principled. **Professional ethics** may therefore be applied to a given profession. They exist to uphold professional standards, protect the integrity of the profession and safeguard the interest of clients. Trade unions and professional associations will often establish a set of professional ethics that members are expected to work within. They may include clauses covering:

* quality of customer care
* representing qualifications and experience honestly
* giving accurate information regarding the scope and limitations of service
* acknowledging contra-indications and seeking medical referral where appropriate
* consistently maintaining or improving professional knowledge and competence
* conducting professional activities with honesty and integrity
* equal opportunities: avoiding unjust discrimination against clients, etc.
* safeguarding the confidentiality of all client information
* gaining a client's informed consent before procedures are carried out

* respecting clients' comfort and modesty
* acting in the client's best interest
* following all legislation, workplace policies, rules and regulations.

Professional ethics may also be referred to as 'codes of practice'.

> **KEY NOTE**
>
> Maintaining 'client confidentiality' is important if you are to build up relationships with clients based on trust. Breaking this trust or becoming a 'gossip' may result in people not wanting to work with you. It is important to safeguard the confidentiality of all client information, whether written or verbally given. The only exceptions to this are when disclosure is required by law or is absolutely necessary for the protection of others.

Providing a high standard of service

Make-up artistry is a service industry. If clients receive a high standard of service they are more likely to want to work with you again. Whether you are working in a big make-up department with other make-up artists, on a photographic shoot with a number of different specialists or as a mobile make-up artist carrying out bridal make-ups or camouflage treatments, the standard of service you provide will largely depend on the following.

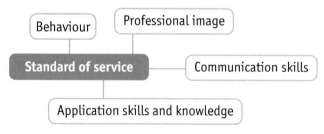

Behaviour

Your behaviour is everything you do or say and as a result is directly observable by other people. Other people will base their opinions about you, both as a person and a professional, on your behaviour. Behaving in an appropriate manner will also encourage others to do the same as 'behaviour breeds behaviour'. We control the way we behave: we are free to make choices about the way we act and speak. It is therefore down to us whether other people will enjoy working with us or not.

It is extremely important to present a professional, considerate and approachable image to your clients. This will inspire confidence, provide support and make them feel welcome. The make-up artist should have the following qualities.

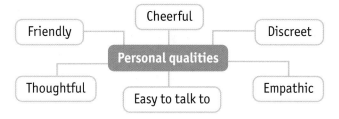

Professional image

In industry, make-up artists are not required to wear uniforms. However, as previously discussed in Chapter 2, it is important that aspects of health, safety and hygiene are considered. To recap:

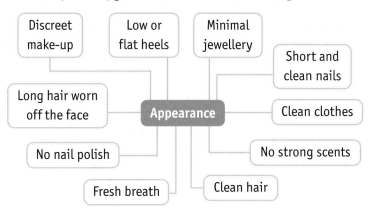

Management will often set standards of appearance, hygiene and conduct and it is the duty of the make-up artist to maintain these standards. If you are working in the fashion industry, it is also important to appear stylish without looking as if you are trying too hard – after all, you are working in an image-conscious industry where individuals will spend time developing a strong sense of style.

Communication skills

Effective communication skills are very important for the make-up artist. Without them you would be unable to relate to clients and colleagues, leading to situations of misunderstanding and frustration for all parties involved. Communication skills may be categorised as written, verbal and non-verbal (body language). Effective communication is clear and understood.

Written communication

You may use written communication when corresponding with clients, suppliers and other contacts. This may take the form of letters, application forms, CVs, emails, etc. In addition, you will certainly be required to complete client record cards and possibly produce aftercare advice sheets. To make sure your correspondence is effective you should:

* ensure your handwriting is clear and readable
* ensure you use appropriate language
* ensure you check your spelling and grammar
* word process where possible.

All written communication should use the right tone, according to whom it is addressed. For example, letters to medical consultants when seeking permission to treat clients would be formal and should be appropriate in style, layout and language. An example of this kind of letter can be found in Chapter 9, page 195.

Verbal communication

We use verbal communication when speaking to colleagues, clients, suppliers and other contacts. It can take place face to face or over the telephone. It is important to remember to:

* speak clearly – do not mumble
* not put your hand over your mouth
* use appropriate language and tone of voice
* choose appropriate topics of conversation
* make eye contact throughout.

As with written communication, it is important to remember to adapt your communication techniques according to whom you are addressing by altering your manner, tone of voice and vocabulary as appropriate.

Formal	Informal
Manager, supervisor	Colleagues
New client, artiste	Existing clients and artistes with whom you have a previously established relationship
At interviews	Friends

If in doubt, it is probably best to use a more formal approach until it feels comfortable to adopt an informal manner. Whoever you are communicating with, it is important to remain friendly and approachable. Using open-ended questions is a useful technique to encourage conversation. Open-ended questions are the opposite of closed-questions in that they cannot be answered with a direct yes or no, for example:

* closed question: 'Do you wear make-up during the day?'

* open question: 'What sort of make-up would you consider wearing during the day?'

There are certain topics of conversation that are considered unsuitable for the workplace and should be avoided. These include:

* sex

* politics

* religion.

In addition to the above, you should never off-load your stresses and problems on a client. You should avoid talking about yourself too much, but listen and appear interested in the other person's contribution to the conversation.

KEY NOTE

Some clients may prefer not to talk during the make-up procedure. It is important to be sensitive to the signals the client is giving out. Chatting incessantly will only irritate such clients.

Listening skills

Listening is a skill that requires you to focus attention on the person speaking. Hearing only becomes listening when you pay attention to what is being said. The following skills will demonstrate that you are listening.

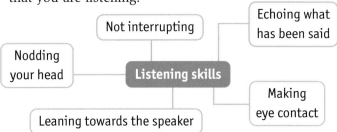

It is important to listen so that you can:

* show your support and help the other person relax

* clarify information

* check assumptions and clear up misperceptions

* encourage conversation

* make the appropriate response.

Responding skills

You also need to practise reacting and responding in positive ways. Responding appropriately is a vital part of communication, and every situation will warrant a different reaction. Possible forms of response may include:

* asking clarifying questions

* summarising facts and feelings to show you have listened and understood

* asking questions to show interest and continue the conversation

* redirecting the conversation if the subject is not appropriate for the workplace

* progressing the conversation with your own input and ideas.

KEY NOTE

Clarifying: When passing on or receiving information, it is useful to clarify the details to ensure that they have been properly understood. The easiest way to clarify is to summarise and repeat back the information so any misunderstandings can simply be corrected straight away.

Non-verbal (body language)

Non-verbal communication or body language refers to the signals and signs given off by posture, expressions and gestures, which can be conscious or unconscious. It affects all face-to-face communication. By learning to observe and interpret this type of communication we can often gain insight into a person's real emotions and thought processes.

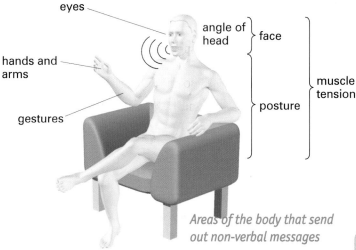

Areas of the body that send out non-verbal messages

Body language can generally be classified as either positive or negative. However, some of this language can be ambiguous and in these cases should not be considered in isolation, for example a person with his or her arms folded may not always be displaying negative body language.

Positive non-verbal communication

This includes gestures, expressions and postures such as smiling, eye contact, nods of the head, adopting open postures such as arms unfolded, and turning or leaning slightly towards the other person.

Negative non-verbal communication

This includes gestures, expressions and postures such as frowning, yawning, avoiding eye contact, adopting closed postures such as arms folded, and turning the body away from the other person.

Barriers to communication

Anything that prevents or hinders effective communication taking place is considered a barrier to communication. Barriers can be both physical and psychological, and include:

* tiredness
* stress
* strong accent or foreign language
* noisy environment
* disabilities such as deafness, speech impediments
* prejudice and preconceptions
* dislike of the other person
* difficult behaviour
* complicated or poorly delivered information.

Difficult behaviour

You may occasionally come across 'difficult people'. However, most of the time, it is not actually the person who is difficult but their behaviour at that time, which can create barriers to effective communication. In the make-up studio this kind of problem may occur, for example, when an artiste arrives early for make-up and is upset at having to be kept waiting.

Listening to the other person without interrupting allows the other person to 'let off some steam'.

↓

Try to adopt positive body language.

↓

Is the behaviour justified? Before any satisfactory resolutions can occur, you need to let the other person know that you understand the strength of their concerns. Using verbal signals can help achieve this, for example: 'I see; I understand; I can see that you feel strongly about that; I can understand how you could see it like that'.

↓

Recognise your own feelings in response to the other person's difficult behaviour, but do not feel you have to express or act upon them as you may later regret an impulsive response given in anger or frustration.

↓

Of course, for the other person to know that you have listened, you must make a controlled and appropriate response that deals with the problem and offers a solution.

↓

Wait for the other person's acceptance of the solution. If you were unable to agree a solution, you should seek advice from a supervisor or manager.

Dealing with difficult behaviour

Application skills and knowledge

It goes without saying that without excellent make-up application skills and knowledge, you will never be able to offer an excellent standard of service to your clients. Application skills and professional knowledge are initially gained via thorough training, but these must then be maintained and improved through a process known as 'continued professional development'. This is particularly important when working in an industry that is developing new techniques and technologies all the time.

Initial training and gaining qualifications
↓
Industrial experience
↓
Continued professional development

You should always strive for professional excellence, working to the highest possible standard. This will give you a reputation as a professional, highly skilled make-up artist who will be greatly sought after by potential clients. Successful continued professional development relies on self-awareness and appraisal, as it is important to be able to evaluate your areas of

professional weakness and take measures to improve them. This is looked at in more detail in Chapter 17.

HANDS ON

Researching products

As previously mentioned, it is important for the make-up artist to keep up to date with the latest make-up application techniques, technologies and products. Trade magazines are useful for researching this information, as well as cosmetic companies. Begin by going to a large department store and spend some time visiting each of the cosmetic houses, trying out their latest products and collecting information. Note any consistent trends in colours and textures and ask the consultants questions about new products. You may wish to keep any literature or pamphlets you collect in a file for future reference when you wish to update your make-up kit.

Client care and support

Because of the variety of working environments available to the make-up artist, the range of clients they may come across is vast. However, for each client it is important to establish and manage a system of support whilst they are in your care.

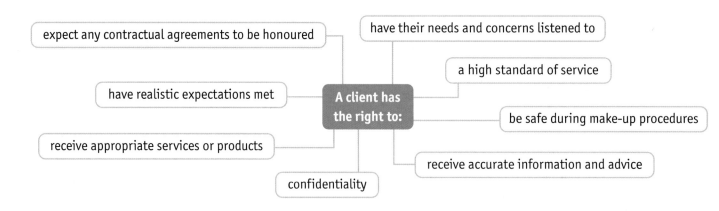

expect any contractual agreements to be honoured

have realistic expectations met

receive appropriate services or products

A client has the right to:

confidentiality

have their needs and concerns listened to

a high standard of service

be safe during make-up procedures

receive accurate information and advice

Generally, on first meeting a client, a make-up procedure will follow the following process.

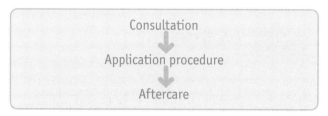

Consultation
↓
Application procedure
↓
Aftercare

Consultation

When you first meet your client it is important to allow plenty of time for the consultation. The client may feel self-conscious or anxious (particularly if undergoing special effect make-up), so it is important he or she does not feel rushed at any point. Creating a professional and relaxed environment is essential and will allow the client to relax and feel comfortable. It is also important to maintain the client's modesty and privacy at all times.

If it is the client's first visit to a make-up department or expert, it is a good idea to outline the limits and boundaries of your duties and responsibilities and the client's rights. This will avoid any misunderstanding as to what the client can expect from you or the department.

It may take some time to build a rapport with the client, but with a friendly approach and effective communication skills most clients will be happy to express their perspectives, concerns and feelings about the forthcoming procedures. Honesty and openness at this stage will help you plan how best to support and manage the client.

It is important to maintain a polite and friendly approach throughout the consultation, and to use effective non-verbal and verbal communication techniques. You will need to discuss or consider the following points during the consultation process. It is important to ensure you show you are listening closely, and respond to the information in an appropriate manner.

* Discuss the client's needs and requirements. Does the client have realistic expectations about the procedure? If not, then it is important to be honest and clearly explain its limits.

* Check for contra-indications. Some conditions will require medical approval whilst others will restrict make-up application. Do you require medical permission before carrying out any procedures? If in doubt, it is best to obtain written permission from the client's GP.

* Gather relevant information from the client that may affect the make-up procedure.

* Establish a rapport with the client. This may take some time if they appear very nervous, stressed or dislike make-up procedures.

* Has the client had this particular make-up procedure before? This will help to establish what level of support is required.

* Discuss and agree a suitable course of action with the client.

During the consultation it is important to make a written record of the information you have collected and agreed with the client. This will act as proof that professional procedures have been followed and consent given in case of future disputes and insurance claims. This is best done on a client record or treatment card, which is then signed and dated by the client and yourself. This record card is then kept in a paper or data-based filing system in line with the Data Protection Act 1998.

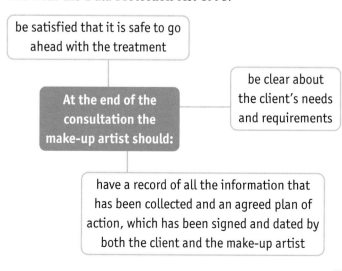

be satisfied that it is safe to go ahead with the treatment

At the end of the consultation the make-up artist should:

be clear about the client's needs and requirements

have a record of all the information that has been collected and an agreed plan of action, which has been signed and dated by both the client and the make-up artist

feel their expectations, needs and concerns have been heard

have realistic expectations of the treatment

feel confident in the make-up artist's ability to carry out the treatment

At the end of the consultation the client should:

be assured that any information given during the consultation will be kept confidential

KEY NOTE

You will not always work with clients that you like or feel comfortable with. Equally, you may find yourself working with famous clients and this may intimidate you or result in you making false assumptions about them. However, it is important to control your reaction and emotional response and remain professional at all times.

Client expectations and needs

Whilst in your care, a client is likely to express a number of requests or 'needs'. These needs may be psychological, social, physical or emotional. Do not assume that the client is being demanding but initially try to respond to the request immediately – it may be important and a quick response may avert a potential problem or incident. For example, a client may feel a product burning on the skin and ask you to remove it: any delay may result in injury. Sometimes it may not be possible to meet a client's need, and you may come across some clients who frequently make unreasonable requests. In these cases, it is important to clearly explain to the client why you cannot carry out their request; it may also be useful to suggest an alternative solution.

Some clients, particularly if they are principal performers on a production, will have specific needs or requests; for example, some actresses will only have a particular brand of make-up applied to their skin. A phone call or meeting prior to production will avoid any embarrassing scenarios or disgruntled clients.

A client will inevitably have expectations of the procedure you are about to perform. It is important that these expectations are realistic and reflect the actual outcome and resource limitations. Clarification of a client's expectations should be sought during the initial consultation or pre-production meetings. If you judge them to be unrealistic, you will need to address the situation with honesty. A client who undertakes a make-up procedure with unrealistic expectations may end up dissatisfied and likely to complain. It is important to ensure that the client is aware of:

* the time involved for the procedure
* the total cost of the procedure
* the required working position for the artiste or model
* possible contra-actions and personal discomfort involved
* requirements for fittings and pre-application procedures
* resource limitations, for example time, space and budget available.

Procedure	Unrealistic expectation
Application of camouflage make-up over port wine stain	Camouflage make-up is a miracle cure and will make the disfigurement 'invisible'– even the make-up will not be noticeable on close inspection
Selling a client an anti-ageing facial cream	The cream will make the client look 20 years younger
Applying an air-brushed tattoo	The tattoo will last a client throughout a two-week summer holiday
Applying full ageing make-up, using prosthetics	The procedure is quick

Examples of unrealistic expectations

Deciding on appropriate make-up services and a course of action

When deciding on appropriate procedures and a course of action for a client, it is necessary to give consideration to the following.

The required outcome / client needs
e.g. application of a tattoo on a principal artiste

⬇

The different types of procedures available to achieve the outcome / client needs
e.g. rubber stamps, transfers, airbrushing, hand painting, etc.

⬇

The advantages and disadvantages of the various procedures
e.g. continuity, length of time for application, durability, finished effect

⬇

Monitoring and reviewing the chosen procedure
e.g. trying out the make-up, evaluating the success of the procedure, making changes where necessary

Application procedure

We have already discussed the health and safety aspects of performing make-up procedures in Chapter 2. To recap, there are a number of steps the make-up artist can take to make the experience more comfortable for the client.

* Ensure the make-up room is at a comfortable temperature.

* Follow the principles of good personal hygiene.

* Ensure effective communication takes place prior to and throughout the procedure – this will help put the client at ease.

* Check the client is seated comfortably, and the neck, back and feet are supported.

* Continue to check throughout the procedure that the client remains comfortable. If required to be in make-up for a long period of time,

ensure the client has frequent short breaks and access to refreshments.

* Use gowns to protect the client against accidental spillages and make-up products soiling their clothes.

* Ensure the client's hair is protected.

* Apply a barrier cream when using known irritants such as skin adhesives and latex.

* Follow safe and hygienic working practices.

* Ensure the work is carried out quickly and to time.

Aftercare

Support for the client will often continue after the make-up procedure has been completed. This support is called 'aftercare' and could include the following, depending on the type of procedure that has been carried out:

* advice regarding the do's and don'ts to avoid premature removal of the products

* ensuring your client is able to remove the products if the make-up artist will not be doing this

* advice regarding recommended frequency of re-application – required for products applied by the client at home, or when planning touch-ups on set

* providing information about alternative sources of support and make-up services that may be of interest to the client

* providing sources of further information and referral to other services as required.

Working with colleagues

Good communication between colleagues will encourage excellent teamwork and positive relationships. When this is apparent in the workplace, it will be reflected by a harmonious atmosphere and productive working day.

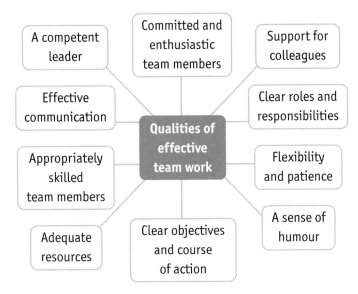

The pie chart shows us how we relate to other people and how they relate to us.

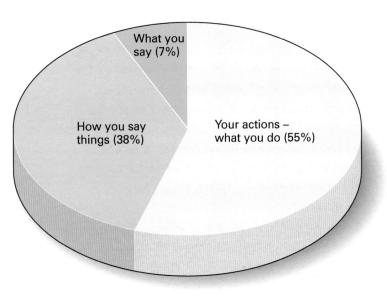

Being an effective team member

* Politely ask for help and information if required.
* Respond to requests for help and information willingly and courteously.
* Use your initiative and offer assistance when you can see a colleague is struggling.
* Perform your roles and responsibilities to the best of your ability.

* Always work to professional standards following workplace rules and regulations.
* Always tidy your work area – do not expect others to do it for you.
* Always ask before borrowing a colleague's equipment.
* Always return borrowed equipment in the same state as it was lent.
* Take responsibility for your actions; do not try to hide mistakes.
* Do not undermine or gossip about colleagues.
* Try to be cheerful, friendly and flexible.
* Treat others as you wish to be treated yourself.

Team spirit could be lost if:

* there is poor management or the team is poorly structured
* there appears to be favouritism within the team
* roles and responsibilities are not clearly defined, leading to confusion and conflict
* there is poor communication
* team members are inflexible and intolerant of others
* the team is overworked or under-resourced
* a member of the team works in isolation without consulting others.

Establish effective working relationships with management

It is important to establish constructive communication with managers and supervisors: you can help this by:

* accepting and acting on instructions willingly
* politely asking for help if you are unsure of how to carry out an instruction
* being honest about mistakes – do not try to hide them
* carrying out your roles and responsibilities to the best of your abilities
* working to workplace rules and guidelines

* only working within the limits of you own authority, and seeking agreement or permission when necessary.

Resolving conflict within the team

If you have a problem with a colleague's behaviour you would need to take appropriate action to resolve the problem whilst allowing you and the colleague to continue to work together without bad feeling. Following the suggestions below will help you to handle the situation professionally and sensitively.

> Do not react in anger, particularly in front of colleagues and clients. Walk away from the situation and calm down first.
>
> ⬇
>
> It is always best to approach the person directly, in a private area away from others. Do not gossip with other colleagues.
>
> ⬇
>
> Explain your feelings calmly.
>
> ⬇
>
> Listen to your colleague's response without interrupting.
>
> ⬇
>
> Offer a solution that is acceptable to both parties.
>
> ⬇
>
> If the problem remains unresolved, you may need to involve your manager or supervisor.

Equal opportunities

Discrimination is the unfair or unequal treatment of people on the basis of:

* race (national and ethnic origin, nationality)
* religion
* sex (gender, marital status, caring responsibilities)
* disability (physical and sensory impairments, learning difficulties, hidden impairments, mental health)
* sexual orientation
* HIV status
* age.

Employers are obliged to promote equal opportunities through various Acts of Parliament including:

* Sex Discrimination Act 1975
* Race Relations Act 1976
* Disabled Persons (Services, Consultation and Representation) Act 1986
* Disability Discrimination Act 1995.

Disability Discrimination Act 1995

According to the law, a person is disabled if they have a 'physical or mental impairment, which has a substantial and long-term adverse effect on their ability to carry out normal day-to-day activities'.

This Act deals with situations when an employer discriminates against a disabled employee or job applicant. An employer directly discriminates against an employee if the employer treats the employee less positively than another employee for a reason that relates to a disability, and if the employer cannot justify his or her behaviour on objective grounds. In addition, an employer discriminates without justification if he or she does not make a reasonable adjustment to the premises or work arrangements as this leaves disabled persons at a substantial disadvantage compared to able-bodied employees or potential employees.

> **KEY NOTE**
>
> What is harassment? Harassment is unlawful when it is on the grounds of sex, race or disability and it affects your working conditions. Harassment is words or conduct that create a hostile or offensive working environment for another individual. Individuals are protected against harassment by various Acts of Parliament.

Knowledge Check

1 Define professionalism and professional ethics.

2 Name three personal qualities required of a make-up artist.

3 List five requirements of a make-up artist with regard to personal appearance.

4 List three ways you could ensure your written communication is clear and understood.

5 List three ways you could ensure your verbal communication is clear and understood.

6 What is meant by an open question?

7 What topics of conversation should be avoided in the workplace?

8 Describe how you could show a client you were listening.

9 What is meant by clarification?

10 Give two examples of non-verbal body language.

11 What are barriers to communication? Give three examples.

12 Describe the procedure for dealing with difficult clients.

13 List three client rights.

14 How would you deal with a client with unrealistic expectations?

15 Describe three ways you could ensure the make-up is more comfortable for the client.

16 List four qualities of an effective team member.

17 Discuss examples of how team spirit may be lost.

18 Give three ways you could improve relations with management.

19 What is meant by equal opportunities?

20 Name two Acts that deal with discrimination in the workplace.

Anatomy and physiology for the make-up artist

 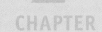

It is important that make-up artists have a full understanding of related anatomy and physiology so they understand the structure of the human body (their canvas) and can work safely and effectively.

Aim and objectives

Aim of this chapter: to provide the underpinning knowledge and skills of related anatomy and physiology required by the make-up artist.

You should achieve the following **objectives**:

* List and position the bones of the skull and shoulder girdle
* Discuss how bone structure determines facial proportions
* List and position the muscles of the face, neck and shoulder girdle and discuss their actions
* Describe muscle tone
* Discuss the structure of the skin, labelling and describing the layers of the epidermis and the structures within the dermis
* Describe the subcutaneous layer and the functions of adipose tissue
* List the functions of the skin
* Describe how skin heals
* Discuss the importance of the acid mantle
* Recognise various skin diseases and disorders
* Discuss the physiological ageing process
* Discuss the structure of the hair, labelling a diagram
* Discuss the role of the blood system, listing its structures.

Bones of the skull

In order to understand how to improve or change the appearance of a face, it is vital that you understand the bone structure beneath the skin.

* The skull protects the brain, eyes and delicate structures of the ear within a hard, bony structure.

* It gives attachment to muscles and teeth.

* It forms the shape of the face and head.

The skull is divided into two parts, the cranium containing eight bones and the face containing 13 bones. The bones are joined by sutures (immovable joints) with the exception of the mandible (lower jaw-bone), which is hinged and therefore moveable.

Bone	Position
Occipital (x1)	Forms the lower, rear part of the cranium – the spinal cord passes through this bone via a large hole
Frontal (x1)	Forms the forehead, top of the eye sockets and front of the cranium
Parietal (x2)	Form upper sides and top of cranium
Temporal (x2)	Form lower part of sides of cranium
Sphenoid (x1)	Positioned in the middle section of the base of the skull – joins with the temporal, parietal and frontal bones
Ethmoid (x1)	Forms the eye sockets and part of the nasal cavities

Bones of the cranium

Bone	Position
Nasal bones (x2)	Form the bridge of the nose
Vomer (x1)	Forms lower part of the septum (bony partition) of the nose
Zygomatic arch (x2)	Form the cheekbones
Maxilla (x1) originated as 2 bones	Forms the upper jaw and part of the roof of the mouth
Mandible (x1)	Forms the lower jaw – the only moveable bone in the skull

Lacrimal (x2)	Delicate bones within the inner eye sockets, form the tear duct
Palatine (x2) (not seen on diagrams)	Form the roof of the mouth and the base of the nose
Turbinator (x2) (not seen on diagrams)	Projections from the lateral wall of the maxilla into the nasal cavity

Bones of the face

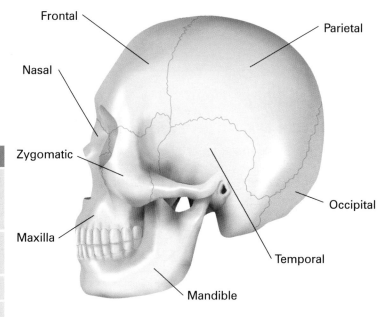

Side view of the skull

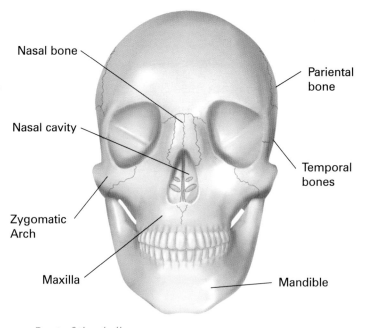

Front of the skull

The skull is attached to the body via the vertebral column, which runs through a large opening in the occipital bone. The bones of the shoulder radiate from the top of the vertebrae.

Bone	Position
Clavicle (x2) – commonly known as collar bones	Radiate from the vertebrae across the chest to each shoulder
Scapula (x2) – commonly known as shoulder blades	Across the back of the shoulder girdle, resting on the rib-cage

Bones of the shoulder

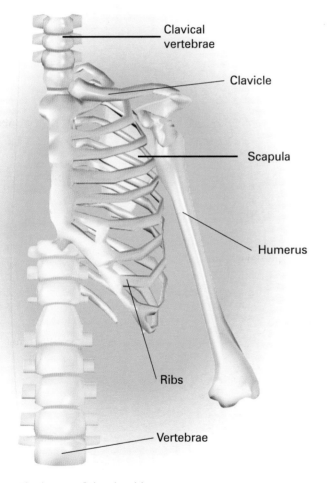

The bones of the shoulder

Bone structure determining face shape

The underlying bone structure will determine the face shape of the individual.

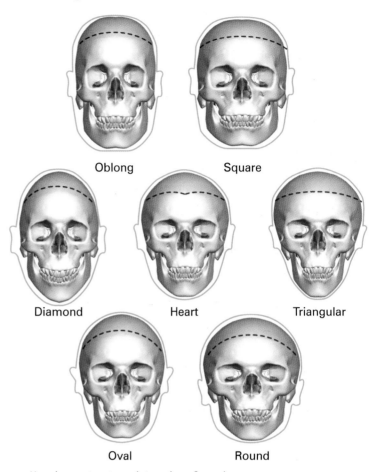

How bone structure determines face shape

Muscles of the head and neck

There are three types of muscle tissue, all of which contract to cause movement:

* voluntary muscle tissue, which is primarily attached to the bone
* involuntary muscle tissue, which is found inside the digestive and urinary tract as well as the walls of the blood vessels
* cardiac muscle tissue, which is found in the walls of the heart.

The position and action of the muscles of the face, neck and shoulders is important underpinning knowledge for a make-up artist.

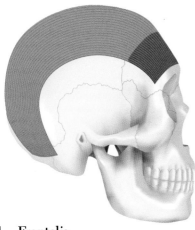

1 **Frontalis**
- Upper part of the cranium
- Scalp moves forward, raises eyebrow

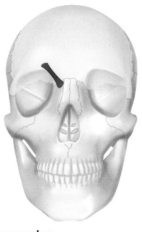

2 **Corrugator**
- Inner corners of the eyebrows
- Draws eyebrows together – as in frowning

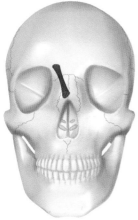

3 **Procerus**
- Top of nose between eyebrows
- Depresses the eyebrows, forming wrinkles over the bridge of the nose

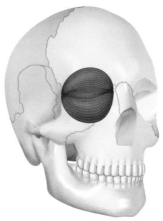

4 **Orbicularis Oculi**
- Surround the eye
- Closes eyes, blinking

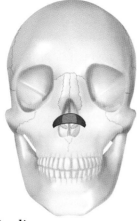

5 **Nasalis**
- Over the front of the nose
- Compresses nose, causing wrinkles

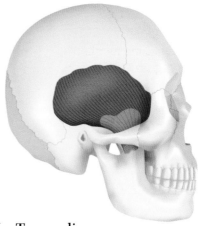

6 **Temporalis**
- Runs down side of face towards upper jaw
- Aids chewing and closing mouth

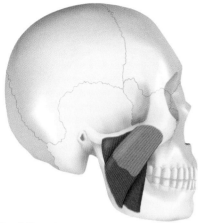

7 **Masseter**
- Runs down and back to the angle of the jaw
- Lifts the jaw and gives the teeth strength for biting

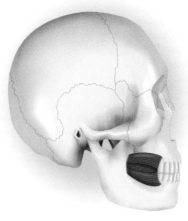

8 **Buccinator**
- Forms most of the cheek and gives it shape
- Puffs out cheeks when blowing, keeps food in mouth when chewing

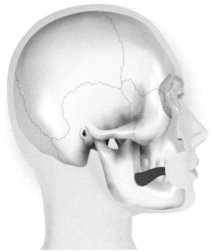

9 **Risorius**
- In the lower cheek. It joins to the corner of the mouth
- Pulls back angles of the mouth – smiling and in grimace

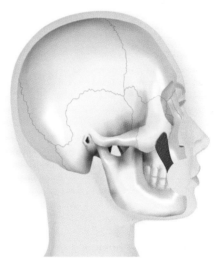

10 **Zygomaticus**
- Runs down the cheek towards the corner of the mouth
- Pulls the corner of the mouth upwards and sideways

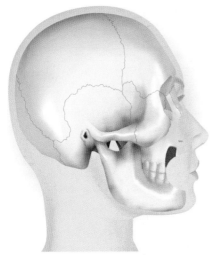

11 Quadratus labii superiorus
- Runs upward from the upper lip
- Lifts the upper lip and helps open the mouth

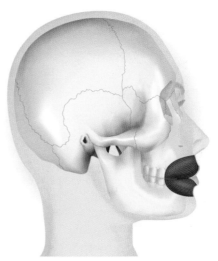

12 Orbicularis oris
- Surrounds the lips and forms the mouth
- Closes mouth, pushes lips forward

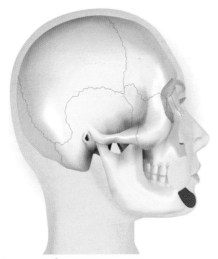

13 Mentalis
- Forms the chin
- Lifts the chin and moves the lower lips outwards

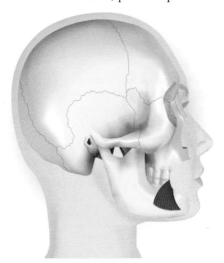

14 Triangularis
- Corner of the lower lip, extends over the chin
- Pulls the corner of the chin down

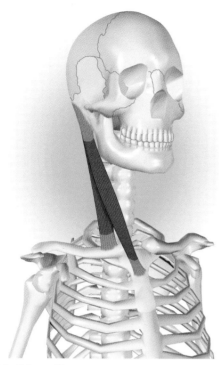

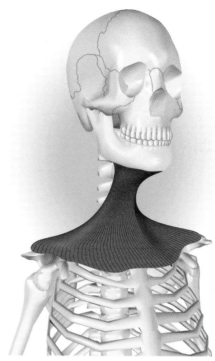

13 Mentalis
- Forms the chin
- Lifts the chin and moves the lower lips outwards

14 Triangularis
- Corner of the lower lip, extends over the chin
- Pulls the corner of the chin down

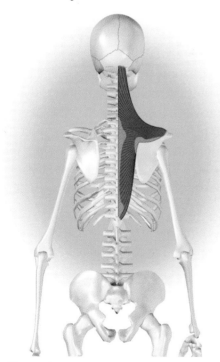

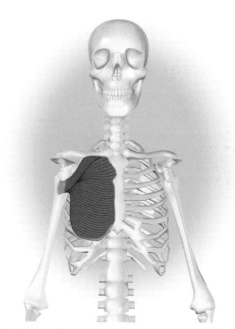

17 Trapezius
- The upper back and sides of the neck
- Rotation of shoulders, draws back the scapula bones, pulls head back, assists in rotation of head

18 Pectoralis
- Front of chest, under the breast
- Pulls arms forwards and assists rotation of the arm

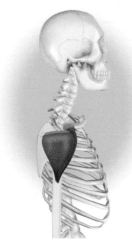

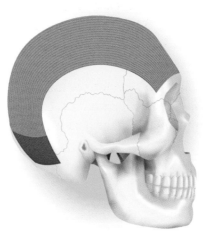

19 Deltoid
- Caps the shoulder
- Raises arm from the side, pulls it back and forward

Muscle tone

Muscle is never completely at rest; it is always in a state of muscle tone, or partial contraction, ready to respond to stimuli. When the muscle is in a partial state of contraction, some of its fibres are contracted and some of them are relaxed. A muscle is in this state when it is tense but not moving. Posture is determined by the degree of muscle tone. A fully contracted muscle will cause movement.

Structure of the skin

The skin is a very important organ to a make-up artist. It is the canvas on which they work, and just as a traditional artist must understand their canvas, so must a make-up artist. An understanding of the structure and functions of the skin is essential for carrying out make-up procedures safely and effectively.

The skin is a large organ, covering the entire body, that varies in thickness on different parts of the body. It is thinnest on the lips and eyelids allowing ease of movement, and thickest on the soles of the feet and palms of the hands to protect against friction. Providing the external covering of the body, the skin is exposed to the elements and can suffer from symptoms of diseases and disorders resulting from damage or irritation.

20 Occipitalis
- At the back of the skull
- Helps with the movement of the head.

Functions of the skin

Thinking of the letters that spell V-SHAPES will help us remember the functions of the skin.

V = **Vitamins:** Ultra-violet light hits the skin resulting in the synthesis of vitamin D.

S = **Sensory:** Within the skin sensory nerve endings allow us to identify pain, touch, pressure, heat and cold.

H = **Heat regulation (homeostasis):** The skin plays an important role in regulating the body's temperature. When we are cold, the hairs in the skin stand on end, trapping warm air and creating an insulating layer. When we are too warm, the skin produces sweat. The sweat evaporates on the surface of the skin, cooling us down.

A = **Absorption:** The skin is capable of absorbing small amounts of products applied to its surface.

P = **Protection:** The skin protects in a number of different ways. Specialised types of cells within the skin called melanocytes protect the body against UV damage by producing melanin. A protective barrier called the acid mantle protects against the invasion if microbes and dehydration. The cushioned layer of the subcutaneous layer of the skin protects the underlying structures against minor trauma.

E = Excretion: Waste products and toxins, such as urea, are eliminated by the skin in the form of sweat, which is produced by the sudoriferous glands.

S = Secretion: The skin secretes sebum onto its surface. Sebum keeps the skin lubricated and plays a part in maintaining the acid mantle.

The structure of the skin

The skin has three main layers:

* the **epidermis**, which is the outer thinner layer
* the **dermis**, which is the inner thicker layer
* the **subcutaneous layer**, which attaches to underlying muscles and tissues.

The epidermis

The epidermis is the outer layer of the skin and is made up of five layers of cells. The lower two layers contain living cells; the three outermost layers consist of cells that have died as a result of the process of **keratinisation**. There is no blood or nerve supply in the epidermis, but the deeper layers are bathed in interstitial fluid from the dermis allowing nutrients and oxygen to pass to the cells in these layers.

> **KEY NOTE**
>
> Keratinisation is the process by which living cells in the stratum germativum move up the layers of the epidermis to become dead, flat, horny cells ready for desquamation in the stratum corneum.

The five layers of cells of the epidermis are as follows:

* **stratum germativum** or basal / germinating layer
* **stratum spinosum** or prickle cell layer
* **stratum granulosum** or granular layer
* **stratum lucidium** or clear layer
* **stratum corneum** or horny layer.

Layer	Characteristics and function
Stratum germativum or basal layer	This is the deepest of the five layers and consists of a single row of cells that meet the dermis. These cells continuously divide to form new cells (mitosis), pushing the upper layers nearer to the skin's surface. This layer also contains specialised cells called melanocytes. It is an active living layer with cells containing nucleii. The lower surface of this layer is ridged by projections in the dermis called dermal papillae.
Stratum spinosum or prickle cell layer	This layer contains rounded cells with short projections that reach out to nearby cells, giving them a prickly appearance. This is an active living layer with cells containing nucleii.
Stratum granulosum or granular layer	These granular cells are almost dead, although some still have nucleii. They lose their projections and become hard and flattened due to the production of keratin.
Stratum lucidium or clear layer	This is a layer of transparent cells that allow light to pass through. It consists of three or four rows of flat dead cells, with no nucleii. This clear layer varies in thickness, being very thin in facial skin but thick on the soles of the feet and palms of the hands.
Stratum corneum or horny layer	This is the outermost layer, consisting of dead, flattened, keratinised cells which have taken between one month and 40 days to travel from the stratum germativum. This outer layer of dead cells, resembling a basket weave, is constantly being shed. This process is known as desquamation and allows room for the cells being pushed up from lower layers.

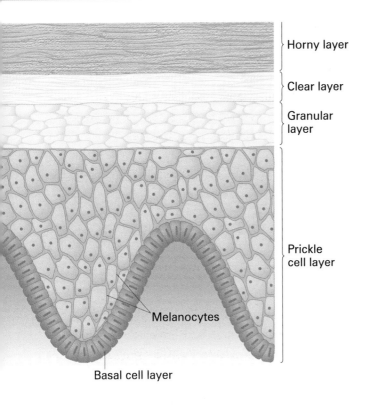

The layers of the epidermis

A healthy epidermis depends on the following:

* the cells in the stratum corneum being desquamated
* the keratinisation of the cells during their journey through the epidermis
* continuous cell division in the stratum germativum pushing the cells upwards.

The dermis

The dermis lies below the epidermis. It is composed of collagen fibres, which provide support and strength, and elastin fibres, which provide elasticity. It also contains a number of important structures. The dermis has two layers:

* a superficial papillary layer
* a deep reticular layer.

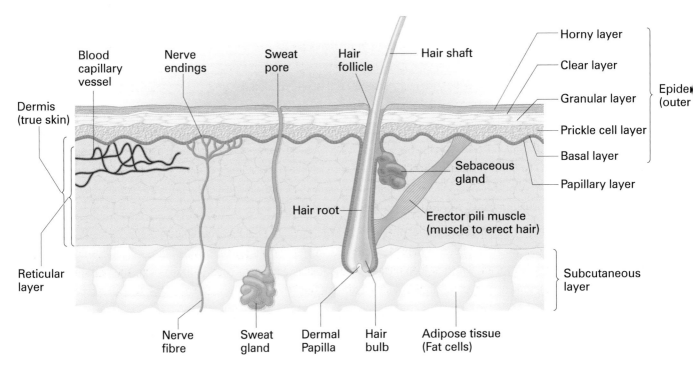

The structure of the skin

The **superficial papillary layer** is composed of adipose connective tissue. It is connected to the underside of the epidermis by projections called **dermal papillae**. The function of these dermal papillae is to aid nutrition of the epidermal cells by increasing the surface area that nutrients and oxygen can travel across from the dermis. The dermal papillae contains nerve endings and a network of blood and lymphatic capillaries.

The **deep reticular layer**, found beneath the papillary layer, is formed of tough fibrous connective tissue. It contains the following features.

Feature	Description and function
Collagen fibres	These contain the protein collagen that gives the skin support and strength.
Elastin fibres	These contain the protein elastin that gives the skin elasticity.
Fibroblasts	These produce dense fibrous connective tissue.
Sensory nerve endings	Numerous nerve endings which are sensitive to pain, pressure, touch, heat and cold are found in the dermis. These nerve endings send messages via the spinal cord to the brain.
Blood supply	A fine network of arterioles (small arteries) and venules (small veins) carry nutrients and oxygen to the dermis, and carry waste products and CO_2 away. These branch into a network of capillaries to reach active structures, such as the hair follicles and the dermal papillae, providing the lower layers of the epidermis with nourishment.
Lymphatic supply	This forms a network throughout the dermis that removes waste and excess tissue fluid. It also supplies mast cells that aid the skin in fighting infection and allergic reactions.
Sudoriferous gland (sweat gland)	These glands consist of a coiled body rising from the deeper layers of the dermis in a tube-like duct. They rise through the epidermis and end at the skin's surface as a pore. Secretions, e.g. urea and salt, are brought to the skin's surface via this pore. There are two types of sweat glands.
	The **eccrine glands** are found all over the body, but in abundance on the palms of the hands and soles of the feet.
	The **apocrine glands** are connected to hair follicles and are situated in the underarm, breast and genital areas of the body. These glands do not become active until puberty. In addition to the usual secretions of urea and salt, an odourless milky substance is secreted. When broken down by surface microbes, this substance causes body odour.
Sebaceous gland	Mainly attached to hair follicles, these consist of secretory cells that secrete sebum. They are found all over the body with the exception of the soles of the feet and the palms of the hand. Sebum is an oily substance that keeps the skin soft, lubricated and to some degree waterproof. It mixes with sweat to form the acid mantle that helps to fight bacteria and infection. Sebum also contains chemical substances that kill microbes. The glands increase in activity at puberty.
Hairs, hair bulbs and hair follicles	Hair follicles are formed when there is a down-growth of epidermal cells into the dermis. At the base of these follicles is a cluster of cells called the hair bulb. When these cells divide a hair is formed, which is then pushed up the follicle as it undergoes keratinisation. The portion of hair within the follicle is referred to as the hair root, and the portion visible above the skin as the hair shaft.
Arrector pili muscle	These are bundles of involuntary muscle fibres attached to hair follicles. When the muscle contracts, the hair is pulled upright and the surrounding skin puckers up to create 'goose bumps'. The muscle is stimulated by nerve impulses triggered by cold or fear.

The subcutaneous layer

This is a thick, insulating layer of fat and connective tissue found below the dermis that supports fragile structures such as lymph and blood vessels. The layer also consists of **adipose tissue**, which plays a role in the formation and storage of fat. The fat cells contained within this tissue help to insulate the body by reducing heat loss, keeping the body warm and forming a protective covering for the body.

Acid mantle

As mentioned before, one of the functions of the skin is to act as a barrier to protect the body against infection. Sebum and sweat mix at body temperature creating a barrier known as the acid mantle. Bacteria thrive in an alkaline environment and the acid mantle forms a slightly acidic barrier, helping to resist the invasion of these microbes.

The degree of acidity or alkalinity of a substance is measured by its pH value. The neutral point on the scale is 7. Anything below 7 is acidic – the lower the number, the stronger the acidity. A pH level between 7 and 14 means that a substance is alkaline – the higher the number the stronger the alkali.

The skin has a value of between 4.5 and 6. Many products now available are pH balanced at 5.5, giving them a very similar pH to that of the skin. Using topical products that are not pH balanced will result in the acid mantle being removed, leaving the skin vulnerable to infection.

The skin and the ageing process

The ageing process is determined by biological changes within the skin: from conception to birth, body cells multiply fast to allow for rapid development and growth. However, from the moment we are born, this process gets slower and slower, with a number of key stages in our development affecting the skin greatly: puberty, pregnancy and the menopause continuing into old age. These changes can mainly be put down to fluctuations in hormonal levels within the body.

Changes during puberty

* Increase in hair growth on the face, chest, abdomen, underarms and pubis.
* The skin thickens and there is an increase in sebaceous gland activity, resulting in more sebum being produced. This makes the surface more oily and prone to skin conditions such as acne vulgaris.

Changes during pregnancy

Each woman will experience the effects of pregnancy in different ways. However, common changes include the following.

* Skin colour may darken, either in patches or all over. Birthmarks, moles and freckles may also darken. Some women develop chloasma – a skin pigmentation disorder (see page 58).
* Hair growth may increase during pregnancy, although some women experience an increase in hair loss. Hair texture may also change, becoming greasier or drier.
* Stretch marks, usually appearing across the abdomen, thighs, hips or breasts, are caused by the breakdown of protein in the skin by the high levels of pregnancy hormones
  They appear as red streaks which will eventually fade to become pale and barely noticeable.
* The skin often appears to develop a 'bloom' due to an increase in the blood circulating around the body.

Changes during menopause and into old age

* The stratum corneum begins to thicken or build up due to a slowing down of the desquamation process. The rate at which these cells are usually shed is significantly reduced; the result is that skin appears dull and less youthful as time goes by.

* Collagen and elastin fibre production slows down, resulting in a general loss of elasticity and firmness in the skin and a gradual thinning of the dermis.

* Collagen and elastin fibres undergo an irreversible process called 'cross-linking', causing fibres to fuse together. This results in puckering and indentations on the skin's surface that we refer to as lines and wrinkles.

* 'Lines of expression' caused by facial movement appear as the skin loses its resilience.

* Blood flow is reduced, lessening nutrition to the cells and resulting in a greying of the complexion.

* The production of sebum slows down, resulting in a drier skin texture.

* Melanocytes clump together in the dermis forming patches of pigmentation, commonly known as age spots.

* Hair loses its colour and condition as the re-growth cycle slows down and the production of sebum slows down, reducing the amount of natural hair oil.

Causes of premature ageing of the skin

The ageing process can be affected by lifestyle and environmental factors contributing to **premature or accelerated ageing**.

* UVA and UVB rays pass through to the dermis causing damage to the cells within. It has been proven that up to 95 per cent of the visible signs of ageing are caused by sun damage.

Visible signs of sun damage include a 'leathery' texture, with evident lines and loss of tone. As a direct result of the skin's attempt to protect itself, melanocytes increase the production of melanin. This forms pigment in the skin resulting in a darkening of the skin colour.

* Lack of skin care or incorrect skin care routines can accelerate the ageing process.

* Poor health or a poor diet affect the condition of the skin. Extreme loss of weight can cause loss of supporting subcutaneous adipose tissue, resulting in loose skin tissue.

* Lifestyle choices, such as fatigue, smoking and stress, all contribute to premature ageing.

How skin heals

1 The damaged surface of the skin becomes inflamed and fills with blood clotting cells (platelets) and cell debris (in the first few hours)

↓

2 White blood cells (phagocytes) and fibroblasts arrive at the wound

↓

3 Phagocytes begin to break down the clot and the fibrocytes create collagen fibres that begin to bind the wound together

↓

4 Epithelial cells arrive and begin to seal the wound by creating a scab (stages 2 to 4 take between three and five days)

↓

5 The scab falls away

↓

6 Layers of epithelial cells continue to grow upwards until the skin regains full thickness

↓

7 There is no longer any inflammation but vascular, fibrous scar tissue may remain, which may take a number of weeks or months to reduce

Skin diseases and disorders

As a make-up artist you should be familiar with certain skin disorders and diseases. There are various terms for the identification of skin lesions:

macule – a flat area of abnormal colour, for example a freckle

papule – a small superficial lump not containing fluid; a large, deep-seated papule is called a nodule – a large papule is a tumour

pustule – a raised lesion containing pus, which often commences as a papule; it usually develops at hair follicles, appearing red and inflamed with a yellow head

vesicle – a small blister (collection of clear fluid)

bulla – a large blister

scales – a build up of flakes of dead skin cells on the skin's surface

crust – scabs of dried secretions: black or brown = blood; yellow = lymph; grey or green = pus.

You will find it helpful to research these lesions, and the skin disorders described below, so that you can recognise them when examining clients.

Disorders of pigmentation

Ephelides (freckles)

These are small pigmented areas of skin and are caused by an uneven distribution of melanin. They become more noticeable when exposed to sunlight and are mostly found on blonde and red-headed people. They do not affect make-up procedures.

Chloasma

Chloasma is a condition of pigmentation commonly associated with pregnancy. It normally forms a 'butterfly shape' area of dark pigmentation and affects the upper cheeks, nose and forehead. It does not affect make-up procedures, but camouflage techniques can be applied.

Vitiligo

This condition causes patches of skin to lose pigment as melanocytes are unable to produce melanin. When it occurs over hairy areas, the hairs become white. Patches must be protected from ultra-violet exposure. It does not affect make-up procedures, but camouflage techniques can be applied.

Lentigo

Often associated with older people, dark areas of pigmentation form that have a slightly raised appearance. They are also known as age spots. They do not affect make-up techniques.

Port wine stain

A port wine stain is a large, irregular-shaped area of dilated capillaries thought to be caused by pressure on the growing foetus. The area can vary in colour from pink to dark red or purple. It is more common on the face and can be disfiguring. It does not affect make-up procedures, but camouflage techniques can be applied.

Strawberry naevus

This is a raised, brightly pigmented area that is red-purple in colour. It is seen at birth or develops soon after. Growth usually stops by 12 months and disappears by the age of 12 years.

Bacterial infections

Boils

Boils are caused by bacterial infection of a single hair follicle, resulting in a swollen lump that is painful and filled with pus. They may leave a scar as the deeper layers of the skin are involved. The area should be avoided during make-up procedures.

Folliculitis

This is bacterial infection affecting many hair follicles. It commences with redness around the hairs and develops into pustules and boils. It often requires a course of antibiotics to clear. The area should be avoided during make-up procedures.

Styes

A stye is an infection of an eyelash follicle leading to inflammation. It usually contains pus. The area should be avoided during make-up procedures.

Conjunctivitis

This is inflammation of the conjunctiva (the thin membrane covering the front of the eyes). The eyes become red, itchy and sore; there is a swelling of the eyelids and a discharge of pus. It is extremely infectious and make-up procedures should be avoided. Conjunctivitis requires GP referral.

Impetigo

Highly contagious, this can be spread by direct or indirect contact. It affects the epidermis and begins as small red spots, followed by the appearance of yellow, itchy blisters. Impetigo spreads rapidly and commonly begins around the mouth. It is extremely infectious and make-up procedures should be avoided. It requires GP referral.

Acne vulgaris

The skin is covered to varying degrees with pustules and nodules. Commonly associated with an oily complexion, the skin appears congested with blackheads and becomes infected with bacteria causing inflammation. It may cause scarring. Make-up procedures can be carried out on mild acne, but should be avoided on severe cases. Do not hesitate to refer to the GP for treatment.

Acne rosacea

A raised, red area covering the nose and cheeks, this is often accompanied by the presence of papules and pustules. It is thought to be aggravated by the consumption of spicy foods and alcohol. Make-up procedures can be carried out on mild acne, but should be avoided on severe cases. Do not hesitate to refer to the GP for treatment.

Viral infections

Herpes simplex (cold sores)

Once the virus has been contracted it remains in the body throughout a person's life. Extremes of temperature, tiredness or the onset of a cold (hence its common name) may cause the virus to become active. Highly infectious, cold sores can be spread by direct or indirect contact. The sores begin as a 'tingling' sensation on the skin. This develops into an erythema, which in turn develops into weepy vesicles. Finally a crust is formed. The area should be avoided during make-up procedures.

Herpes zoster (shingles)

A painful condition, this affects the nerves of the skin. It causes a painful rash of small, crusting blisters. Even after the rash heals, the pain may persist for many months. Make-up procedures should be avoided when the rash is present.

Verruca vulgaris (common warts)

Highly contagious papules that vary in size, these appear most frequently on the hands, although they can be found all over the body. They tend to disappear of their own accord. The area should be avoided during make-up procedures.

Verruca plantaris

This belongs to the same family as the common wart, but rather than growing outwards, the wart grows inwards. It may become painful as it becomes larger. The surface of the skin has a rounded area of dry skin with a black dot (or dots) in the centre. It requires treatment for removal.

Fungal infections

Tinea (ringworm)

Ring-shaped, reddened, scaly patches develop into pustules on the skin. For its full name, the word tinea is followed by the Latin term for the affected part of the body. For example, **tinea pedis** affects the feet, **tinea corporis** affects the body and **tinea manus** affects the hands and nails. Tinea is highly contagious and cross-contamination can occur from person to person, from animals or from objects. Make-up procedures should be avoided. Tinea requires GP referral.

Skin imperfections
Dilated capillaries

These are ruptured blood vessels that appear on thin, dry, sensitive skin types and occur most commonly across the nose and cheeks. They are caused by repeated contraction and dilation (opening and closing) of the capillaries, resulting in a loss of elasticity in their walls which makes the capillaries visible on the surface of the skin. The condition can be exacerbated by severe weather conditions, spicy food and alcohol. Vitamin P combined with Vitamin C can help to strengthening the walls of the capillaries. They do not affect make-up procedures, but camouflage techniques can be applied.

Spider naevus

This is a central dilated blood vessel with smaller capillaries radiating from it like the legs of a spider. The spider naevus usually develops in adult life, particularly during pregnancy because of hormonal changes. It does not affect make-up procedures.

Milia

Milia appear as white, pearl-like lumps under the skin and are formed when sebum becomes trapped. They are commonly found on dry skin types and around the eyes. They can only be removed by 'breaking' the skin's surface using a sterile probe or diathermy. Milia do not affect make-up procedures.

Comedones

Comedones are commonly known as blackheads because of their dark colour. They are usually found on oily skin, as they are caused by excess sebum secretions blocking the entrance to the sebaceous gland. The dark colour of the blackhead is due to surface debris turning black when it comes into contact with oxygen (oxidisation). They do not affect make-up procedures.

Verruca filiformis (skin tags)

Skin tags are commonly found on areas exposed to repeated friction, for example collar lines, armpits and bra strap lines. They have a soft fibrous tissue form, which looks like a loose extension of the skin, and are attached to the surface by a 'stalk'. The colour may be grey or hyperpigmented. They can be removed by diathermy or by a GP under local anaesthetic. They do not affect make-up procedures.

Long-term skin disorders
Eczema and dermatitis

These start as a very dry, scaly, itching red area with tiny vesicles which progress in severe cases to weeping sores. This is a tissue reaction involving the epidermis and upper layers of the dermis and is caused by:

* external contact with a substance to which the skin is allergic – **dermatitis**
* internal stimuli via the blood stream (systemic) – **eczema**.

Medical advice is often required to determine which of these is present, as the surface skin reactions are much the same. It is not infectious. Make-up procedures can be carried out on mild conditions, preferably using hypo-allergenic products, but they should be avoided on severe cases.

Psoriasis

Psoriasis is non-infectious and commonly affects the elbows and knees, but can be found anywhere on the face and body. It develops as red patches with distinct edges, with flaky-silvery scales on the surface. The cause is unknown, but sufferers have reccurring attacks throughout life which have been linked to stress. Make-up procedures can be carried out on mild psoriasis, but should be avoided on severe cases. Camouflage techniques can be applied.

Skin infestations

Scabies

This is a skin infestation caused by the female itch mite, which burrows into the skin where she lays eggs. Scabies is highly contagious. It is visible on the skin's surface as small, grey, scaly swellings, and is usually found between the fingers, on the wrists, genitals and in the armpits. It may progress into red lumps on the limbs and upper body. The visible symptoms are accompanied by itching, often resulting in scabs and sores. It requires medical attention and make-up procedures should be avoided.

Lice

Small, wingless insects lay a daily batch of tiny, pale eggs (nits). After approximately seven days they hatch, feeding on human blood and living for up to several weeks. There are three types of species, each living on different areas of the body – the head, the body or the pubic area. Hairstyling and make-up procedures should be avoided until treatment has been carried out.

Skin cancer

Basal cell carcinoma

Commonly known as a rodent ulcer, this is thought to be associated with long-term exposure to sunlight and often affects areas of the body that have had repeated exposure, such as the face. It is visible as a nodule, which later breaks down becoming an ulcer. This type of cancer is locally invasive but seldom spreads. All suspicious skin areas should be reported to a doctor.

Malignant melanoma

This is another type of cancer thought to be caused by exposure to UV light. It usually originates as a blue-black mole that gradually increases in size. Although a relatively rare type of cancer, there has been an increase in its occurrence over the past couple of decades, thought to be due to an increase in the ozone level. If an existing mole increases in size, changes colour, or ulcerates and bleeds, medical attention should be sought immediately. This type of cancer can spread quickly. All suspicious skin areas should be reported to a doctor.

Squamous cell carcinoma

Again associated with UV skin damage, this tumour starts as a small, firm, painless lump or patch. Commonly affected areas are the lips, ears, nose and back of the hands. It gradually enlarges, resembling a wart or ulcer. Without treatment, the tumour may spread to other parts of the body and prove fatal. All suspicious skin areas should be reported to a doctor.

Structure of the hair

Hairs are found in hair follicles. Hair follicles are formed when there is a down-growth of epidermal

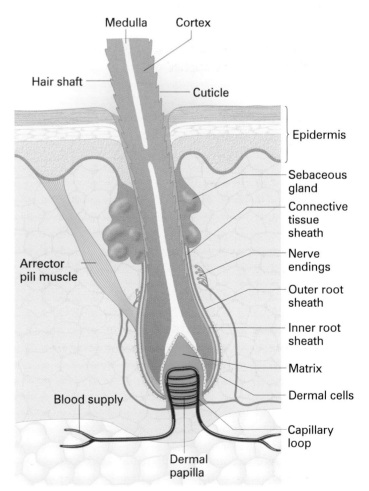

A vertical cross-section of hair in its follicle

cells into the dermis. These follicles are made up of an inner sheath and an outer sheath. At the base of these follicles lies a cluster of cells called the matrix, which is contained within the hair bulb. When these living cells divide a hair is formed, which is then pushed up the follicle. It dies as it moves away from the source of nourishment (dermal papillae) and undergoes keratinisation. The portion of hair within the follicle is referred to as the hair root and the portion visible above the skin as the hair shaft. The hair is a dead structure composed mainly of the protein keratin.

The hair has three layers:

* cuticle: the outer layer, covered in protective scales, which protects the cortex and gives the hair elasticity
* cortex: the middle layer, which gives the hair strength and pigment (it contains melanin)
* medulla: the inner layer consisting of air spaces between keratinised cells, which gives the hair shine as light passes though the air spaces.

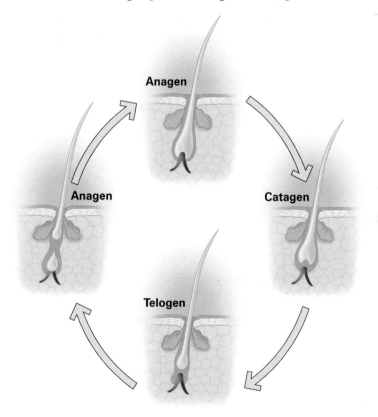

Hair growth cycle

Hair growth cycle

Hair growth begins on a foetus at around the third month. Throughout life hormones, the ageing process, illness and diet all affect hair growth. The growth pattern is a continuous cycle, which varies according to the area of growth: an eyelash hair takes approximately three months to complete the cycle, a hair on the scalp anywhere between four and eight years. The growth cycle follows three stages:

* anagen – the growing stage
* catagen – the changing stage
* telogen – the resting stage.

Anagen

The hair is receiving nourishment from the dermal papillae, allowing the cells in the matrix to reproduce (by mitosis). The hair grows and moves upwards out of the hair bulb, forming its different layers and structures. Cells undergo keratinisation, and the hair eventually moves out of the inner root sheath, emerging at the surface of the skin.

Catagen

The hair separates from the dermal papillae and becomes loose in the base of the hair follicle, slowly moving upwards to rest just below the sebaceous gland. It still receives some nourishment from the follicle wall. A hair in this stage is sometimes known as a club hair, as it does not have a bulb.

Telogen

The final, shortest stage is known as the resting period. The hair follicle remains in this stage until hormones stimulate the follicle to return to the anagen stage, when the hair is shed to make way for a new hair.

Types of hair growth

There are three types of hair growth:

lanugo – hair found on a growing foetus
vellus – soft, downy hair found over most of the body except the soles of the feet and palms of the hand
terminal – strong hairs containing pigment, found on the head, pubic regions, eyebrows etc.

Blood system

It is useful for the make-up artist to understand the blood system, particularly when planning casualty effects. Blood is essential for human and animal life. It is the transport system for the body, delivering nourishment to cells in the body and removing waste and toxins. Blood is carried under pressure in blood vessels and is moved around by a continuous pumping action provided by the heart. In a resting human body the heart pumps five litres of blood every minute; this is increased substantially during strenuous exercise.

Blood is a sticky substance that is made up of:

* 55 per cent plasma
* 45 per cent blood cells (99 per cent are red blood corpuscles (erythrocytes) which contain the blood colour, haemoglobin; 1 per cent are white blood corpuscles (leucocytes) and platelets).

Functions of the blood

Transport

* Oxygen is carried from the heart and lungs to the cells of the body.
* Carbon dioxide is carried from the cells back to the heart and lungs.
* Nutrients are carried from the digestive system to the cells.
* Waste products are removed from the cells to be excreted.
* Hormones are carried from the endocrine glands to the organs.

Defence

* White blood cells are carried around the body to fight against infection and disease.
* Platelets are specialised blood cells that clot to prevent blood loss when the skin becomes damaged.

Regulation

* The blood regulates body heat, which has been produced by the liver and muscles, by carrying it around the body.
* The blood regulates the body's pH levels.
* The blood also regulates the water content of the cells.

Blood vessels

These are the vessels that transport the blood around the body.

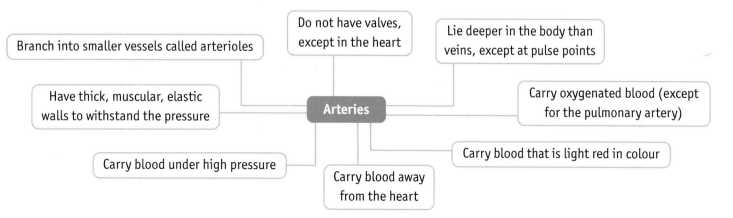

Branch into smaller vessels called arterioles

Do not have valves, except in the heart

Lie deeper in the body than veins, except at pulse points

Have thick, muscular, elastic walls to withstand the pressure

Arteries

Carry oxygenated blood (except for the pulmonary artery)

Carry blood under high pressure

Carry blood away from the heart

Carry blood that is light red in colour

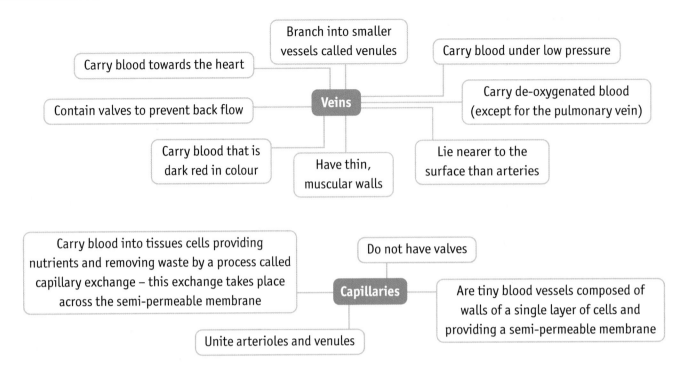

Carry blood towards the heart

Branch into smaller vessels called venules

Carry blood under low pressure

Contain valves to prevent back flow

Veins

Carry de-oxygenated blood (except for the pulmonary vein)

Carry blood that is dark red in colour

Have thin, muscular walls

Lie nearer to the surface than arteries

Carry blood into tissues cells providing nutrients and removing waste by a process called capillary exchange – this exchange takes place across the semi-permeable membrane

Do not have valves

Capillaries

Are tiny blood vessels composed of walls of a single layer of cells and providing a semi-permeable membrane

Unite arterioles and venules

The heart

The heart is a large, muscular organ that is responsible for pumping blood around the body to maintain a constant circulation. It is divided into three layers of tissue:

* pericardium: the outer layer
* myocardium: the middle layer
* endocardium: the inner layer.

The heart is divided into two sides – the right and left – by a partition called the septum. Each side is further divided into atriums (at the top) and ventricles (at the bottom) by valves: the tricuspid on the right and the bicuspid or mitral on the left. These valves prevent the regurgitation of blood between the atriums and ventricles.

The circulation of blood

The heart receives de-oxygenated blood from the body via two main veins – the superior and inferior vena cava. This blood is delivered to the right ventricle through the tricuspid valve. The blood then leaves the heart via the pulmonary arteries and is carried to the lungs where carbon dioxide is removed and oxygen levels are

replenished. The oxygenated blood is carried back to the heart via the pulmonary veins entering through the left atrium and passing into the left

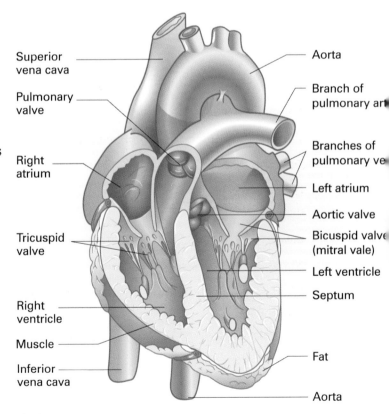

Superior vena cava

Pulmonary valve

Right atrium

Tricuspid valve

Right ventricle

Muscle

Inferior vena cava

Aorta

Branch of pulmonary art

Branches of pulmonary ve

Left atrium

Aortic valve

Bicuspid valve (mitral vale)

Left ventricle

Septum

Fat

Aorta

The heart

ventricle via the bicuspid (mitral) valve. The blood is then pumped out of the heart via the aorta and into the systemic circulation, to be transported to all parts of the body (except the lungs).

> **KEY NOTE**
>
> **Blood pressure** is the force with which the blood is pumped around the body. It is measured in millimetres of mercury and takes into account the maximum (systolic) and minimum (diastolic) pressure during a heart beat. It can be affected by stress, excitement, fitness and lifestyle choices such as smoking. **The pulse** is a pressure wave that can be felt in the arteries with every beat of the heart.

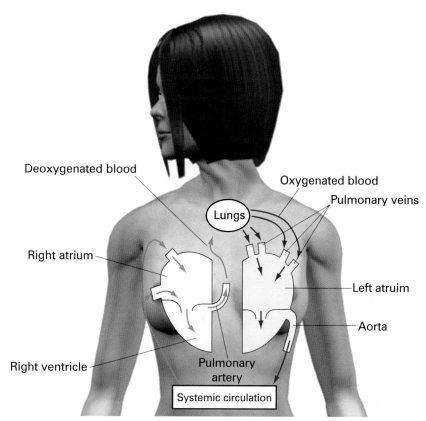

Blood circulation

Knowledge Check

1. List the eight bones of the cranium.
2. Name the bones that form the shoulder girdle.
3. Which is the only moveable bone in the skull?
4. Describe muscle tone and how it can vary.
5. Describe the position of the corrugator muscle and its action.
6. List the five layers of the epidermis.
7. Name the protein in the epidermis.
8. What is the function of melanin and where is it found?
9. How do cells regenerate in the epidermis?
10. What is the function of the dermal papillae?
11. What is the function of the sensory nerve endings?
12. What is the function of the subcutaneous layer?
13. List the seven functions of the skin.
14. Describe how skin is affected by the ageing process.
15. Describe the skin condition vitiligo.
16. Describe the skin disease impetigo.
17. Name the three layers of the hair.
18. Where are new hair cells produced?
19. What are the stages of hair growth?
20. Describe the differences between veins, arteries and capillaries.

Developing the artistic eye

Sometimes people forget that a make-up artist is just that – an artist who uses make-up as a medium and the body as a canvas. The more 'naturally artistic' a student is, the easier it will be for him or her to pick up many of the skills required of the make-up artist. However, many make-up artists would consider themselves as being creative rather than artistic in the traditional sense.

Aim and objectives

Aim of this chapter: to provide you with the artistic fundamentals required to progress with many make-up techniques.

You should achieve the following **objectives:**

* Discuss the tools required for various mark making in make-up application
* Create various marks on your canvas using a variety of tools
* Discuss the importance of keeping a workbook and creating a reference file
* Discuss the basics of colour theory
* Demonstrate competence in mixing a variety of colours and tones
* Create form using light and shade
* Imitate a variety of textures using marks and materials

* Draw the human head, giving consideration to proportion, anatomical structure and individual characteristics
* Transform sketches into workable designs for make-up and hair
* Professionally present your ideas to clients
* Create design sheets
* Use your imagination and find inspiration from a variety of sources.

Equipment and products

In order to complete the activities in this chapter you will need the following equipment in addition to your standard make-up kit.

* Pencils in a range of grades from HB to 6B. The grade of a pencil refers to the softness or hardness of its lead.

* Paper – an A3 sketch book and A3 pad of watercolour paper are advisable. It is important to use watercolour paper when working with water-based paints as this will prevent the paper from wrinkling. Paper is available in a number of different textures from smooth to rough – for the exercises in this chapter a smooth paper is preferable.

* A longish ruler.

* An eraser.

* A selection of water-based paints in red, blue, yellow, black and white.

* Tracing paper and acetate.

Mirrors and lighting

When you create a make-up for film, television or photography you are essentially creating an image that will be viewed on a two-dimensional medium. Using a mirror will help you 'see' how your make-up will be viewed two-dimensionally. In addition, cameras use mirrors to record images they receive through the lens, so viewing your make-up in the same way will help you view your work as a camera would. Mistakes in your work, which could otherwise be missed, become glaringly obvious in the mirror. It is particularly useful for checking symmetry in your make-up.

It is also important that your mirror is adequately lit. Lighting has a direct effect on make-up application, affecting colour and strength. The best type of lighting is daylight balanced; any other type of light will affect how you view the make-up. This is discussed in more detail in Chapter 6 'Professional studies'.

Tools and mark making in make-up application

Brushes

Your make-up brushes are indispensable. Buy the most expensive brushes you can afford and they will reward you by offering durability, ease of care and excellent application. Natural fibres, such as sable hairs, are usually preferable to synthetic fibres as they can be sanitised more effectively. There is little difference between good quality, sable haired traditional artists brushes and the brushes on sale in make-up stores. Most make-up artists will have a combination of both in their kits. Always test brushes on the back of your hand; if they scratch or irritate the skin don't use them. Try to collect a good variety of sizes and shapes – brushes with fine points, flat brushes, round brushes, firm brushes, soft brushes. The bigger the selection, the more tools you have to choose from.

Sponges

Make-up wedges are a popular tool for applying make-up, particularly bases, to the skin. They are also useful for blending make-up. They are commonly made from latex, although alternative materials are available for those with an allergy. A firmer texture is preferred and they can be tested by soaking them in water – if the wedge goes floppy and misshapen it will be difficult to work with. Make-up wedges are available in a variety of sizes and shapes.

Stipple sponges are useful for creating texture effects. They are available as fine or coarse.

Natural sea sponges are useful for applying natural textures to the skin as they offer irregular natural patterns. They can also be used to apply an ultra-fine, natural looking base.

Make-up pencils

Pencils can be used to apply various marks onto the skin. They are available in soft and hard textures and a variety of sizes, for example Kajal pencils are thick and very soft.

Holding the brush

There are various ways to hold a brush. It is best to experiment and find a position that is comfortable and gives you the greatest control. Unless you are painting fine detail, move your arm rather than just your hand to create strokes that 'flow'. This avoids 'stiff' looking strokes that are created when the brush is used as a pencil. For greater control it is sometimes useful to rest your little finger lightly on the canvas. Some make-up artists will use a clean powder-puff under their working hand to avoid contact with the model's skin. It is very important not to lean on the model.

The width of the brush strokes will depend on how much pressure is applied to the brush. For fine strokes the tip of the brush should glide over the canvas; to make wider strokes, press down on the brush. The length of the brush hair will also affect the type of stroke that is created – longer lengths of hair will create looser, more flowing strokes than shorter ones. The firmness or softness of the hair will also affect the brush stroke.

Creating lines

You can practise this technique on the inside of your arm or on a model. You will need two crème-based make-up colours – one that matches the skin tone and another significantly darker. Begin by applying a base to the area that matches the skin tone using a make-up wedge.

* Using a fine pointed or flat, narrow, square-edged brush, angled at 90° (right angle) to the skin, stroke the darker colour onto the skin creating a straight, even, crisp, narrow line. Practise this several times ensuring your pressure remains constant and the line remains the same in appearance from start to finish.

* Then create some additional straight, crisp, narrow lines, but this time vary the pressure. Reduce the pressure as you move along to create a line that fades.

* Next, create some curved lines using the above techniques.

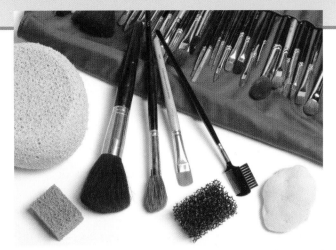

From left: large and small synthetic sponges, a selection of brushes, a course stipple sponge and a natural sea sponge

* Calligraphic lines are characterised by variations in width along the length. Try creating some of these lines by varying the pressure and angle of the brush against the skin.

* Repeated lines are also useful. Try painting several lines next to each other, ensuring they look identical and the width between them remains constant.

Feathering lines

Used to soften one side of a line, feathering lines create a gradual change of tone. The result is a line with an edge that starts as dark and hard and then softens and blends into the surrounding skin tone. Again, begin by applying a base to the area that matches the skin tone. Make one straight, even, crisp, narrow line. Place a clean, flat, narrow brush on the top of the line and drag away sideways, reducing the pressure as you go and keeping the original edge of the line crisp. Continue in this manner down the length of the line. You should end up with a wide line that graduates in tone from side to side.

Blending

A very important technique that forms the basis of most make-up applications is blending. It is vital that you learn to blend cleanly and accurately. Begin by painting several repeated lines over a make-up base, as described earlier. Take a make-up wedge and work across the lines with a 'patting' motion, blending the lines so they merge. Keep working the area until you end up with a shadowed area that graduates in tone from dark in the centre to lighter at the edges, eventually blending into the surrounding skin tone. Avoid 'rubbing' the area as this can 'dirty' your make-up.

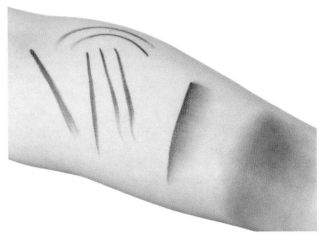

Creating lines, feathering lines and blending repeated lines to create a shadow

Mixing highlights and shadows for skin tones

All skin tones are derived from tints and shades of the three quaternary colours (see Colour Theory section from page 70). From the darkest to the lightest skin tones, each one of us will have one of these three basic brown shades underlying our complexion. Shadows and highlights in the skin are therefore variations of these mixes.

When applying shadows and highlights to the skin it is important to ensure there is a significant tonal difference between them and the base colour, otherwise they will be lost. You can test this in a couple of ways. Apply some of the shadow and highlight colour, blend lightly, step back and squint at the tones (use your mirror if your workstation has one). If they fade into the base colour you will need to strengthen them; if they look very harsh you may need to reduce their strength.

The easiest way to mix shadows and highlights is to take some of the base colour and add the appropriate colours. This will ensure your shadow and highlight will share a common colour range with the base, creating a natural-looking result. Use the tables below to help you mix correctly.

Shadows

Tonal range	Colours found in black skins	Colours found in white skins
Two to three shades darker than base	Purple, blue, and for very dark skins a touch of black	Greyish-brown or brownish-grey, red-brown for darker areas of definition

Highlights

Tonal range	Colours found in black skins	Colours found in white skins
Two to three shades lighter than base	Muted orange and yellows	Pale pink and pale yellow, cream, and for very light skins a touch of white.

HANDS ON

We can learn much from looking at how artists use colour in their portrait painting to depict shadows and highlights in the skin. Look in books or on the Internet for examples. For instance, Rembrandt's 'Self-portrait with beret and turned up collar' (1659) shows use of colour in depicting shadows and highlights in skin.

Keeping a workbook

A workbook is a useful place for keeping a record of your ideas and thoughts about potential designs. Sometimes ideas will come to you at the most unexpected times and often, if you do not write them down you will forget them. The more you use your workbook the more imaginative an artist you will become. You can also use your workbook for the following:

For **practising** skills and techniques you are shown and **experimenting** with new ideas, or trying out different ways to compose or colour your make-ups. Some of the new ideas you try out may not work, but you won't know until you try. Some may turn out to be so successful that you can then develop them into workable designs and a final piece of work.

For **notes and records**. It is also a place to keep a record of sources of inspiration. Magazine clippings and pictures you come across, articles about products, etc. can all be a source of inspiration for future designs. An idea jotted down on a page or a clipping from a magazine may later prompt you to turn it into a finished design.

For **curing 'designer's block'**. A make-up artist's workbook is a great builder of confidence. Even experienced make-up artists are sometimes intimidated when faced with a new brief. Working out ideas in a sketchbook gives you the chance to practise and try out ideas before you start on the real thing.

Finally, the workbook is a place to develop your creativity and style through collecting clippings of ideas and images that interest you and jotting down ideas that come to you. In this way, your sketchbook will become a record of how you develop as a make-up artist.

Keeping a reference file

A reference file is a valuable tool for a make-up artist. Collecting pictures for this file should be an ongoing process, so be on the constant lookout for potentially useful images. Newspapers and their supplements, magazines and brochures are all valuable hunting grounds. As you progress through this book, you will be encouraged to source various images. However, the earlier you start to collect reference material the better prepared you will be for your make-up designs and application.

How you file your reference material is down to personal preference, but whatever method you choose, it should be well organised. There is no point in having a picture that you cannot lay your hands on when required.

Your reference file could contain the following:

* images of artwork and sculptures you find interesting
* images of high fashion (make-up and hair)
* a variety of full frontal, head, neck and shoulder images of women of different ages, and social and ethnic backgrounds
* a variety of full frontal, head, neck and shoulder images of men of different ages, and social and ethnic backgrounds
* facial expressions and emotions
* children
* obesity and emaciation
* nose shapes
* styles of facial hair
* casualty injuries
* skin diseases and disorders
* corpses
* baldness and alopecia
* images of people photographed at different ages, demonstrating the ageing process
* hair styles and wigs
* examples of fictional characters, for example fairies, Dracula
* examples of historical characters, for example Winston Churchill, Cleopatra, Geishas
* historical fashion
* make-ups from television, film and theatre
* images from nature – flowers, animals, textures, etc.

Colour theory

As a make-up artist, it is important to understand the principles of colour theory.

The principles of colour and light

In 1676, the British physicist Isaac Newton used a triangular prism to demonstrate scientifically how colours are formed and to show the existence of an entire colour spectrum. To do this, he shone a ray of sunlight onto the prism, placing a white screen in front of the ray as it passed out from the prism. The prism produced a range of colours from red to orange to yellow to green to blue to indigo and violet on the screen.

There are three basic colours – red, yellow and blue. All other colours are combinations of these three. Mixing red and blue produces violet, blue and yellow produce green, red and yellow produce orange and so on.

If you isolate one colour from the spectrum – red, for example – and mix the rest of the colours the result will be green. This is because green is the complement of red, the colour we have isolated. If, on the other hand, you isolate yellow, the remaining colours will produce its complement, which is violet. So every colour in the spectrum is the complement of the colour resulting from the mix of all the others – a scientific fact used by artists every time colours are mixed on a palette.

This quirky saying will help you remember the colours and their order in the spectrum: Richard (Red) Of (Orange) York (Yellow) Gave (Green) Battle (Blue) In (Indigo) Vain (Violet).

Colours are produced by light waves, which are a particular type of electromagnetic radiation. We measure wavelengths in microns. The light waves that we can actually see are those between 400 and 700 microns in length. But there are also colours that we cannot see because their wavelengths are beyond our range. As well as being formed of waves, light also has the property of being particles of energy called photons. Colour is therefore a type of energy, and it has a direct physical effect on us. Many blind people are able to identify colours using their fingertips alone.

Colour is communicated to objects by light hitting them. The light is partially absorbed and partially reflected. The colour of the surface is determined by the degree to which each colour of the spectrum is absorbed. For example, the atomic structure of the skin of a red tomato will reflect red light waves (which is what we see) and absorb the others. Grass will reflect green light waves and absorb the others. Black absorbs all light waves and white reflects them all.

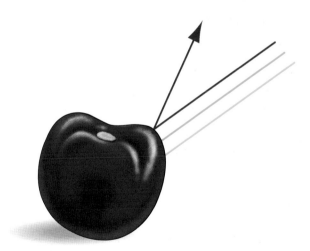

Light reflecting on the surface of a tomato

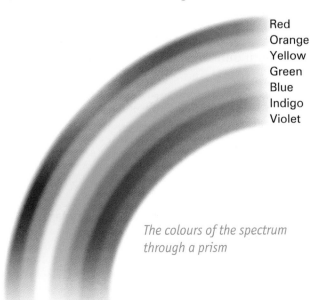

Red
Orange
Yellow
Green
Blue
Indigo
Violet

The colours of the spectrum through a prism

There are only a handful of basic words to describe colour in the English language, and yet there are millions of colours. Computers can give us approximately 16 million colours and the human eye can distinguish an even larger number. After the basic words, we use words borrowed from other sources to describe shades of colour, such as 'olive green'.

There are two colour systems – the **additive system** that refers to colour created by light and the **subtractive system** that refers to colour created by pigments. As a make-up artist you need to familiarise yourself with both, but in this chapter we will be looking at the subtractive system in more detail.

The basics of colour harmony when using colour pigments

Colours can be combined in many ways. As a make-up artist you will need to understand the basic principles of colour harmony when using colour pigments. The colour wheel is used to explain the following principles of colour harmony. Because pigments, unlike light, are not pure it is sometimes difficult to mix the exact colour we want. Knowing just what you can mix from your colours is often a case of trial and error and will differ from product to product and from manufacturer to manufacturer.

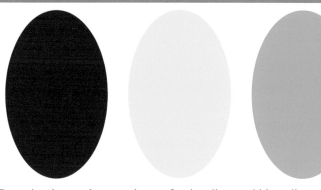

From the three primary colours of red, yellow and blue all additional colours are created

Mixing all three primary colours together in equal quantities will create a **neutral colour**, resembling very dark grey. If you change the proportions of each primary colour in the mix, a variety of neutral tones can be achieved.

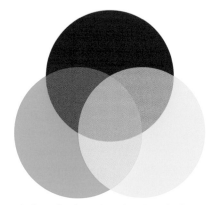

Three overlapping circles of primaries showing dark grey at centre and secondary colours

Mixing equal amounts of two of the primary colours creates the **secondary colours:**
yellow + blue = green
red + yellow = orange
blue + red = violet

Tertiary colours are achieved by mixing a secondary colour and a primary colour in equal amounts, for example blue-violet, yellow-green.

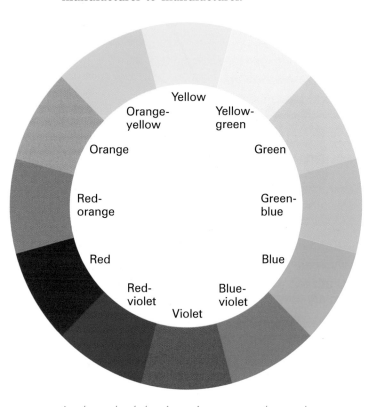

Yellow
Orange-yellow   Yellow-green
Orange   Green
Red-orange   Green-blue
Red   Blue
Red-violet   Blue-violet
Violet

A colour wheel showing primary, secondary and tertiary colours

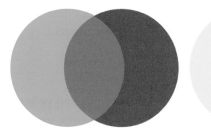

Tertiary mixes

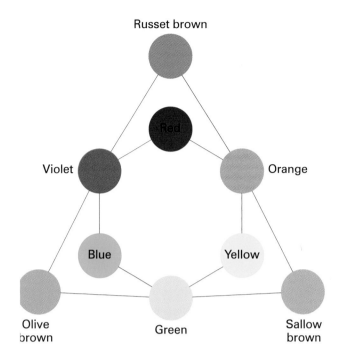

Quaternary mixes

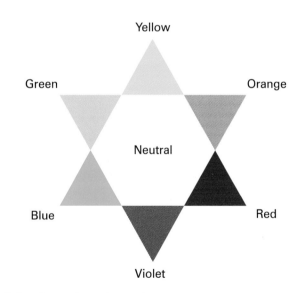

Pairs of complementary colours

Quaternary colours, a series of three distinct tones of brown, are created by mixing two secondary colours together.

Orange + violet = russet brown
The russet brown is made up from red and yellow (orange) and red and blue (violet), thereby creating a mix of two parts red, one part yellow and one part blue. This gives the brown a reddish hue.

Orange + green = sallow brown
The sallow brown is made up from red and yellow (orange) and blue and yellow (green), thereby creating a mix of two parts yellow, one part red and one part blue. This gives the brown a yellowish hue.

Green + violet = olive brown
The olive brown is made up from blue and yellow (green) and red and blue (violet), thereby creating a mix of two parts blue, one part yellow and one part red. This gives the brown a bluish hue.

If you look at the colour wheel, you will see that a secondary colour is always directly opposite a primary colour. These opposite colours are said to complement each other, for example, as we have seen, red complements green, yellow complements violet and blue complements orange.

When mixed in equal quantities **complementary colours** will neutralise each other, creating a greyish, neutral tone. To understand why, let's take one set of complementary colours – red and green. Green is a secondary colour made up by mixing yellow and blue in equal quantities. Its complementary colour – red – is the only colour not used to make green. We have already discussed how mixing the three primaries creates a greyish tone. By mixing red and green we are effectively mixing red, blue and yellow together, hence the neutral tone produced.

When using cosmetics, we can simply transfer this colour theory. A ruddy complexion with lots of red undertones can be neutralised by applying a thin layer of a pale green colour-correcting product. A heavy beard shadow that appears bluish can be camouflaged with an orange-toned product. Alternatively, a sallow complexion (lots of yellow tones) can be enhanced by a lilac colour-correcting base. However, too much coverage in all these cases would produce an unattractive grey-toned complexion.

Quality of colour

Below is a review of colour terms.

Hue	A colour as the eye perceives it. We have learned to identify colours by names as we see that colour. Red is seen as red. The hue is the name of the colour.
Intensity and luminosity	Refers to the amount of light that a coloured surface seems to reflect; the brightness or dullness of a colour. A hue of strong intensity – such as yellow – seems vivid, while a hue of weak intensity – such as violet – seems dull.
Saturation	Refers to the amount of the colour present or the strength of the hue.
Value and tone	The lightness or darkness of a colour. Every colour has what is known as its own 'local tone' – the actual tone of the colour as seen under neutral lighting conditions. For example, yellow is naturally light in tone, and violet is naturally dark. However, adding black to a colour darkens it, or shades it, while adding white lightens, or tints it. Both tints and shades therefore describe tone. It is important to remember that different colours can share the same tone, and one colour can represent a range of tones if you tint or shade it. Lighting conditions will also affect the tonal value of a colour: a colour seen in strong light will appear lighter, whilst the same colour seen in deep shade will appear darker.

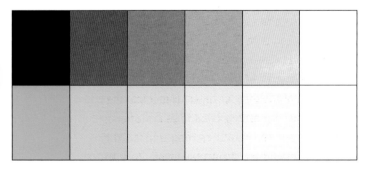

Illustration showing tints and shades of a hue

Colour interaction: what colours do

* **Colours advance and recede.** Bright colours advance and make the area covered appear larger. Dull and dark colours recede and make the area covered appear smaller. This colour rule can be applied to conceal or to create an illusion. Light emphasises; dark minimises.

* **Colours reflect other colours.** Some colours tend to reflect back more colour than they take away. For example, a red scarf near a ruddy complexion will make the face appear redder. A bright yellow would tend to emphasise the yellow in a skin with a sallow tone. Shadows tend to reflect the colour of the object causing the shadow.

* **Colour will steal colour.** Bright blue placed beside light or pale blue will make the pale colour appear less colourful. Thus, the darker and brighter colour will steal colour from a lighter colour. A person with blue eyes can intensify the eye colour by wearing a lighter blue than the blue eye colour. A darker blue worn near the face would make the eye colour appear lighter in contrast.

* **Colour has temperature.** Colours are classified as warm or cool. Some colours can be both warm or cool depending on the lightness, darkness or intensity of the colour. If you place yellow at the top of the colour wheel, the yellow and red-based hues are said to be warm, whilst the blue and green-toned hues are said to be cooler. Violet and yellow can be either cool or warm depending on their mix, for example a yellow with a hint of blue will be cooler than a yellow with a hint of red. Cold colours tend to make objects appear to be further away, whereas hot colours bring objects forward.

* **Colour reacts with other colour.** Individual hues are also affected by the colours that surround them. For example, if you place a greyish colour against a violet background, the grey will have a slightly yellow tone; if you put grey against a green background, it will look slightly red. This is because grey is essentially

the combination of two complementary colours and one of the complementary colours is drawn out by the presence of the other in the background. The character of a colour can also be changed by the colour that is positioned next to it. For example, a yellow can appear cold or hot depending on whether it is placed next to a warm or cool colour. Op-Art, popular in the 1950s and 1960s, used the principle of placing pure colours of the same tonal value next to each other. This causes a visual vibration or pulsation where the colours meet.

* **Colours are affected by light.** Colour will also be affected by the light it is seen in. Daylight gives off a bluish tone, tungsten artificial lighting gives off a yellow tone and fluorescent gives off a green tinge. How much the colour is affected will depend on the material that the coloured surface is made of.

Colour schemes

You may choose to use one of the following colour schemes in your make-up designs.

Monochromatic colour scheme

This is a combination of tints and shades of one hue only.

Complementary colours

Complementary colours lie opposite each other on the colour wheel. When placed next to each other complementary colours tend to 'fight' each other for attention. This makes for a striking effect. Artists sometimes use this theory to add vibrancy to a painting, particularly when painting shadows. For example, if painting an orange (the fruit) on a white surface, an artist would add blue to the shadow created by the fruit.

Analogous colours

Related colours are called 'analogous' colours and are often used to convey a certain mood or feeling. In most cases you can create analogous colours by changing their tint or shade, or adding another hue, such as its complement.

HANDS ON

Mixing colour

For all these exercises it is best to use paint and watercolour paper (this will prevent your paper from wrinkling).

1 Creating a colour wheel

Make a colour wheel showing primary, secondary and tertiary colours. Try to use as pure a colour as possible for your three primary colours and mix these together to produce the secondary and tertiary colours. No cheating – you must mix the colours yourself! Remind yourself which colours are warm, which are cool, which are complementary and which are harmonious.

2 Tints and shades activity

* This is a useful exercise to train yourself to see colours in terms of tone.

* Divide your paper into six columns. Paint a row of six squares across the top of the paper, one in each column. Start with pure white, then make each consecutive square a progressively darker shade of grey. The final square should be almost black.

* Place the following colours onto a palette: pale yellow, orange, red, light green, dark green, sky blue, violet, mid-brown, pale pink. You may add more colours if you wish.

* Paint a square of each colour in the column that represents the tonal value of the colour most closely.

* A good tip is to squint at the hues; this helps you see them as tones rather than colours.

* You can check how good your judgement is by taking a black and white photograph of your tone chart and seeing how accurately the coloured squares match the top row.

3 Analogous chart activity

Create a chart with three columns and six rows. Paint yellow, orange and red in the three columns of the first row. In each of the columns gradually add more and more of the complementary colour into the original hue. For example, in the yellow column gradually add purple. Keep adding until the hue changes into the complementary itself. You can always add more rows if you need to.

Harmonious colours

Harmonious colours lie next to each other on the colour wheel. Blue harmonises with violet and green, yellow harmonises with green and orange, etc.

The psychology of colour and colour symbolism

Colour is light, and exists everywhere. We respond to it instinctively and unconsciously. The colours within our immediate environment will affect our mood and ultimately our behaviour. Think about how you feel when spring arrives – the skies lose their greyness, yellow daffodils and green foliage spring up around us. We instinctively feel brighter, more cheerful and have more energy. Our response to individual colour is subjective, but reactions to colour combinations can be predicted with startling accuracy. Science has always recognised the link between colour combinations and mood or behaviour.

The various wavelengths strike our eyes in different ways, affecting our senses. Within the eye, the retina converts these waves into electrical impulses, allowing the brain to decode this visual information. This information is passed to the hypothalamus, the part of the brain governing our endocrine system producing hormones, and hormones affect our mood.

Every basic colour has underlying negative and positive psychological properties regardless of what shade or tint you are using. However, the effect created will always depend on the other colours it is being combined with.

Colour symbolism refers to the conscious associations that we are conditioned to make through cultural references. Red is the colour of blood and is therefore seen as aggressive and strong.

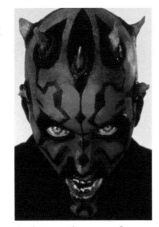

An interesting use of colour psychology in this make-up design for Darth Maul, Star Wars, Episode 1

When applied to the lips it has strong sexual connotations. Western wedding dresses are traditionally white, symbolising the purity and innocence of the bride. There are many more examples – see if you can observe them around you. Refer to the Make-Up Artistry website for a detailed evaluation of the psychological properties of colours.

HANDS ON

Colour psychology activity

Research how various artists have used colour to portray emotion and feeling within their paintings. Explore the use of white and pure colour to create space and freedom in the paintings of the Impressionist period. Look at how Picasso explored the theory of using colours that were dulled by the addition of greys to produce a solemn or tranquillising effect in his Cubist still-life paintings. Mark Rothko, the leader in colour field painting, uses colour to impact on the senses. Don't forget the Op-Artists and their use of pure colours to create 'pulsating' effects in their images.

Then, using your knowledge of colour theory and your own responses to colour, create an **abstract** coloured painting (no smaller than A3). You may use any medium you like. The painting should be in response to an emotion or an event in your life. Your painting must **not** be figurative. The idea of this exercise is to explore your own reaction to colour as a way of demonstrating something of importance to you. You should then give your painting a title. The following may give you some ideas as a starting point: *Depression, Sunday Mornings, The Argument, Saturday Night Out, Listening to Music, Love Affair.* Think carefully about the colours you choose. You may like to include shapes or textures to enhance your painting.

KEY NOTE

Figurative art – art that represents a human, animal or object's form by means of a symbol or figure.

Abstract art – any art in which real objects in nature are represented in a way that wholly or partially neglects their true appearance and expresses it in a form of sometimes unrecognisable patterns of lines, colours and shapes.

Creating form using light and shade

Chiaroscuro (creating form using light and shade) is a fundamental skill for the make-up artist. The technique will form the basis for many make-ups that you will create and it is important that you understand its basic principles.

Study the tints and shades chart earlier in the chapter and you will notice the lighter tones seem to advance from the page whilst the darker tones seem to recede. This is the fundamental principle of tone: **Light advances and shade recedes.**

Used alone, line can only imply form on a given surface. Tone is required to 'model' and capture an object's three-dimensionality and true structure. Tone is really the modelling used to express the way light falls onto an object.

When light hits an object with angular planes, each plane will be a distinct tone, the lightest being nearest to the light source and the darkest being the furthest away.

t source

Light falling on an angular object

t source

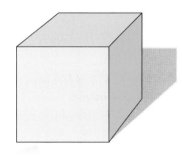

When light falls on a curved surface, the tonal change from light to dark is gradual and progressive. Leonardo da Vinci noted that light falling on a curved object caused five varying tonal ranges, although these are indistinguishable to the eye as they merge together indiscernibly. The area nearest to the light source will be the lightest (highlight), next to that will be a mid-tone, then a dark tone

Light falling on a curved object

(shadow), and at the very far edge away from the light will be a small area of reflected light. The fifth and darkest area will be the shadow caused by the object on the surface it is resting (cast shadow).

The drawings below illustrate how the form and structure of an apple can be rendered using tone. The artist starts off by shading in the mid-tones, and then lightens them with an eraser to show highlights and darkens them by applying more pressure to show shadows. Other mediums would require a different technique, for example with water-based paints the artist would start off with the lightest tones, building up the darker tones progressively with layers of wash or opaque colour.

1 The shape of the apple is filled in with a mid-tone.

2 The shadowed areas of the apple are darkened.

3 The lighter parts of the apple are worked on with an eraser.

4 Highlights are added (these are caused by reflections of light, where the shiny surface of the apple catches the light). These highlights bring the apple 'to life', creating a true three-dimensional effect.

5 A shadow is added to indicate where the apple sits on a surface (otherwise it will float on the page). Notice how this shadow's tone graduates as it moves away from the base of the apple.

6 Finally a highlight is added to the shadow on the apple at the furthest point from the light source to take account of light reflected off the surrounding surface.

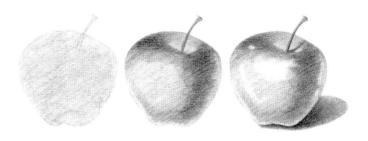

Illustrations of an apple modelled with tone

Once you feel confident modelling using tone on paper, you can move onto the face as your canvas for the following exercise.

HANDS ON

Creating the illusion of obesity using light and shade

This exercise requires skilful application and a thorough understanding of the use of light and shade. You are trying to create an illusion of obesity that is satisfactory whilst the face is seen from the front. The make-up itself has many limitations but the exercise of creating it is very useful for developing skills that you will be using time and time again. The effect of the make-up will be more successful if you choose a model with a 'roundish' face shape (see Chapter 8, page 154, if you are unsure what is meant by this).

It is always useful to have pictures as a reference whilst you are working, so begin by collecting images of people with heavy features for your reference file.

Don't forget to use a lighted mirror, and continually check your progress, making adjustments to the make-up as you go along. Refresh your knowledge of application techniques discussed earlier in this chapter – you will need to use them in this exercise.

The procedure below is a guide. Remember to look at your model and try to assess what will work for him or her. You are not trying to create a subtle, realistic effect; this is more of a stylised make-up. Your model will look like they are wearing make-up.

The following equipment is required:

* clips or a head band to secure hair away from the face
* gown or towel
* selection of clean brushes
* couple of make-up sponges or wedges
* crème-based foundation colour, matching the skin tone
* crème-based highlighting colour (two to three tones lighter than the skin tone)
* crème-based shading colour (3 shades darker than the skin tone)
* crème-based colour for adding definition (2 shades darker than the shading colour)
* a powder puff
* translucent powder.

1 Begin with a clean skin that has been lightly moisturised. Ensure the model's hair is secured back from their face and protect their clothes with a gown or towel.
2 Arrange the four crème-based colours on a palette.
3 Apply the foundation, using a make-up wedge. The application should be thin and blended carefully (also cover the lips). Keep any remaining base on your palette – you may need it later.
4 Follow the face chart as illustrated below, carefully blending the highlights and shadows as shown. Lines of definition should not be blended, but kept fine during application.
5 When you are happy with your application, set the make-up by gently pressing translucent powder onto the skin. Remove the excess with a large brush.
6 Don't forget to take a photograph as a record of your work.

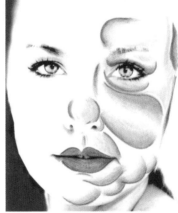

Obesity make-up design sheet by Julia Conway

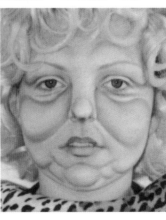

Completed obesity make-up

Creating texture

Using texture in your work will create more interesting and realistic make-ups. However, mastering the skills required to imitate a variety of textures is perhaps one of the more daunting aspects of make-up application. There are millions of different textures in our world and probably hundreds of artistic techniques for recreating them on a canvas. For many artists, success has come after much experimentation. The first step when approaching the challenge of texture is observation. It is important to really look at what you are trying to recreate, get a feel for its structure and then choose an appropriate technique.

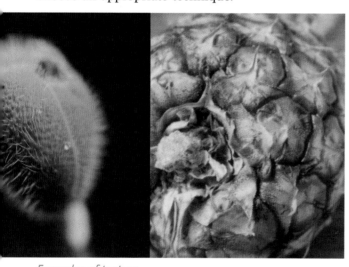

Examples of texture

You can create an illusion of texture in a variety of ways:

* by using various markings and brushstrokes

* by imitating strong tonal patterns that textures create

* by bringing out the way different surfaces reflect light, suggesting a shiny or matt finish. If you are to translate textures into artwork successfully, it is important to consider the full range of techniques and 'mark making' available to you. Mastering the techniques listed below will get you started and hopefully inspire you to experiment further.

1 Strokes: these may be vertical, horizontal, long, short, curved, straight, angled, light, dark – the list is endless.

2 Cross hatching: this can create a variety of effects depending on the pressure of the strokes. To create a very dense effect, cross hatching can be applied over cross hatching.

3 Stippling: this can be achieved with a 'stipple sponge', which is highly textured and will leave broken-up marks on the surface. Alternatively, a similar effect can be achieved by applying lots of small dots.

4 Splattering: an old toothbrush is useful for this. Load it with the paint and agitate the bristles with your thumb. Ensure you protect any areas you do not wish to be 'splattered'. The effect will differ according to whether the canvas is wet or dry.

5 Wet on wet: soft feathering marks can be achieved if you apply wet paint onto a wet surface.

6 Dry brush: applying paint onto a dry surface using a dry, stiff brush will create rough, hard marks.

7 Frottage: interesting textures can be created with this technique of rubbing a cloth, a sheet of crumpled paper or other textured surface over wet paint. The effect will differ according to the thickness of the paint.

8 Printing: textured surfaces (leaves, for example) can be painted and pressed onto the canvas to leave interesting marks.

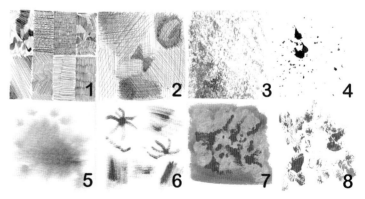

1. strokes, 2. cross-hatching, 3. stippling, 4. splattering, 5. wet on wet, 6. dry brush, 7. frottage, 8. printing. Techniques by Julia Conway

Experimenting with texture

Using textures in make-up

The following exercise will get you using and thinking about texture in make-up.

* Begin by researching a face paint that is highly textured (animals, flowers or wood, etc. are good starting points).
* Think about how you are going to imitate the texture of your design source using make-up.
* Practise creating the texture using paint or make-up in your workbook.
* Complete a face chart of your make-up design.
* Create the face paint on a model, concentrating on texture using paint effects.

Drawing the human head

Proportions

According to classical ideals of proportion (established in ancient Greece), the human head is divided into three equal parts. These ideals were rediscovered during the Renaissance period by artists such as Leonardo da Vinci, who attempted to divide the entire human body into ratios and proportions, and Albrecht Dürer, who attempted to divide the body into various sub-proportions. Each artist was striving to establish a divine principle behind the construction of the human body. Leonardo da Vinci's *Male Head with Proportions* (c. 1490) is a good example. The profile head contains notes on proportion such as 'the size of the figure is eight heads'. Leonardo produced not only studies of the proportions of the human head, but also a table in which he recorded all possible types of noses. In addition, he combined various forms of foreheads and chins as well as different types of noses and mouths.

According to the Greeks, in a beautiful face, the brow should be one-third of the way down from the hairline, the tip of the nose another third down from the brow and the chin one third down from that. The width of the face should be two-thirds of the length. Eventually, the face was divided into a mathematical formula – the perfect face had a ratio of 1:1.618. However, we recognise a face by combining two important sources of information – the proportions and relationships of the features and the pattern of light and shade on the face, caused by facial planes.

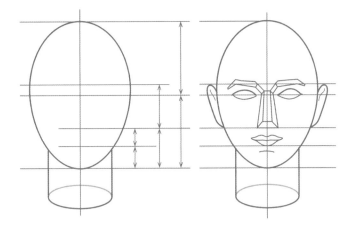

Drawing the human head

Few subjects challenge the artist more than the human head. Although no two heads are exactly alike, it is useful to start by familiarising yourself with basic head proportions.

Here is a list of standard facial proportions, but measurements will vary from face to face and across different ethnic groups.

* The eyes are halfway between the top of the head and the chin.
* The bottom of the nose is halfway between the eyes and the chin.
* The mouth is halfway between the nose and the chin.
* The corners of the mouth line up with the outside of the iris.
* The tops of the ears line up with the eyebrows.
* The bottom of the ears line up with the bottom of the nose.
* The eyes are approximately one eye width apart.

Once you are familiar with the proportions of the head it is useful to grasp an understanding of how the structure of the skull and muscles of the face affect what we see on the outside. Refer back to Chapter 4 to remind yourself of the anatomical structure of the face. You can use the illustrations to help you with the following activities.

HANDS ON

Exploring your face to create a skull effect
The following equipment is required:
* a head band or clips to secure hair away from the face
* two brushes
* black water-based make-up colour
* white water-based make-up colour.

Begin by exploring the structure of your face with your fingertips, noting areas of prominence and depression. Start in the middle of the forehead, work your way across to the temple area, down to and around the eye socket, across the cheekbone to the top of the nose, down the nose, outwards under the cheekbone, down to the jawbone and across to the chin.

When you feel familiar with the underlying structure, go back to the forehead and this time paint each area as you go along, applying black to areas that feel hollow and white to areas that feel raised or prominent. At the end of the activity your face will resemble the skull you have been studying. You may wish to paint on teeth (these will run from the centre to just in front of the ears) to complete the effect.

HANDS ON

Exploring muscles of the face

Sit in front of a mirror and observe your face as you slowly pull the following expressions. Try to be aware of the muscles as they move.

You should now be familiar with the proportions and structure of the head. The final stage is to try to understand what gives a face character and makes it individual.

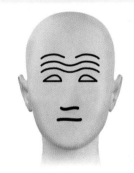

Frontalis
Attention, astonishment

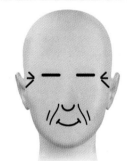

Zygomaticus
Laughter

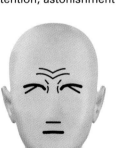

Corrugator
Sorrow

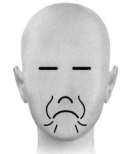

Triangularis
Dislike, disapproval

Illustrations of muscles and expressions

Portrait work

1 Capturing a likeness

These exercises are designed to develop your skills of observation. The idea is to try to capture a likeness. What distinguishes this person from the next? A caricature artist finds the distinguishing features in a person and then exaggerates these features. You can use a model or your own reflection for these exercises. The first exercise will give you a new perception and allow you to draw what you see without being influenced by your own built-in assumptions about facial proportions. You are not attempting to create beautiful pieces of art; the process is more important than the finished result.

* Take a large sheet of paper (A3 is ideal) and pencil. Place the pencil somewhere in the middle of the paper. This is the last time you will look at the paper for the whole of this exercise. Without removing your eyes from the face in front of you, begin to draw the outline and features you see. Try not to lift the pencil completely from the paper or you will lose your place. Allow yourself no more than five minutes to complete the exercise. You will probably end up with a rather 'cartoonish' image, which will hopefully give an 'impression' of the face in front of you.

* Take another sheet of paper. Working quickly and giving yourself no more that 15 minutes to complete the exercise, you are going to attempt to capture a likeness of the face in front of you, this time looking at the paper when you choose. Really

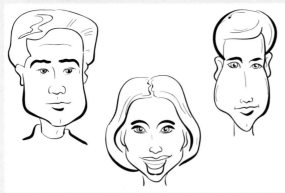

Examples of caricatures

look at what makes this person unique, concentrate on finding a distinguishing characteristic and exaggerating it. You should end up with a piece of work resembling a caricature, which with any luck captures 'something' of the face you worked on.

2 Creating a self-portrait

Give yourself two to three hours at least to complete this activity. The aim of the activity is to create a self-portrait with a good likeness. If you feel confident, lose the ruler and use your eye to judge of proportions.

i Position yourself in front of a mirror with a ruler to hand and a selection of pencils. Pull back your hair from your face. For simplicity keep to a full frontal view of the face.

ii Start by measuring the length of your face from the top of your head to your chin. Draw a faint line this length on your paper.

iii Measure how far your hairline drops from the top of the head. (Remember to keep your head straight – perspective plays a part here.) Mark this on your drawing with a faint horizontal line.

iv Measure how far the highest point of the eyebrows, eyes, tip of nose and lips (top and bottom) are from the hairline. Mark them all on your drawing with faint horizontal lines.

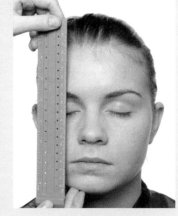

Measuring the face

v Measure the width of the face across the top of the eyebrows, then across from the tip of the nose and lips. Mark these measurements with faint vertical lines.

vi Check your measurements. Do they look right?

vii Continue to mark on important proportions. How far are the ends of your eyebrows from the edges of the sides of your face? How far apart are the inner corners of the eyebrows? How wide is your mouth? How wide apart are your eyes? How wide are your eyes? Keep going until you have a clear map of your features on the drawing.

10 Draw in the outline of your face and your hairline, and then begin to fill in the shapes of your features, using the marks as guidelines. Look carefully at yourself in the mirror and try to find idiosyncrasies that make you who you are – is your bottom lip much fuller that your top, or do you have an uneven top lip line? Look carefully at the shape of each eye.

11 Next, start to fill in some tones indicating where shadow falls on your face. This will help give your picture form and will make your portrait more recognisable. You may find it helpful to light your face more strongly from one side.

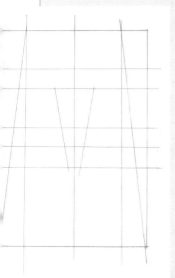

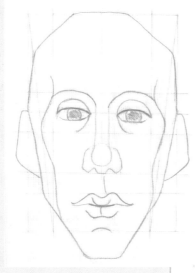

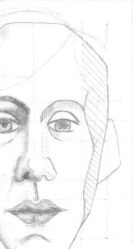

Three stages of a self-portrait by Mark Barrett
1. *Marking on the measurements*
2. *Drawing the outlines and shapes*
3. *Filling in the tones*

Transforming sketches into workable designs

Your ideas and designs will often start as simple sketches and notes in you workbook. When you hit an idea, you then need to consider how you are going to develop it

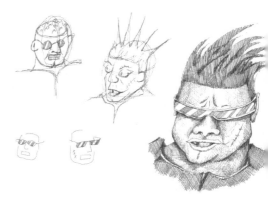

Design sketches by Paul Conway

into a workable design. Ultimately you will need to give some thought to how you are going to transfer a two-dimensional sketch onto a three-dimensional canvas. There will also be other practical considerations such as budgets, availability of products, time and expertise in techniques. Is the design realistically achievable as it stands or will you have to make compromises?

Presenting designs to clients

Once you have a workable design, you will need to present it to the client ('clients' may include art directors, directors, photographers, or if you are working within a training environment your tutor or examiners).

In industry, you will normally be given the opportunity to deliver your ideas during a 'design meeting'. 'Mood boards' are a useful tool for presenting designs to clients. It is often easier for people to comment on ideas that are presented to them visually. The mood board should be viewed as a prompt to demonstrate the design process that resulted in the final make-up design.

Mood boards are a collection of sketches, pictures, words, even textures or colours. For example, a range of pictures depicting a particular type of character could be used to explore various approaches to characterisation, or a selection of images could be used to show sources of inspiration

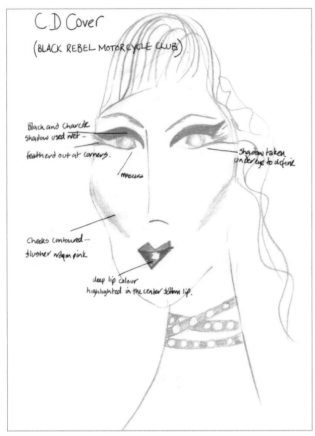

Design sheet by Amanda Duxbury

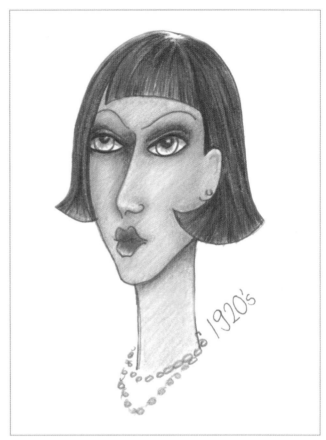

Design sheet by Kristen Tunley

behind the characterisation. Materials and products can also be demonstrated here, showing how texture and colour play their part in the final design.

The mood board will also be accompanied by a final image presenting the design in its entirety. If the make-up is head, neck and shoulders then this will often take the form of a design sheet.

Stylising make-up design sheets

It is useful to create your own design sheets that reflect your individual creative style. They can be an important part of your portfolio, and should be approached with the same professionalism as the make-ups themselves. Even those who are not confident in their drawing and painting skills on a paper canvas can achieve attractive design sheets by following the suggestion below.

1   Begin by selecting a full frontal or three quarter head shot. The image should be at least A4 size – if it is any smaller you will find it more difficult to work with. Magazines are a useful resource.

2   Take a sheet of acetate paper and trace the outline of the face and features with a fine permanent transparency marker – this is your template.

3   Take a sheet of tracing paper and trace the outline on the acetate sheet of paper. Transfer this outline onto a sheet of paper (remember to use watercolour paper if you intend to paint your design sheets).

4   You will now have a faint outline you can work with. A faint line is useful as you may wish to change the position or shape of certain features, for example the eyebrows or nose.

5   Draw in your basic design elements. It is useful to indicate the hairstyle to complete the design.

6   Choose your medium and begin to add form and colour to your design. Let your individual style come through. Don't worry about creating

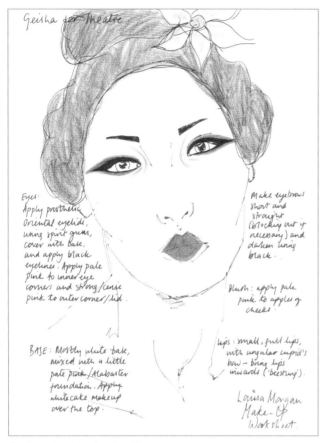

Design sheet by Louisa Morgan

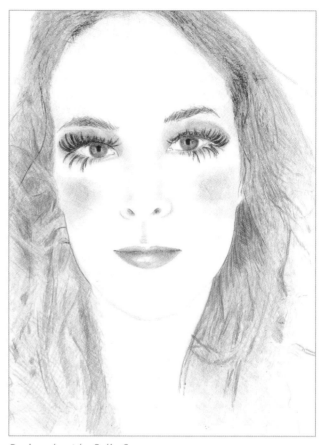

Design sheet by Julia Conway

a perfect piece of fine art; some students feel more comfortable developing a caricature or cartoon style.

It is a good idea to have three or four different templates that you can transfer your designs onto. The templates should include male and female as well as varying head positions.

Finding inspiration and using your imagination

One of the hardest things to teach is imagination. We all use our imagination to different degrees and some of us find it easier to tap into this natural resource than others. Try the exercise on the next page with four friends to 'loosen up' your imagination.

The harder you find this activity, the more you will need to work on releasing your inner creativity and imagination!

Children use imagination more readily than the average adult. In some ways we need to begin to view the world around us with a 'child's eye' to find inspiration for design. Many of us have lost the knack of really looking around us as we go through our day-to-day lives. Potential sources of inspiration are often lost in over-familiarity and habit. Try making a journey (preferably walking) that you are very familiar with – perhaps a route you take to walk the dog or go to work or college – but this time take a camera with you. Now, really look around you and observe everything – textures, colours, shapes and people – taking pictures of

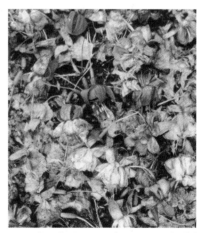

Decaying flowers produce a wonderful effect of colour and texture

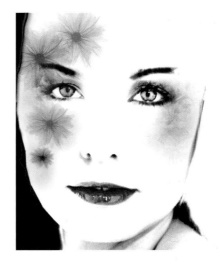

Design sheet by Julia Conway, inspired from photo of decaying flowers

HANDS ON

Creating an alien doodle

Take an A4 sheet of paper.

1 The first person draws an 'alien' head and neck at the top of the paper. No one else must see what is being drawn. Encourage the first person to use his or her imagination and to be as outrageous as possible. If the person is struggling, get him or her to think about aliens from a film or television for inspiration. The first person then needs to fold the section of paper with the drawing back, so it is no longer visible. Two marks need to be made at the 'new' top of the paper, indicating where the neck finishes. This ensures each section of the body of the alien meets the next.

2 Without looking at the head and neck, the next person, using the marks as a starting point, continues to draw the torso and arms of the alien. The second person should stop at the waist. The paper is then folded back again to hide this section. Again, two marks are made at the 'new' top of the paper, indicating where the next person should start drawing.

3 Continuing as above (remembering not to look at the previous drawings), the next person draws from the waist to the top of the thighs.

4 The next person draws the legs.

5 The last person draws the feet.

6 When the final part of the doodle has been completed, unfold the paper to reveal your alien. Now comes the fun part. Give your alien an identity by considering the following.

* Give your alien a name.
* What planet does it come from (this can be made up)?
* Does it have any special powers?
* What does it eat?
* Does it have any other unusual characteristics?

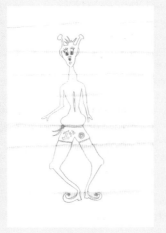

anything that catches your eye. You will be amazed at how much you 'see' that you don't usually notice. Once you have developed the film, stick some images in your workbook and begin to think about make-up designs that may evolve from them.

Inspiration for creativity can come from a wide variety of sources. As starting points for their designs, make-up artists have suggested the following:

* nature – flowers, foliage, shells, decay, landscapes

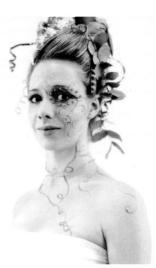

Make-up inspired by the fairytale 'Princess and the Pea'

* animals, fish, insects
* artwork, modernism, surrealism, photography, etc.
* other make-up artists' work
* pop and rock artists, movie stars

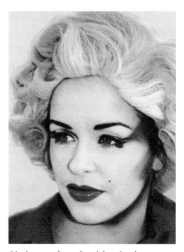

Make-up inspired by Andy Warhol silk screen prints of Marilyn Diptych (1962)

* fashion – designers, runways, textiles
* film, cinema
* historical influences
* books – fairy tales, cartoons.

Presenting your portfolio

Poorly presented work will not do justice to your talents. It is worth investing in a professional 'display book' or portfolio. A wide variety is available from good art stores and your choice will be determined by personal preference and budget. However, do not go for too large a portfolio as you are going to have to carry it around. Below are some general suggestions you can follow to ensure your work is professionally presented.

* Design sheets and photos should have neat, straight edges. Rather than using scissors, a scalpel knife, cutting board and ruler should be used to achieve this.

* If photos and design sheets require mounting (usually if they are smaller than the portfolio page) ensure you use a suitable adhesive. Spray mount offers good adhesion and re-positioning, and gives a clean finish. Make sure you use it in a well-ventilated area and follow the manufacturer's instructions. Avoid getting glue on any visible surfaces and ensure you mount 'straight'.

* Black and white photos and drawings are best mounted on black, white or cream mounts. Colour photos and paintings should avoid black mounts and any colour that will distract from the image itself. It is probably best to stick to one or two mount colours throughout the portfolio for a unified, professional effect.

* If you use labels, make sure you check your spelling and legibility. If your handwriting is untidy, consider using other forms of text. Any text should be discreet and informative.

* Ensure the plastic pages of your portfolio are clean and free from fingerprints.

* Images in your portfolio can be placed back to back. Make-ups with accompanying design sheets should preferably be displayed so they can be seen together (i.e. on an open double page).

* Ensure you portfolio is labelled with your name and phone number. A business card is useful for this.

Spending time ensuring your portfolio is presented well is very important. A professional looking portfolio will give a good impression of your approach to work and encourage prospective clients and examiners to spend time looking through your designs.

Knowledge Check

1 What are the primary colours of the subtractive colour system?

2 What are the secondary colours of the subtractive system and how do you mix them?

3 Define what is meant by the following terms: hue, tone, value, intensity.

4 Describe four ways colours interact.

5 Describe the following colour schemes: monochromatic, contrasting, complementary, analogous, harmonious.

6 Describe the theory of light and shade in the art of chiaroscuro.

7 Suggest three ways of creating texture with mark making in make-up.

8 Why is it important to keep a workbook?

9 List three suggestions for preparing a professional portfolio for presentation.

10 Describe the importance of quaternary colours in make-up.

CHAPTER 6

Professional studies

This chapter will help you become a well-rounded make-up artist, able to function in various professional environments. It takes you through subjects such as lighting, the design process, production environments and processes, selecting and ordering materials, budgets, continuity, maintaining records, promoting products and services. It should be read in conjunction with Chapter 1, which describes roles and responsibilities and general working conditions of the make-up artist.

Aim and objectives

Aim of this chapter: to provide you with an understanding of the requirements of various production environments, which will affect your work as a make-up artist.

You should achieve the following **objectives:**

* Discuss the principles of the colour theory of light
* Describe the optimum lighting set-up for a make-up room
* Identify how various light sources affect make-up
* Evaluate the considerations of applying make-up for various sizes of stage
* Define the team structures for various production environments
* Review the production schedules for theatre, television or film and fashion environments
* Break down a script and produce recommended schedules

* Define continuity and produce continuity schedules
* Discuss the benefits of digital technology for the make-up artist
* Evaluate the process of promoting products or services to clients or customers in a retail environment
* Identify the features and benefits of products
* Review techniques to close a sale
* Review consumer legislation
* Contribute to the design process by researching, preparing and presenting designs
* Identify the main considerations when selecting and obtaining supplies for a production

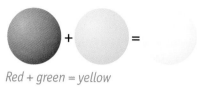

Lighting

Lighting is critical to the work of a make-up artist, whatever medium he or she works in. It is important because it has an effect on:

* perception of colour
* form – it can help to model the face.

Principles of coloured light

Colour theory is split into two systems:

* the subtractive system (or coloured pigments, as discussed in Chapter 5, page 72)
* the additive system (or light colours).

Light colours behave differently from coloured pigments. This chapter looks at the additive system.

Primary **light** colours are called 'additive primaries'. These are:

* red   * blue   * green.

Combinations of these three primary light colours will produce further colours called 'subtractive primaries'. These are:

* cyan   * magenta   * yellow.

This can be demonstrated be shining three primary coloured lights of equal brightness onto a white surface.

If we merge the red and blue spotlights together, a single spotlight of a magenta-coloured light will be produced.

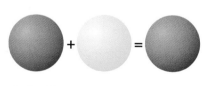

Red + blue = magenta

If we merge the blue and green spotlights together, a single spotlight of a cyan-coloured light will be produced.

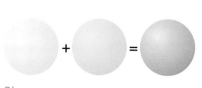

Blue + green = cyan

If we merge the red and green spotlights together, a single spotlight of a yellow-coloured light will be produced.

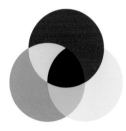

Red + green = yellow

Finally, merge the three primary spotlights together. A single spotlight of white (clear) light will be produced.

If coloured lights of the subtractive primaries were projected and they overlapped, black would be produced. Where cyan and yellow overlap, green would be produced; where magenta and yellow overlap, red would be produced; where magenta and cyan overlap, blue would be produced.

The theory of subtractive primary coloured light

Types of lighting

Light is measured in degrees kelvin (K), which relates to the temperature of its colour. Light with higher kelvin ratings produces a bluish cast; light with lower ratings produces a red-orange cast.

Candle flame	1,850ºK
150 watt tungsten (household) bulb	2,900ºK
Studio tungsten light	3,200ºK
Exterior arc lamp	5,000-5,500ºK
Daylight (on a cloudless day)	5,400-5,800ºK
Make-up room lighting (CRI approx 100)	5,500ºK
Studio flash	same as daylight

Lighting the make-up room

It is important that the make-up room is adequately lit. Make-up mirrors should be lit to allow the make-up artists to fully view their work with a frontal light source. The lighting will need to be the same as during production so the make-up artists can judge the colour; in most cases this will be daylight. Daylight bulbs are fluorescent lighting, but they should be chosen carefully as there are a number of varieties of fluorescent bulbs. Most give out a yellow-green colour cast as they have very little red in their colour spectrum; the exception are those with a CRI (colour rendering index) of 100, which is closest to daylight and ideal for colour matching. Make-up not applied under the correct lighting conditions may result in the following.

Lighting for make-up application	Result when viewed under daylight
Tungsten (gives off an orange-yellow colour cast)	Make-up looks heavy and too warm in colour temperature
Fluorescent (without a CRI index of 100 so giving off a yellow-green colour cast)	Make-up may look washed out and cool in colour temperature

When the make-up is applied in daylight-balanced lighting but will be viewed under studio tungsten lighting, warm colours will appear lighter and cool colours will appear darker in the studio.

Amount and placement of light and the effect on make-up

Lighting in the studio or on stage relies on a number of lights set up to create a variety of effects. Most lighting set-ups will consist of the following components:

* key light – the main light
* fill light – a secondary light, usually less powerful than the key light, that is used to define the features
* back light – this lights the background, separating it from the subject
* hair light – this is shone on the back or side of the subject to create a halo and highlight the hair.

Any light sources used to illuminate areas of the 'set' or 'scene' are referred to as set lighting. Lighting arrangements on set are either **high key** (bright, with few shadows) or **low key** (subdued, lots of contrast and shadows).

Different lighting effects rely not only on the use of different light sources, but also on the direction of light. A series of possible lighting arrangements are illustrated below.

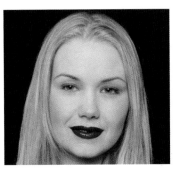

Frontal lighting is the illumination of the subject from the front. The light may be hard or soft.

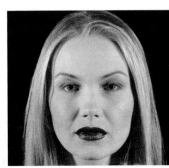

Cross lighting is the illumination of the subject with two light sources from opposite angles but at an equal distance from the subject. Cross lighting emphasises texture on the face.

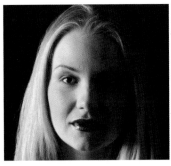

Side lighting is the illumination of the subject with one light source from the side. It has the effect of illuminating one side of the subject, whilst leaving the other side in shadow.

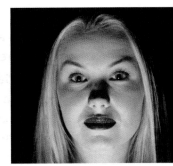

Under lighting is the illumination of the subject from underneath. It creates unnatural shadows and an 'eerie' effect.

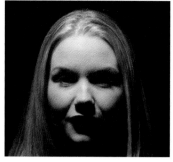

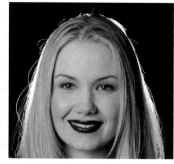

Overhead lighting is the illumination of the subject from above. It creates shadows around the eyes, under the cheekbones and under the mouth and jaw line. Make-up application should be avoided in this lighting arrangement but should be carried out under a more general frontal illumination.

Rim lighting outlines the subject's profile in light. A direct light source is placed behind the subject.

KEY NOTE

Light may be direct, creating a hard 'contrasty' light, or reflected, creating a softer effect.

Different lighting arrangements for specific production environments are discussed in the following sections.

Working in the theatre

Lighting considerations

On stage everything is affected by lighting. The main considerations are as follows.

* The stage is normally lit from overhead and from footlights. This often creates a flattening effect on the performer's features. Contouring the features with make-up will help to counteract this.

* The lights are usually very intense and can make skin tones and other make-up colours look washed out. Warmer make-up shades should be used to counteract this.

* The colour temperature of the lights is not critical on stage as filters (also called gels) are used to create desired effects. The coloured filter

absorbs all the colours in the light spectrum except the colour of the filter. For example, a red filter placed over a light will only allow the red light waves of the spectrum to pass through; therefore a red light is produced. Generally, stage lighting is a combination of cold and warm neutrals, which do not affect make-up colours. However, some filters, which are used for creating special lighting effects on stage, will produce colour changes in make-up shades.

Colour	Effect on make-up of filter	
Peach	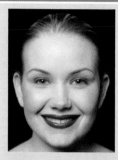	Warms the skin tone without altering any other colour in the make-up design.
Blue	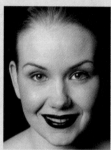	Changes red tones, making them appear darker. Blue or green shades appear lighter. The skin tone becomes cool.
Red	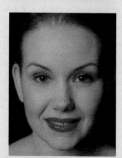	Red tones appear lighter. Green shades appear darker. Blue becomes darker and greyer.
Green	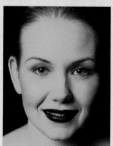	Will darken red lipstick. Shades of green appear lighter. Blue appears dark green. Shades of purple become very dark.

The effect of lighting filters on make-up colours

KEY NOTE

Neutral shades of make-up (black, brown and grey) remain the same under any colour of lighting, except for an indistinguishable change in tonal value.

The size of the theatre

Make-up for stage will vary significantly according to the size of the theatre. Large theatres, where a large proportion of the audience will be sitting some distance from the stage, require quite different considerations from small theatres or theatres in the round. However, regardless of the size of the theatre, the make-up must never be crude or heavily applied, as even in the largest theatres a poorly blended application will be obvious to those in the front rows.

Make-up for large theatres

In large theatres it is generally accepted that make-up is applied for the benefit of the first fifteen rows of the house (these are the most expensive seats and where the critics usually sit). Much of the make-up effect will be totally lost on the rear of the house; instead, the audience here will rely on the overall representation of the characters through costumes, facial hair and wigs or hairstyles. Postiche work is therefore very important in the theatre.

In some large theatres, particularly where the orchestra pit is positioned directly in front of the stage, even the first few rows of the audience sit some distance from the stage. In these theatres the make-up has to be stronger than in other mediums, and both colour and facial definition have to be emphasised. There are no close-up shots, so do not waste time on fine details, but bear in mind that the make-up must still look precise and professionally applied.

Consideration	Adaptation to make-up
Overhead and footlight lighting, which may flatten the performers' features	Increase the strength of contouring make-up to sculpt the face, counteracting the flattening effect.
Intensity of light sources, which may drain the colour of make-up	Make-up needs to be warmer, particularly on lighter skin tones. On darker skin tones make-up does not generally need adjusting.
Greater distance of the audience from the stage, resulting in a lack of definition of the facial features	Features generally need to appear larger – follow make-up application suggestion on the next page. The shape of hairstyles and wigs becomes very important in creating an overall impression to the audience.
Colour of lighting	Liaise with the lighting technician about the use of filters and adjust make-up accordingly. Consider using neutral shades on the eyes to avoid problems.

Adaptations of make-up application for the large stage

STEP-BY-STEP | Straight make-up for large theatres

The final effect of this make-up should appear stronger than that for television, film or small theatres, but remember that stronger does not mean heavily applied. Your application should still be precise and products should be applied with a light touch. It is the choice of colour and placement and the intensity of highlights and shadows that will give the make-up strength and the performer's face definition.

Example of straight make-up for the female on a large stage

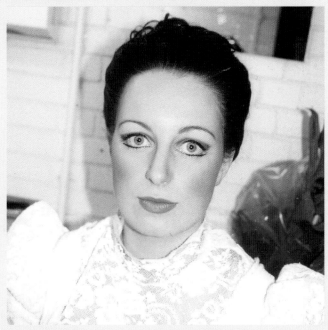

Straight make-up for the female on a large stage

1 Apply a thin base all over the face. For light skins it may be necessary to warm the skin with a darker or warmer colour than the natural skin tone. Blend the thin base well.

2 Apply cream-based contouring make-up to define the features (see Chapter 8). You are aiming for a stronger effect than for television, film or photographic work.

3 Powder generously. Dust off the excess.

4 Define the eyebrows. Do not over-emphasise.

5 Apply a light eye shadow – take account of any coloured lighting on the set) across the entire eye area. Blend to nothing on the brow bone.

6 Apply dark-blue eye lines (rather than black or brown, to achieve more brightness in the eye area). Continue across the entire top lid, extending past the outer corner of the eye and fading to nothing at the ends. Apply lower eye lines just below the bottom lashes. Extend past the outer corner keeping parallel to the top eye-line. Apply a highlighting colour on the outer corner of the eye, between the top and bottom eye lines and between the natural lower lashes and eye line; this will open up the eye area.

7 Use a darker toned eye shadow of your choice in the socket line. Intensify the colour at the outer corner and sweep upwards. Apply highlighting colour on the brow bone.

8 Add false lashes.

9 Apply a strong-coloured but blended blusher to the cheeks.

10 Apply a strong, bright-coloured lipstick – a clear red usually works best. Brown or plum tones tend to make the mouth look smaller from a distance. You should make full use of the mouth area.

11 Check the effects of your make-up on stage. Add more definition where required.

12 Dress the hair or apply a wig (for larger stages, a coarser hair lace on wigs is more economical and often preferred).

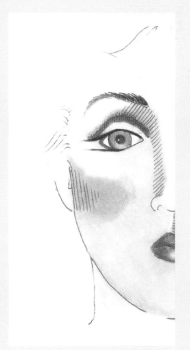

Make-up for the large stage

Example of straight make-up for the male on a large stage

Stage make-up for men should look natural to the audience, even those in the first few rows.

1 Apply a light base all over the face. For light skins it may be necessary to warm the skin with a darker or warmer colour than the natural skin tone. This is not necessary for tanned or dark skin tones. Blend well.

2 Apply cream-based contouring make-up to define the features (see Chapter 8). You are aiming for a stronger effect than for television, film or photographic work. Men often like their jaw line to be emphasised.

3 Powder generously. Dust off the excess.

4 Fill in any gaps in the eyebrows. Do not make them too heavy.

5 Apply fine dark-blue eye lines. Continue across the entire top lid, extending slightly past the outer corner of the eye and fading to nothing at the ends. Apply lower eye lines just below the bottom lashes. Extend past the outer corner keeping parallel to the top eye-line.

6 Apply a little bronzer to the lower part of the cheeks if required.

7 Apply a nude-coloured lip liner and blend with a little Vaseline to define the mouth.

8 Check the effects of your make-up on stage. Add more definition where required.

9 Dress the hair or apply a wig (for larger stages, a coarser hair lace on wigs is often preferred).

For Gilbert and Sullivan operetta and ballet make-up, it is acceptable for the men to appear more made-up.

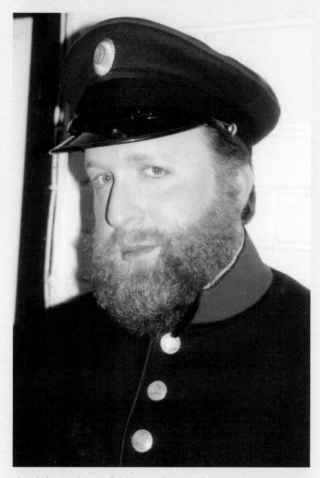

Straight make-up for the male on a large stage

KEY NOTE

Pure white make-up can appear blue on stage, so 'off white' should be used. Add a little pink to the white for females and a little beige for males.

Small theatres and theatres in the round

Smaller theatres require less intense lighting and the audience often sit very close to the stage. Therefore, the make-up requirements for this type of theatre reflect television and film requirements. Performers often apply their own 'street make-up' for modern productions, but may require a make-up artist for more elaborate make-ups. Postiche used in a small theatre requires a fine lace so that it is not visible to the audience.

The theatrical production team

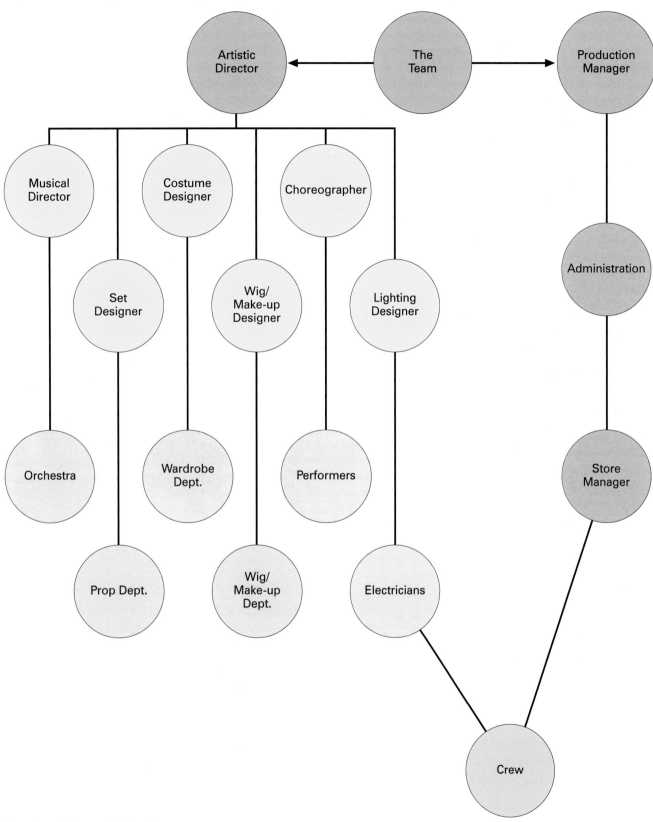

Structure of the production team

The theatrical production schedule

The production schedule is generally split into four time periods.

Pre-production (period of planning and preparation)

⬇

Production (generally covering rehearsal period)

⬇

The run (first night to last show of a production)

⬇

Post-production (short period after last show)

Pre-production

This period of planning and preparation normally involves the wig / make-up designer and sometimes the wig / make-up mistress or master. During this period they are required to:

* meet other members of the team and ensure they are aware of their roles and responsibilities

* familiarise themselves with the synopsis, structure and text of the production so that they are able to enter into discussions during meetings with other team members

* attend pre-production design meetings to discuss production genre and style. The artistic director, production manager, costume designer and set designer will usually attend these meetings

* research and produce designs acceptable to the production team – designs should reflect the chosen style of the production

* negotiate budgets and ensure they are realistic in realising the hair and make-up designs

* hire a team of wig / make-up specialists to meet the requirements of the production

* research, negotiate with suppliers and order general materials and equipment

* check dressing room facilities to ensure there is sufficient space, lighting and ventilation. Any issues should be reported to the production manager as soon as possible.

Excellent preparation and planning during the pre-production stage will allow more time to deal with issues and responsibilities arising during the production process.

KEY NOTE

The genre and style of the production will affect your make-up and wig designs. Popular styles include:

* realism: sets, costumes, hairstyles and make-up are as historically accurate as possible.
* neo-realism: ideas based on realism but adapted or exaggerated to suggest plots and themes to the audience.
* abstract: themes and plots are portrayed through creative elements of the production, for example in the gambling scene of the opera *The Queen of Spades* the gentlemen's faces are made to look skull-like, illustrating their obsessive and destructive behaviour.

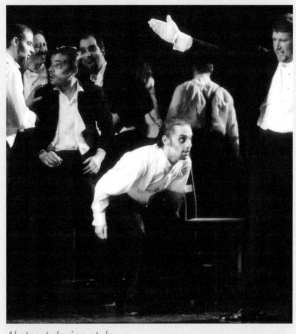

Abstract design style

Production

The length of the production period will vary from theatre to theatre and from production to production. On average, the production period may refer to the six weeks prior to opening night, during which time the wig and make-up team will be required to:

* attend production meetings to discuss script cuts, running times, changes in the schedule, etc.

* attend the read through to present the make-up and wig designs to the performers, discuss the make-up application process and possible contra-actions of any special effects, and answer any concerns or questions

* produce make-up and wig schedules – negotiate call times, quick changes and responsibilities within the make-up and wig team

* organise make-up application training sessions for performers if necessary

* attend rehearsals regularly, and liaise with the artistic director as to how often would be appropriate

* liaise with stage management and ask to be kept informed of any changes

* take measurements for postiche fittings

* carry out allergy patch tests as required

* order postiche

* check stock and chase orders if they have not arrived

* buy hair accessories and decoration as required

* try out make-ups and postiche on principal performers

* attend the technical rehearsal to view make-up and wigs under lights; make alterations as required to colour and definition in consultation with the artistic director, set or lighting designers and costume designer

* attend the run through or full dress rehearsal and make final adjustments.

KEY NOTE

Sometimes you will be required to apply make-up and wigs for a publicity photo shoot. In this case the application will have to be adapted to make it suitable for television or photographic purposes.

The run

The 'run' describes the actual performances from opening night until the last show. During this time, individuals should perform their duties and responsibilities as laid down in the make-up / wig schedule. Make-up artists should be aware of running times and ensure they are in the right place at the right time. Stage wings (left or right of stage, out of view of the audience) are good places to wait for and perform quick changes.

Checks on stock should be made frequently and items re-ordered if low. Postiche should be maintained and cleaned after each performance.

Wig / make-up schedules

To enable the wig / make-up master or mistress to produce working schedules for the department, he or she will need to gather the following information:

* cast list (it is often a good idea to photograph the principal performers for reference)

* list of principal covers (covers are stand-by performers, in case the main actor is not able to perform)

* list of the wig / make-up team with contact telephone numbers

* list of allocated dressing rooms for performers (this will need to be negotiated with the costume department and performers)

* the script with a breakdown of acts and scenes.

From this information, the following can be produced to ensure the smooth running of the department:

* design sheets for make-up and wigs

* list of call times (the amount of time a performer is required to attend to hair and make-up prior to curtain up)

* rota of duties and responsibilities for each make-up artist

* breakdown of make-up and hair for each of the principal characters, including changes throughout the performance.

Make-up artist	Prior to performance (dressing room)	Act 1, Scene 1 Park	Act 1, Scene 2 Liza	Act 2, Scene 1 Ball
Emma	Bald cap Countess (25 mins)	Countess – remove hat and check wig (right stage wing)	Countess – add hair piece and comb (dressing room)	FLOAT
Julia	Ageing Countess (45 mins)	FLOAT	Children into characters at ball – Gods, Plutus, servants, etc. (dressing room)	FLOAT
Stephanie	Hermann, Tomsky, Yeletsky (1 hr 15 mins)	FLOAT	FLOAT	Mid Scene Tomsky into Plutus Add hook on beard and blush (4-5 mins) (left stage wing)
Nyla	Liza – hair and make-up (1 hour)	FLOAT	Liza – change lipstick, add a touch more blush and add comb to hair (left stage wing)	FLOAT
Robert	Governess – make-up and wig (1 hour)	FLOAT	Add combs to hair for ball for governesses and change lipstick (left stage wing)	FLOAT
Jo	Chloe – fit wig and make-up (30 mins)	FLOAT	No 62. Major Domo (add chin beard and darken moustache) (dressing room)	FLOAT

Example of make-up schedule

Remember, a theatrical production is 'live'; the purpose of make-up schedules is to ensure everyone knows when and where they are supposed to be throughout the performance itself.

Post-production

The wig master or mistress is sometimes employed on larger productions for a short period (or in larger houses on a permanent basis), post-production. During this period the following will take place.

* Wigs will be cleaned and returned to the supplier if hired or stored if bought.
* Any remaining make-up stock will be recorded and stored.

* Research material and designs will be filed for future reference.

Working in television and film

Lighting considerations

The type of lighting used in film and television depends on whether the filming is interior or exterior. Exterior shots use the sun as the key light. However, when the sky is cloudy, additional light sources or fill light are provided by large arc lamps. In television studios, lighting is generally fixed on the set and consists of numerous overhead, side and floor lights.

Interval 20 mins (dressing room)	Act 2, Scene 2 Bedroom	Act 3, Scene 1 Barracks	Act 3, Scene 2 Canal	End of evening duties
Check countess' make-up and wig	Countess, mid scene – change wig to balding wig (right stage wing)	Countess – fit white wig, apply white powder and silver lipstick (dressing room)	FLOAT	Countess – remove wig and bald cap
FLOAT	Countess, mid scene – remove lipstick, whiten eyebrows and powder face to reduce make-up (right stage wing)	FLOAT	Countess – check wig and make-up (left stage wing)	Clean and block Countess' wigs.
Remove false beard and reduce blush – return to Tomsky	FLOAT	Hermann – add dark shadows under eyes and perspiration (right stage wing)	FLOAT	Remove and clean facial hair
Emaciation on chorus	Liza – Change lipstick, powder to reduce blusher, remove hair ornaments (dressing room)	Liza – Fit and secure hat (right stage wing)	Emaciation (dressing room)	Remove and clean facial hair
Remove Empress and Chloe wigs, clean and block	FLOAT	Emaciation on chorus (dressing room)	Emaciation on chorus (dressing room)	Remove, clean and block wigs, remove hair pieces
Remove hair combs from hair and change lipstick on dancers	FLOAT	Emaciation on chorus (dressing room)	Emaciation on chorus (dressing room)	Check stock and artists' make-up bags

Example of make-up schedule (continued)

Nowadays, lighting for film and television is usually adjusted to suit performers' skin tones, ensuring that the face is properly lit for a scene and make-up artists no longer have to worry about colour correction. However, certain make-up textures, for example shimmer products, can still create problems. Collaboration between lighting and make-up is the key to success. Occasionally in film, it is possible to light a scene specifically so the make-up artist can view the make-up and make any necessary alterations.

Make-up for television tends to be stronger than for film, as the lighting is 'flatter' and some definition is lost in the shadows and highlights.

However, the introduction of digital video technology, giving film quality definition and colour rendition to this medium, has reduced the need for stronger make-up.

Film magnification and digital technology

Performers' faces are magnified up to 200 times on screen, so make-up application has to be perfect as even minor mistakes will be very noticeable. Beauty for film is based on symmetry; screen stars who are considered to be beautiful or handsome usually have extraordinarily symmetrical faces, making them 'pleasing to the camera'. However, the make-up artist is often called upon to enhance or improve nature by making the features appear as symmetrical as possible. The other concern for the film make-up artist is what is termed as 'flesh impact' – that is the skin must look healthy and natural, even when special effects have been employed.

> **KEY NOTE**
>
> It is generally accepted to be good practice to view the make-up during application in a lighted mirror. This will give the make-up artist an accurate representation of what will be viewed on screen.

The introduction of digital technology has vastly improved the two areas of main concern to make-up artists:

* colour rendition
* picture clarity.

Digital technology is now being used in all areas of screen work from commercials to pop videos, television and film work. It requires make-up artists to work to film standards – that is cleanly and finely, taking extra care to make postiche lace invisible and to make sure edges to prosthetics are lost on screen. However, this should hold no fear for the competent make-up artist who should already be working to these high standards, assisted by the on-going development of excellent products and techniques designed to meet the challenges of the digital age.

The team structure – an overview

A comprehensive breakdown of roles and job descriptions in the television and film industry can be found by following the links from www.heinemann.co.uk/hotlinks to the Skill Set website.

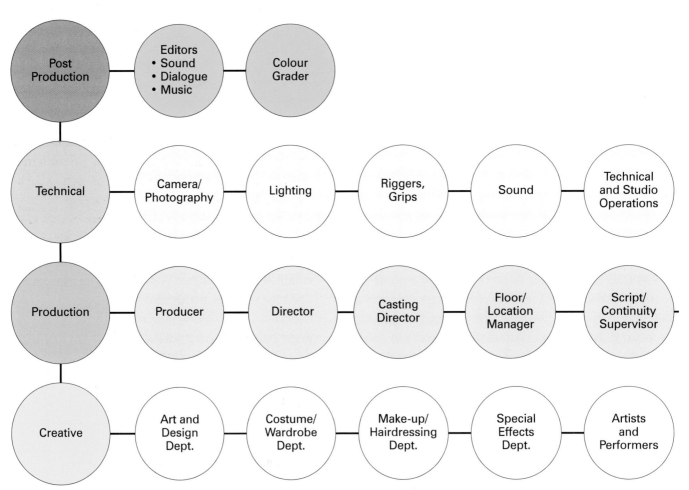

Structure of the television and film team

The television and film production schedule

Pre-production

This period of consultation, planning and preparation normally involves the hair / make-up designer and the hair / make-up supervisor. During this period they are required to:

* meet other members of the team
* familiarise themselves with the script so that they are able to enter into discussions during meetings with other team members
* attend pre-production design meetings to discuss the creative approach to the production
* break down the script and produce character breakdowns and continuity schedules
* research and produce designs acceptable to decision makers: director, performers, producer

* negotiate budgets and ensure they are realistic in realising the hair and make-up designs
* hire a team of hair, make-up and special effects artists to meet the requirements of the production and send them a copy of the script
* research, liaise with suppliers and order general materials and equipment
* check dressing room facilities and ensure there is sufficient space, lighting and ventilation – any issues should be reported to the production manager as soon as possible
* contact performers to establish needs, allergy patch tests, etc.
* arrange postiche fittings and place orders
* arrange make-up tryouts
* dress postiche.

Unlike theatrical productions when there is a rehearsal period, the pre-production period will lead straight into filming so the make-up department must be prepared for this: wigs must be dressed and any potential problems with the hair and make-up ironed out before the first day of filming. The pre-production period can therefore be very stressful, particularly if you are working with a director who is indecisive or frequently changes his or her mind. Towards the end of the pre-production period each department will be issued with a **shooting schedule**, detailing the anticipated scenes that will be filmed on each day. However, this schedule is likely to undergo many changes throughout the production period, so be prepared to be flexible.

Breaking down a script

Breaking down a script to establish make-up and hair requirements is an important part of pre-production preparation. Only by reading a script can a make-up designer enter into discussions regarding the characters' appearance and begin the design process. The best approach to breaking down a script is one of logical progression. Below is a suggested sequence of actions.

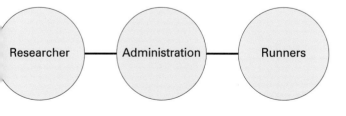

Read the script as a story. Your first experience of the script should be as a member of the audience. Just read it through as you would any other story.

↓

Identify all of the characters in the story and produce a **cast list**. When you know who is in the story you can start to build a picture of how you can make them look in the film. A cast list will enable you to give each cast member a number that will correspond to the number allocated by the shooting schedule. This will enable you to see at a glance which characters you will be dealing with in each scene.

↓

Mark up the script. With a highlighter pen mark all the pertinent information that is relevant to hair and make-up in the script.

→

Produce a **script breakdown**. This will enable you to see what is happening in each of the scenes. Information required is scene number, character, story day, including day or night, interior or exterior shooting and action.

↓

Produce a **continuity schedule** for each character. Write down the make-up requirements for each scene that the character appears in.

↓

Produce a **daily make-up schedule and scene breakdown** in accordance with the shooting schedule. Be prepared to amend this as the shooting schedule will almost certainly change during the production period.

Cast lists

Casts lists should be broken down to show characters and performers' names and their allocated number from the shooting schedule. The characters can also be grouped as follows:

* principal characters: stars of the production – the actor's name usually appears above the title of the film on publicity material

* bit characters: actors with small speaking parts

* extras and background artists: actors with no speaking parts.

KEY NOTE

A 'double' is a person who is made-up and costumed to appear as an actor in a scene. Stunt doubles will carry out dangerous stunts on behalf of the actor. A 'stand in' is a person hired to stand in for the actors whilst menial tasks are carried out such as lighting a set (they do not require make-up).

CONTINUITY SCHEDULE
Ellie

Scene 1	Hair and Make-up requirements
1	Straight corrective natural day make-up (see design sheet). Hair pulled back in loose ponytail.
2	Sexy, heavily made-up eyes, glossy lips (natural colour – kissing scene coming up). Sexy hair – wavy, tousled and down (see design sheet)
3	As Scene 2
4	Not in scene
5	As scene 3, looking slightly dishevelled as she is drunk
6	Make-up minimal – perhaps slightly smudged mascara (just got out of bed). Hair down and loose, slightly untidy.
7	As Scene 6
8	As Scene 7
9	Straight corrective natural day make-up. Hair in loose French pleat.
10	Straight corrective natural day make-up. Hair pulled back in loose ponytail.
11	As 10
12	Not in scene
13	Straight make-up but with red lipstick and hair loose
14	As 14
15	As above plus special effects – blood (see design notes)

Continuity schedule

SCRIPT BREAKDOWN
City Bells Episode 15

Scene No.	Cast	Story Day & Detail	Action
1	Ellie	Day 1, Interior	Ellie on phone to Fern
2	Ellie, Joe, Scott, Arthur Fern, clubbers	Night 1, Interior	First meeting, Ellie and Joe go to the dance floor
3	Ellie, Joe, Clubbers	Night 1, Interior	They talk and dance provocatively
4	Arthur, Fern, Scott, passers by	Night 1, Exterior	They talk and leave
5	Ellie and Joe, cab driver	Night 1, Exterior	They stumble into cab and kiss
6	Ellie, Joe	Day 2, Interior	They wake up in Ellie's bedroom by knocking at the door
7	Ellie, Joe, Scott	Day 2, Interior	Ellie lets Scott in, Ellie and Scott argue, Scott leaves
8	Ellie, Joe	Day 2, Interior	Joe gets dressed and leaves
9	Ellie, Fern	Day 2, Interior	They talk over coffee, mobile phone rings
10	Ellie	Night 2, Interior	Alone in flat, drinking wine & watching TV, knock on door
11	Joe, Ellie	Night 2, Interior	Joe arrives, beaten up, they talk
12	Scott, Arthur	Day 3, Exterior	Scott working on car, while Arthur tries to talk to him, Scott gets angry
13	Ellie, Scott, Arthur	Day 3, Exterior	Ellie arrive at garage, Arthur leaves
14	Ellie, Scott	Day 3, Exterior	They argue and move inside
15	Scott, Ellie	Day 3, Interior	Scott hits Ellie over head with wrench

An example of a script breakdown

DAILY SCENE BREAKDOWN – MAKE-UP/HAIR DEPARTMENT

Production: City Bells

Date: Monday, 11th November 2004

Episode & and Scene Nos: Episode 15, Scenes 2, 3, (+ pick-up scene 11)

Production Notes: Closed set, scene 9, absolutely no visitors

Scene 2 (Night / Interior, Story Day 1)

Character	Make-up / Hair Breakdown
Ellie	Sexy, heavily made-up eyes, glossy lips. Sexy hair – wavy, tousled and down (see design sheet)
Joe	Straight, corrective make-up, hair tidy
Scott	Straight, corrective make-up, hair pulled back in ponytail
Arthur	Straight, corrective make-up, hair tidy
Fern	Trendy, evening make-up (consult with costume), hair to be worn in straight bob.
Clubbers	Trendy, club make-up and hair

Scene 3 (Night / Interior, Story Day 1)

Character	Make-up / Hair Breakdown
Ellie	As scene 2
Joe	As scene 2
Clubbers	As scene 2

+ Pick-Up, Scene 11 (see records from Friday 8th November 2004)

Daily scene breakdown

KEY NOTE

When a scene is '**picked up**' it means a scene or part of a scene is re-shot because the first take was later deemed unsatisfactory. The re-shoot may happen several days (or even weeks) after the original take and therefore extra care must be taken to ensure accurate continuity.

HANDS ON

Breaking down scripts

Get hold of a script: you can download them from the Internet or purchase them from good bookshops.

Following the suggestions in the daily scene breakdown on the previous page, break down the script and produce the schedules as listed. This is an excellent training exercise as it will help you understand the format of scripts and the concept of continuity.

The production period

Schedules, referred to as **call sheets**, are produced on a daily basis by the production team in collaboration with each department and given to the crew and performers the day before the day to which they refer. The call sheet contains all the information to ensure the smooth running of the next day's shoot.

As you can see from the call sheet below, the performers are given a make-up and hair call time. If a performer is consistently late for the call it may be worth mentioning it to the make-up supervisor, who may in turn report it to the production team. The make-up and hair styling will usually be applied in the make-up rooms, where equipment and correct lighting conditions will be available. Acceptable timescales for make-up and hair styling application will vary, but a rough guide is given below.

Male straight make-up and hair	30 mins maximum
Female straight make-up and hair	45 mins maximum
Male period make-up and hair using facial postiche	1 hour maximum
Female period make-up using wig	1 hour 30 mins maximum
Minor casualty effect	20 mins maximum
Fantasy make-up using special effects	1 to 2 hours depending on design
Make-up using special effects and prosthetics	2 hours + depending on design

A rough guide to timing in make-up

Once the make-up has been completed and approved by the performer and the make-up designer or supervisor, the make-up artist will usually accompany the performer to the set and report to the assistant director. Some directors prefer to check the make-up themselves before shooting begins. At this stage, it is not practical for the make-up artist to bring the entire kit to the set, therefore he or she will carry a **set bag**, which is a smaller kit (some make-up artists like to use a bum-bag or apron with pockets for uncomplicated make-ups) containing essential materials. A typical set bag for a straight make-up may contain:

* compact powder (it is best to avoid taking loose powder onto the set)
* a few brushes
* a small palette of camouflage and concealers
* lipstick
* tissues
* cotton buds
* a sponge
* hairspray, brush and comb
* a camera for continuity information.

CALL SHEET NO: 62

Production: City Bells, Episode 15

Date: Friday, 13th June 2004

Director: Alan Pictor

Unit call: 8.00 am

Set: Studio 10

Scene Nos: 4, 10, 11, 15

Production Notes: Closed set scene 15 – absolutely no visitors

Artiste	Character	Dressing/ Room	Pick Up Time	M/Up, Hair and Wardrobe	On Set
Paul Nichols	Scott	3	7.00am	7.30am	8.00am
Ben Omar	Joe	4	6.30am	7.00am	8.30am
Steven Black	Arthur	5	7.00am	7.30am	8.00am
Claire Tallis	Fern	6	6.30am	7.00am	8.00am
Sandra Sanders	Ellie	7	7.00am	7.30am	8.30am
Samantha Wright	Stunt double for Ellie	Required at studio from 9.00am			
Anne Last	Stand-in for Ellie (Ms Sanders)		6.30	7.15am	8.00am
Extras x 7	Passers-by			10am	12.00noon

Props: As per script, flowers, glasses, trolley, telephone, ornate vase, tools

Special Effects: Blood bladder, blood, wrench required from 8.00am, as arranged with FX Supplies

Make-Up / Hair: Artistes to be made up / hair in Rooms A, B and C (New Block)

Wardrobes: Artistes to be costumed in their dressing rooms

Prod / Stunt Co-ordinator: R. Clayton required on set from 8.00am

Prod / Asst. Directors: Artistes dressing Rooms, make-up/hair rooms to be open and practical from 6.00am

Catering: 9.30am and 3.30pm trolley outside studio 9 for approximately 50 persons

Lunch: 1.30 – 2.30pm unless otherwise advised

Rushes: 6.00pm – 7.00pm in Theatre 9

Medical: First Aid Department in New Block, Extension 246

Transport: See separate sheet

A call sheet

The make-up artist should try to ensure he or she has everything that is required to maintain the make-up on set. The make-up artist should never leave the set without first informing another member of the make-up team or an assistant director.

One of the most daunting situations that a new make-up artist will face is walking onto a set for the first time. Film sets and television studios can be very frantic places and it is often difficult to find a place to stand where you feel you are not in the way. Always remember that you are on set to carry out a job, and you need to stand in a position where you can do this most effectively without interfering with others or causing disruption. There are many monitors on set and in the control room, each with a particular purpose. The one of relevance to the make-up artist is the **line monitor**, which shows the actual image that will be screened and is therefore colour corrected. The make-up artist should study his or her work on this monitor during scene rehearsals and note any required changes to the make-up or hair. It is always best to be honest about the length of time changes are likely to take. If the changes are complicated it may be necessary to return to the make-up room with the performer.

Once filming begins it is best to remain on set – a good place to stand is behind a camera (but stand well back in case the camera person decides to suddenly reverse) – and remain as quiet as possible.

It is essential to find out from the director whether he or she wants you to maintain the make-up and hair between each take or wait for instructions. If the latter is the case, the make-up artist will wait to hear 'checks' or 'make-up' called and then will immediately walk over to the performers and re-touch the make-up and hair as quickly as possible.

It is the make-up artist's responsibility to observe his or her allocated performer as closely as possible, both on and off camera. However, it is best not to stare at the performers directly during filming as this may distract or annoy them. Whilst they are performing, it is more appropriate to view them via a camera or monitor. The make-up artist must constantly be on the look-out for required make-up or hair adjustments, repairs and continuity errors; this is generally referred to as **maintaining** the make-up and may include adding more lipstick, powdering, blotting perspiration or smoothing the hair. Changes are much easier to make at the time of shooting rather than later, when a scene may have to be re-shot (or picked-up) because of an unspotted error.

Continuity

Continuity is central to film and television work and it is up to all make-up artists to maintain continuity in their work. Film and television productions are usually shot out of sequence; that is, filming will jump from one scene to another, which may be either much further on in the script or story or back near the beginning. This causes problems for the make-up and hair department, who have to ensure that the performers' appearance:

* meets the requirements of the script or story and of the design specification for the production and achieves realism and credibility on camera

* is seamless from one scene to the next where the story timeline is continuous, and that the make-up and hair 'match' the preceding and following shots

⁎ alters logically to follow the developing action in a script, even when scenes are shot out of sequence.

> Passing of time (progression of illness or disease, healing of wounds, hair growth, ageing)

> **Aspects of a script affecting the continuity of a performer's appearance**

> Weather conditions (perspiration, skin colour, breaking down hair)

> Emotion (perspiration, shock, tears)

The continuity process begins at the pre-production stage. As discussed earlier, once the make-up designer has read and broken down the script, he or she will produce a continuity schedule for each character. This information is then transferred onto scene breakdown schedules that are produced for each day's shooting.

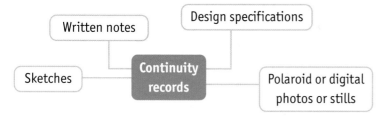

In order for the process to work, each make-up artist within the department must ensure accurate continuity records are kept. These records may be kept in several ways.

The continuity records can be pinned to the wall so that the make-up artists can refer to them as they work. It is vital that they are then filed at the end of the day and kept for future reference.

The most common method of documenting a performer's appearance is by taking photographs and making written notes on the reverse. Photos should include frontal, side and back views of the performer to ensure the make-up and hairstyle can be recreated accurately from all angles. A photo should be taken to record:

⁎ a performer's appearance at the beginning of a scene

⁎ a performer's appearance at the end of a scene or when there is a direct cut

⁎ changes to a performer's appearance mid-scene.

The notes on the back of the photo may include information about the colours and brands of products used, a description of any hair accessories, details about application techniques of special effects, etc. The make-up artist must provide sufficient information to ensure the make-up and hairstyle can be recreated in the future by any of the team.

Polaroid versus digital

Many make-up departments are switching from Polaroid cameras to a digital continuity system.

> **KEY NOTE**
>
> Whichever method is chosen it is important to ensure the equipment is in good working order and the camera is loaded ready for use when on set. The make-up artist should also ensure there is plenty of film stock available at the start of the shoot.

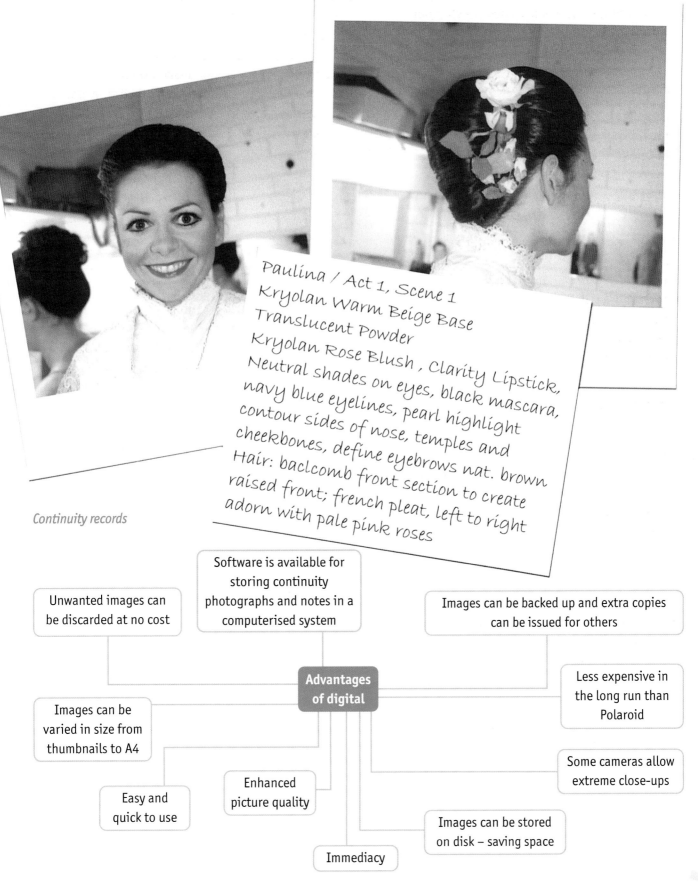

Continuity records

Paulina / Act 1, Scene 1
Kryolan Warm Beige Base
Translucent Powder
Kryolan Rose Blush , Clarity Lipstick,
Neutral shades on eyes, black mascara,
navy blue eyelines, pearl highlight
contour sides of nose, temples and
cheekbones, define eyebrows nat. brown
Hair: baclcomb front section to create
raised front; french pleat, left to right
adorn with pale pink roses

Unwanted images can be discarded at no cost

Software is available for storing continuity photographs and notes in a computerised system

Images can be backed up and extra copies can be issued for others

Images can be varied in size from thumbnails to A4

Advantages of digital

Less expensive in the long run than Polaroid

Easy and quick to use

Enhanced picture quality

Some cameras allow extreme close-ups

Images can be stored on disk – saving space

Immediacy

Storing continuity records

Make-up records should be stored in an efficient filing system to allow easy access for those who need to refer to them, for example a make-up artist may need to refer to continuity records for a scene that is being re-shot. Filing systems will vary from production to production according to the make-up supervisor's preferred method of working, but it is generally accepted as good practice to install a centralised system, which might perhaps be kept in the make-up room, rather than separate records being held by individual make-up artists. Consideration should be given to storing the following information:

* the shooting schedule
* call sheets
* scene breakdowns
* script
* continuity records.

KEY NOTE

If a make-up artist is unable to attend the set in person, he or she must ensure arrangements are made for someone else to record continuity details. This may be a reliable colleague within the department, perhaps a make-up assistant. Alternatively, some productions will have a continuity supervisor responsible for overall continuity of the production, who may be able to assist.

Working in fashion and photographic environments

Lighting considerations

Most professional still films are daylight balanced, meaning they are colour corrected for use with lighting temperatures between 5,400° K and 5,800° K. If the photographer wants to shoot in colour using tungsten lighting, there are two options: the photographer can use a blue tinted filter that will counteract the yellow / orange colour cast thrown off by tungsten lighting, or purchase special still film which is balanced for tungsten lights. This problem of colour correction only applies when shooting in colour film.

Still film photography can be exposed using the following light sources:

* tungsten studio lighting
* electronic flash, which is a very intense and rapid flash of light activated by a high voltage source
* daylight on external shoots, which is sometimes supplemented by fill-in electronic flash.

REMEMBER

Studios are dangerous places, filled with trailing wires and expensive high voltage equipment. Never touch or attempt to move studio lights unless you are absolutely sure it is safe to do so.

Different photographers will vary in their working styles and preferences, and it is down to the make-up artist to work flexibly and adapt to fit in with the photographer's lighting. Generally speaking, the stronger the light, the more it bleaches out the make-up. Shiny and glitter products should be used with caution and always in consultation with the photographer, as they may cause problems with some lighting set-ups.

The team on a fashion shoot

Team member	Role
Photographer (and sometimes an assistant)	To get 'the picture'. The photographer is probably under the greatest pressure of any of the team members.
Stylist	To plan the presentation of the clothes and ensure they look immaculate, paying attention to detail. The stylist must also ensure the clothes are styled to suit the shoot's design brief.
Models	To look good and perform to the camera with the aim of selling the clothes or product.
Client: editor, designer or advertising agency	To establish the brief for the photo shoot and oversee its implementation.
Art director	To successfully bring together all the elements of the shoot.
Hairstylist (on large budget shoots)	To translate the concept of the brief into a hairstyle.
Make-up artist (on smaller budget shoots the make-up artist is also expected to undertake the role of hair styling)	To translate the concept of the brief onto the face and sometimes body.

The process of the fashion shoot

Pre-production

The client determines a brief and the creative parties – the photographer, stylist, hairdresser, make-up artist and sometimes the art director – discuss ideas and concepts. The storyboard, location, clothes, props and models are chosen and it is the role of the make-up artist to translate the original concept onto the face (and sometimes body) of the models. It is important to be thoroughly prepared for a photo shoot, although sometimes you may find yourself hired for a job at very short notice. Ensure you find out as much information as possible about what will be required and make sure you have the necessary equipment in your kit to carry out the job. Make certain you keep an eye on consumable stock levels such as sponges, and *always* make sure you turn up for a job with clean brushes, powder puffs and palettes.

For big budget fashion shoots or shows, hair and make-up artists are usually booked through agencies. The artists are chosen in a similar way to the models – from their portfolios (also called books) containing pictures of their work. Once the job has been confirmed, the make-up designer will assess how many assistants will need to be hired. This will depend on the number of models and the complexity of the work. You will certainly be required to attend design meetings, during which in-depth discussions will take place about the make-up and hair concepts. Following this the make-up designer will come up with make-up design sheets or mood boards to communicate his or her ideas.

Once the designs have been approved, the make-up team must purchase equipment and materials and prepare special effects such as wigs or hairpieces. It is also a good idea to contact the models either directly or through their agency to ensure they do not have any known allergies to products or brands. The make-up and hairstyle should be planned in as much detail as possible. The make-up designer should consult with the photographer to establish whether technical aspects, such as lighting or the type of film being used, will affect the approach of the make-up design.

* High-speed grainy film: some definition will be lost. Make-up application may need to be stronger than usual.

* Cross-processed film: this will alter the colours of the make-up application. Discuss the implications with the photographer.

* Black and white film: ask whether the shoot will be mixed with colour prints or shot entirely in black and white. Black and white photography requires a different approach by the make-up artist because the placement of light and shade and the tonal range of colours become more important than colour (see Chapter 8).

Production

The make-up and hair artists will usually arrive at the same time as the models (on big make-up shows this may be about four or five hours before the show is due to start). Male models will arrive later unless they are having an intricate design applied. On arrival, the head of the make-up team will view the clothes, discuss the running order and construct a plan of action with the stylist, designer and show producer or photographer.

Once the make-up has been applied and the hair styled, you will need to maintain it throughout the photo shoot or show. On shoots, most photographers like the make-up artist to stay close to the camera but remain unobtrusive, in case the make-up or hair requires re-touching. Re-touching will almost certainly be required after a model has changed outfits or had a break and eaten or drunk. Studio lights may cause a problem with perspiration, and on external shoots consideration will need to be given to environmental conditions, for example sun protection will be needed in hot climates.

On test shoots you may be required to undertake several make-up and hair changes on a single model. Often, the model or photographer will want to show the diversity of a model's look and this will require some dramatic changes to the hair and make-up with several outfit changes. In consultation with the photographer and stylist it is always preferable to begin with a minimal make-up application and work in a logical order, finishing with the most dramatic look. You will be required to work very fast and simply will not have time to begin each make-up from scratch. On average, you may have thirty minutes to apply the make-up and hairstyle for the initial application and a further twenty minutes for each change. The examples below show the progression of a model's make-up and hair application throughout a test shoot. The make-up and hair was simply adjusted and built on for each change of look.

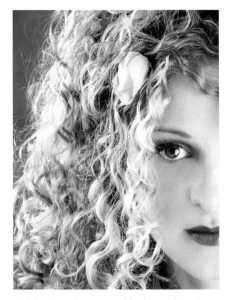

Original make-up and hair application for the first look on a test shoot

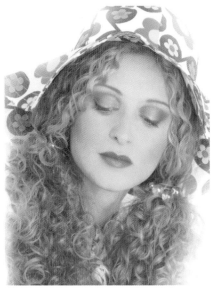

Adapted make-up and hair application for the second look on a test shoot

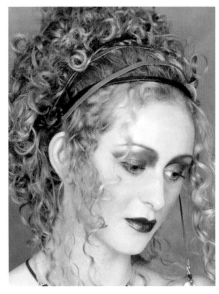

Third make-up and hair changes for the final look on a test shoot

**Adapting the make-up to change
the model's appearance**

Working with one model, begin by applying a minimal make-up. Take a photo and then adapt the make-up to create a stronger effect, perhaps experimenting with colour. Take another photo, and finally adapt the make-up to create a dramatic and glamorous application, perhaps by adding more eye make-up, false lashes or a change of lipstick colour. Take a photo.

Post production

After the job has finished the make-up artist should obtain pictures of the shoot to add to his or her portfolio. This is important so you can show potential clients examples of your experience and capabilities. Sometimes it can take much chasing to obtain these pictures, but perseverance is necessary if your portfolio (or book) is to be kept up to date.

Working in retail

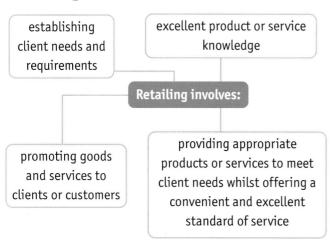

establishing client needs and requirements

excellent product or service knowledge

Retailing involves:

promoting goods and services to clients or customers

providing appropriate products or services to meet client needs whilst offering a convenient and excellent standard of service

Successfully promoting products and services to clients will bring financial reward to the company and its staff and will promote good will with customers if their needs and requirements are met.

Establishing client needs

If you are going to sell to a client it is important you begin by establishing the client's needs and requirements so you can promote a product or service that will interest the client and bring him or her some benefit. You could identify the client's needs by:

* assessing the client through observation
* questioning the client
* *briefly* informing the client about a range of products to see if their reaction is one of interest.

Once you have established a client's requirement, you are reliant on your expert knowledge to successfully match the need with the appropriate product. Without this knowledge you will be unable to make the sale, so it is vital that you are up to date with the *features* and *benefits* of the range of products you are promoting.

Product knowledge

Product knowledge can be achieved through:

* working with others
* asking questions and checking information
* product training
* product literature
* reading trade magazines.

Features and benefits of products

Products may be described in terms of their features and benefits. Features are product characteristics that deliver benefits; clients will often purchase products once they acknowledge their benefits.

* Features are product characteristics such as ingredients, design, texture and colour.
* Benefits are the reasons why a client will purchase the product; they answer the client question: What will it do for me?

The following table demonstrates the difference between features and benefits, using Clarins Gentle Eye Make-up Remover Lotion as an example.

Feature	Benefit
Based on ingredients of cornflower and rosewater	Soothes and refreshes without stinging
Ultra-gentle	Suitable for sensitive eyes and contact lens wearers
Contains soya proteins	Helps to strengthen lashes

Some benefits are more difficult to define, particularly the benefits of some cosmetic products that may offer emotional rewards to the client, allowing him or her to feel better in some way. For example, buying a new lipstick may boost the client's morale and wearing it may give him or her more confidence. Likewise, buying products not tested on animals offers the client an opportunity to be socially responsible. To identify a product's benefits, you must consider the client's viewpoint and requirements.

Understanding your product features and benefits allows you to:

* describe the product in a way that is most relevant to the client
* explain how your products differ and compare favourably with those of competitors.

HANDS ON

Features and benefits

Visit a local make-up store and ask for some literature on their product range. Using a couple of products as examples, make a list of their features and potential benefits to clients.

Promoting goods and services to clients or customers

Once you have matched the product to the client, you should begin the process of promoting it to the client in order to make a sale. A number of opportunities may arise enabling you to promote products, including the following.

* A client looking at product displays. Product displays should be eye catching to attract passing trade and be kept clean to encourage the client to browse and sample tester items. Some cosmetic houses will leave disposable brushes, cleaners and cotton wool or tissues for the client to use whilst trying out various products. Whilst clients are browsing, the retailer has an opportunity to promote the products.

* Using posters and publicity material to promote the company image and products to clients, who will often be seduced into buying into 'the image' of a product range. Some cosmetic houses will keep a portfolio or book of press clippings promoting their products by the front displays. Alternatively, some clients will spot a particular colour used in a publicity picture, and many cosmetic houses insist their retail staff wear the products they are promoting, hoping the client will notice the products.

* Carrying out a make-up application on the client enabling the retailer to demonstrate the potential of the products. This is one of the most successful ways of promoting cosmetics, providing you apply the make-up in a way that will suit and please the client. Remember to listen to the client and establish her likes and dislikes – applying a bright green eye shadow on a client who doesn't like colour on her eyes will defeat the object and lose you a sale. Discuss with the client what you intend to apply and use the opportunity to talk to her about the product's features and benefits as you apply the make-up.

* Giving the client special offers or free samples if available. This enables the client to try out the products and may lead to a full purchase in the future.

* Using link selling. If a client is a returning customer and knows what he or she wants to purchase, you could use the opportunity to promote a product that complements the one the client has already chosen.

When promoting products or services it is important to give accurate, balanced and sufficient information to the client, who should be encouraged to ask questions. It is against the law to give misleading or false information.

You should always be positive and helpful when making a sale. There is nothing more off-putting than an over-zealous, pushy sales person, so do not be too persistent or pressure the client into making a purchase. In addition, customers must never be rushed into making a purchase. They must be given time to make up their minds. Remember to use effective communication skills (as discussed in Chapter 3).

Closing the sale

An experienced sales person will recognise the signs that a client is ready to purchase. But by listening to the client, even a relatively inexperienced retailer should be able to spot the signals. Clients may use expressions such as:

* I like this colour best.
* This is just what I've been looking for.
* Does it come in different sizes or colours?

Once you have established that the client is interested in making a purchase, you should begin the process of closing the sale.

Summarise the benefits to the client of making the purchase.

Offer an incentive, such as a free sample or tester of a product that complements the purchase (this will also encourage future purchases).

Offer the client alternatives. This is based on the fact that people like to have choices. They don't like to be given what may sound like an ultimatum to either buy it or not buy it. To apply this technique, you can structure your close by saying, 'Which of these products would you prefer, A or B?' You can also give him or her choices with regard to payment and packaging, for example, 'Would you like it gift wrapped?' or 'How would you like to pay?'

You should conclude the sale by checking the client's understanding of how to use the product and then obtain his or her agreement to take payment.

Delivery of products

If the product the client requires is out of stock, it may be necessary to order it and either put it to one side for collection or arrange delivery. If this is the case, you must ensure that you offer an efficient service to the client. In order to achieve this you must make sure you have all the information you require: the client's name, address, contact telephone number, etc. The client will probably want to know an estimated delivery date and it is important to let the client know immediately if any problems arise with meeting this date.

Closing negotiations when the client shows no interest

If the client shows no interest in the products you are promoting, you need to ask yourself the following questions.

* Have I understood the client's needs accurately?
* Do the products I am trying to promote meet the client's needs?
* Am I clearly explaining the benefits of the products to the client?
* Am I using effective communication skills?

If you can confidently answer 'yes' to the above questions, then you should not pursue the sale any further in case you come across as an insensitive, pushy sales person. Politely tell the client to ask for further help if required and leave the client to browse.

Referrals

If you are unable to assist a client because of inexperience or lack of knowledge, it is important to acknowledge this and ask for help from a colleague. If the client requests a product or service that you are unable to provide, it is important to be professional and try to assist the client by referring them to an alternative source. Clients will always remember a helpful and polite service and may be more likely to return to you for a different service or product in the future.

The selling process

Introduction and greeting – retailers must always greet customers in a cheerful and polite manner.

Finding out the customer's needs - it's no good trying to sell products to a customer who already has them, does not want them or will never need them.

Promotion of the product and giving knowledge to the client - retailers should make sure they know all the products well and should be able to inform the client about suitable products as well as being prepared to answer any questions, queries and concerns a client may raise about a product. They must be able to put the customer's mind at ease about quality, payment, competitiveness, safety and so on.

Readjustment of needs or realisation of suitability of product – this takes place when the client realises the product will be of benefit.

Closing the sale – after advising the client of the cost and payment methods, the client decides to make a purchase.

After-sales follow up – some companies will check whether the product has matched the customer's needs and expectations. This may be part of the organisation's aftercare service and may take the form of a survey or questionnaire.

KEY NOTE

Sales targets: management will often try to improve productivity by setting sales targets for members of staff or for the entire team. Staff are encouraged to meet these targets by being offered commission on sales. Commission is a percentage of the product's selling price, which is added to their basic salary. If sales targets are not met then the company may make a financial loss, resulting in a loss of job security for all staff.

Consumer legislation

In addition to the legislative Acts described below, you will need to recall the following information from previous chapters.

* health and safety legislation (Chapter 2)
* the Data Protection Act (Chapter 2)
* equal opportunities and disability discrimination (Chapter 3).

The Consumer Protection Act 1987

There are three main areas to this Act. The first area is concerned with **product liability** and protects the consumer against death or injury caused by using defective consumer goods. Since 1987, the consumer no longer has to prove a manufacturer's negligence prior to suing for damages. The consumer can now claim against any supplier (including the manufacturer or importer), rather than simply the person from whom the goods were purchased, as was formerly the case.

The second area of the Act institutes a **general safety requirement** calling for all domestic goods to be reasonably safe, bearing in mind all the circumstances. Powers under the Act allow suspect goods to be 'suspended' from sale for up to six months, whilst checks on safety are conducted. If faulty, the goods may be destroyed.

The third area of the Act regulates against businesses giving **misleading price indications** for products or services. A guide to good practice has been published by the Department of Trade and Industry, which if followed may protect a trader against prosecution.

The Sale and Supply of Goods Act 1994

This Act updated both the Sale of Goods Act 1979 and the Supply of Goods and Services Act 1982. It affects the sale of all goods, regardless of where the sale took place. According to the Act the retailer must ensure that the goods or service provided are of satisfactory quality. This is defined as a standard that any reasonable person would consider as satisfactory with regard to the fitness for purpose, appearance, durability and safety of the goods or service.

If the goods or service are found to fall below satisfactory levels of quality the retailer should:

* refund the money paid for the goods or service (if there is no receipt, retailers can offer an exchange)

* make a complaint to the supplier.

Consumers have a right to expect products and services to be of merchantable quality and fit for the purpose for which they were sold as described in advertising literature. If this is not the case their rights are protected under this Act.

Trades Descriptions Act 1968 (updated in 1987)

This Act applies to business transactions and makes it a criminal offence to:

* apply a false description to any goods or services, whether it be written or verbal

* produce misleading advertisements

* make misleading statements about the price.

Cosmetic Products (Safety Regulations) 1996

This Act sets strict guidelines affecting the packaging and composition of cosmetic products. To summarise the Act, the following information should be marked on the container or packaging and sometimes both:

* the name and address of the manufacturer

* the best before date (where necessary)

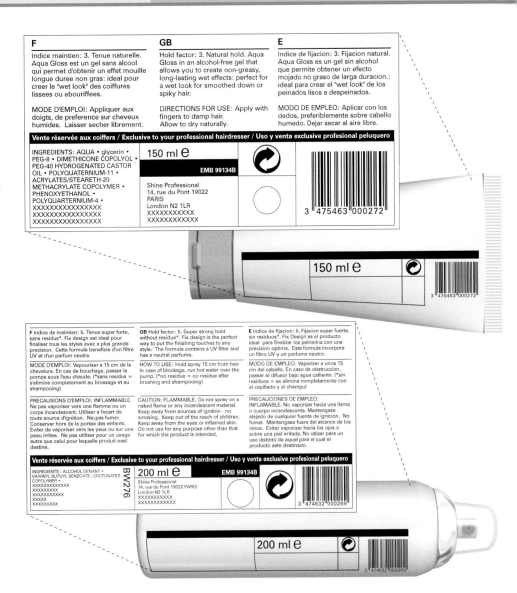

Typical information found on cosmetic product packaging

* the product's function (where necessary)

* specific information and precautions

* ingredients listed in descending order

* batch identification.

Where this is impractical, a leaflet should be enclosed or attached to the product, and the consumer should be informed of its presence on the container or packaging.

Contributing to the design process

The degree to which you will be involved in the design process for make-up and hair work will depend on your experience, your role within the department and how responsibilities have been delegated by the make-up supervisor or designer. It is important that you fully understand and clarify what will be expected of you. If you are unsure or feel unable to undertake an assigned responsibility, it is important to let the supervisor or designers know as early as possible. It is far better to be honest, so that help or alternative responsibilities can be given without major disruption to the production schedule.

Once you have established and agreed your contribution, it is important you approach and carry out your responsibilities efficiently and effectively to promote the smooth running of the design process. Colleagues will undoubtedly have

The script / text / storyboard / brief is received, reviewed and analysed.

⬇

Design meetings are attended to establish style / genre of the production or photo shoot.

⬇

The script / text / storyboard / brief is broken down and the appearance of characters or models is considered.

⬇

Make-up and hair designs are researched.

⬇

Make-up and hair designs are prepared.

⬇

Make-up and hair designs are presented to decision makers with approximate costs.

⬇

Make-up and hair designs are agreed with decision makers.

⬇

Make-up and hair materials and equipment are selected to realise designs and fit in with production requirements.

⬇

Suppliers are sourced and contacted according to selection criteria.

⬇

Make-up and hair designs are implemented.

⬇

Documentation is filed for future reference.

their own responsibilities to undertake, and although you should feel able to ask questions and consult with colleagues, you will be expected to work on your own initiative.

The process of designing

The design process itself will vary somewhat according to the environment in which you are working. However, listed below is a general overview the various stages:

The first three steps are discussed earlier in this chapter, so we will begin by looking at the fourth step, researching designs.

Researching designs

If you are required to carry out character research for a make-up or hair design, there are a number of useful sources you could use.

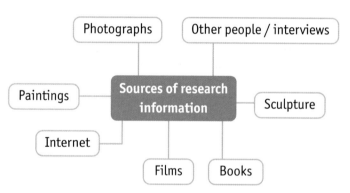

Remember, you are often not researching simply for historical accuracy but also to portray characterisation. Therefore it is important to make sure you are not simply looking at correct time periods but also at the correct social class, etc. Traditional portrait paintings were generally made of the upper classes, so it is far more difficult to research hairstyles of the poorer classes prior to the twentieth century. In addition, paintings will usually only give detail of the front or side view; it is very unusual to find paintings of the rear view of the head. This is where sculpture is useful as it represents a three-dimensional form, enabling the researcher to view hairstyles from every angle. If you are researching time periods from the late nineteenth century onwards, you should be able to source photographs of all social classes.

You will not always be carrying out research for historical accuracy. You may be required to research the actual or perceived appearance of particular characters, perhaps over different periods of their life. This may involve researching how different designers have portrayed them in the past. It is always useful to keep research information for future reference.

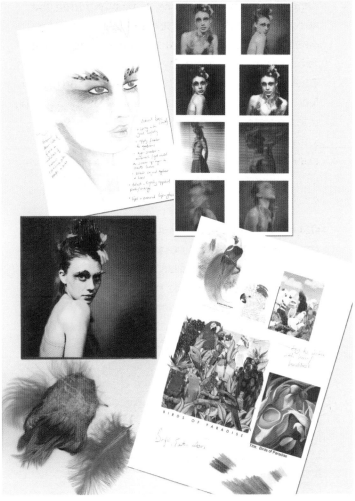

Mood board showing research photos, and photo of final design, inspired by the theme: 'Birds of Paradise'

HANDS ON

Researching a character

Using the sources suggested, research the character Queen Elizabeth I as she appeared throughout her life. Try to include images of how make-up artists have portrayed her in various productions. Using the information and images you collect, create a mood board of the character.

KEY NOTE

Richard Corson's books *Fashions in Hair* and *Fashions in Make-up* are invaluable resources when carrying out historical research. They contain detailed sketches and written text describing the changing fashions in make-up and hair from ancient times.

Preparing, presenting and agreeing make-up and hair designs

Once the research has been undertaken, the designer must find a way of communicating his or her ideas to others; this is usually done in the form of design sheets and mood boards. Information regarding the artistic process of preparing design sheets and mood boards can be found in Chapter 5.

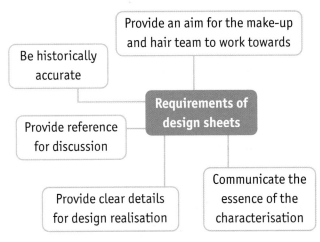

- Provide an aim for the make-up and hair team to work towards
- Be historically accurate
- Provide reference for discussion
- **Requirements of design sheets**
- Provide clear details for design realisation
- Communicate the essence of the characterisation

The completed make-up and hair designs should be clear and provide accurate information that can be easily translated by decision makers during the presentation process and by artists and stylists at the realisation stage.

The designs should include as much information as is required. On some productions the designer is only responsible for creating a concept and communicating the character's personality through appearance. In these cases the designs can be more vague and focus on creating an overall impression. On other productions the designer is responsible for creating both the concept and detailing the process of realisation: in this case the design sheets will contain more detailed information. Budgets will also be discussed at this stage of the design process and the designer will have to consider these when working on designs.

Detailed information on a design sheet may include sketches, notes, research source details, photographs and samples of materials. It is worth giving some consideration to the visual presentation of designs, which are best displayed on neutral-coloured mount card and covered with tracing paper to protect them against damage.

When presenting designs it is important to use effective communication skills (see Chapter 3) and appear enthusiastic about the designs themselves. In some ways the designers are 'selling' their ideas to the decision makers (directors, clients, performers, producers or other designers) and the better the product, or design sheets / mood boards, the easier this should be. The designer should also be prepared to answer questions about the designs and approximate costings. It is important to listen to others' opinions, taking on board suggestions and ideas if they are valid. Sometimes, the designer will need to go away and make changes to the designs before agreement to proceed can be reached. It is very important that agreement is reached before the design process moves forward.

Selecting make-up and hair materials and equipment

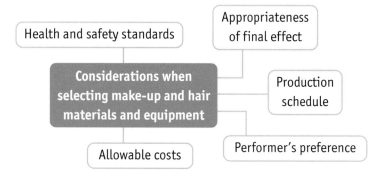

Allowable costs versus appropriateness of final effect

A budget will have been agreed with the client or production team and this will have the biggest influence on the selection of materials. It is important to explore all the options available to find a balance between cost and quality of effect on screen, stage or print. If a particular material is considered essential to the success of the

realisation of the design but exceeds the set spending limits, it is important that you approach the decision makers with justifiable reasons and gain approval before materials are ordered.

Health and safety standards

It is important that selected materials meet standards set by legislation and the production company (if applicable). Suppliers are required to ensure their products are safe and fit for use under specific legislative Acts (see page 112).

Production schedule

When selecting materials, the timescale of the production will need to be considered. It is important to decide on materials as early as possible and to check availability with the supplier to ensure they can meet delivery deadlines before an order is placed. The shorter the timescale, the more limited the options are in the choice of materials.

Performer's or model's preference

It is always best to obtain a performer's approval when selecting materials. Principal performers or models may have a particular liking for specific brands, or they may have a history of allergies to certain products. Consideration should always be given to the performer's or model's safety and comfort. Providing their preferences are not unreasonable and fit in with budget and production requirements, the make-up artist should try to accommodate them where possible.

Sourcing and contacting suppliers according to selection criteria

* **Research a number of suppliers.** It is always best to research a number of suppliers to ensure the one you finally select is competitive in terms of quality, cost, choice and delivery schedule.

* **Ensure potential suppliers understand the purpose of your material and equipment requirements, so that they can advise accordingly.** It is important to give the suppliers a full briefing of your intentions. If possible show them the designs and working notes. It may also be useful to refer to past jobs

they have been involved with. It is vital you communicate in a clear manner and check the supplier's understanding by using clarifying techniques (see pages 35-6).

* **Ensure the selected suppliers are able to supply the materials and equipment to meet your requirements.** Your requirements may include quality, quantity, type, size, cost, time schedules, and health and safety regulations. To ensure suppliers will meet these requirements you could:

  * ask around – do they have a good reputation within the industry
  * check the terms and conditions of any contracts
  * ensure they fully understand your requirements
  * try to obtain any agreements in writing
  * ensure documentation is clear and detailed.

* **Ensure that the selection and cost of materials and equipment are sanctioned by the production team or client.** It is very important that you gain approval of expenditure before placing any orders with suppliers. You should also obtain approval to use the selected supplier. Production companies and clients will want to ensure that the supplier meets company standards and may also wish to check out any past business transactions with the supplier.

* **Negotiate and agree terms and conditions with suppliers.** To ensure you are in a strong position when negotiating terms and conditions it is important to shop around and know exactly what you want to order. You will then be less likely to be talked into buying unnecessary materials. It may also be worth checking previous terms and conditions if the supplier has been used before. Sometimes a promise of further orders may help in negotiating costs and terms. It is important to agree:

  * costs
  * delivery timescales and return policies
  * methods and conditions of payment
  * insurance
  * retentions

* fitting arrangements
* exchange and refund policies.

* **Prepare clear and specific documentation for the supply of materials and equipment.** Suppliers will often provide their own paperwork for you to complete when placing orders. If they do not, you will need to create your own. Documentation must be clear, easy to read and contain sufficient information for the supplier, including any special instructions. It is good practice to check the order ensuring the correct codes, sizes, quantities and colours are recorded before it is placed. If you place your order verbally it is advisable to follow this up in writing. A quick phone call should be made to the supplier a couple of days later to confirm the written order has been received. Orders may be placed by post, email, fax or telephone.

Order form supplies

* **Deal with problematic timescales and suppliers.** It is important to be organised and order supplies as soon as possible to ensure problems with delivery dates are kept to a minimum. If you are working to short timescales, you may have to work around the materials that are immediately available from suppliers. It may also be useful to offer suppliers the opportunity to supply alternatives if the original request is unavailable. If the production timetable is tight through no fault of your own, it may be necessary to negotiate a bigger budget with the production team or client to pay for a premium on quick deliveries. If a supplier's service turns out to be problematic, refer to the terms and conditions that were agreed at the time of placing the order. Do not forget your rights under consumer legislation (see page 112) and if necessary seek alternative suppliers.

* **Keep and file documentation appropriately.** It is important to keep and file documentation for easy reference. Documentation may be required in cases of discrepancies with the supplier, to claim expenses or reimbursement, for VAT purposes or to check against delivery of the supplies. Documentation may include:

  * invoices
  * delivery notes
  * receipts
  * contracts
  * agreements.

Knowledge Check

1 What is the main light on a studio set called?

2 Describe what is meant by cross lighting and what effect it has.

3 Give two uses of back lighting.

4 In external location shots what acts as the key light?

5 What two types of lighting does still film use?

6 Should stage make-up be warmer or cooler in tone, and why?

7 Describe the effects of daylight on make-up.

8 Describe the effects of tungsten lighting on make-up.

9 Describe the effects of fluorescent lighting on make-up.

10 Describe the effects of halogen studio flash lighting on make-up.

11 List three responsibilities a make-up artist may undertake in the post-production period of a theatrical production.

12 Define continuity.

13 Describe what is meant by a 'pick-up' in a film or television production.

14 What should a set-bag ideally contain?

15 What do we mean by the features and benefits of a product?

16 How can you establish a client's needs in the retail environment?

17 List three legislative Acts that provide consumer protection.

18 List five sources when researching designs.

19 List four considerations when selecting make-up and hair materials.

20 Why is it important to keep records of orders and supplies?

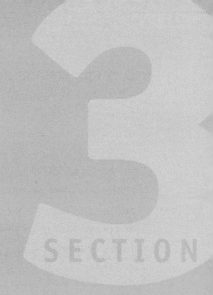

SECTION 3

Practical Skills

Cosmetic techniques

Before make-up artists can begin to apply colour to the face, it is important they have a full understanding of the basic cosmetic techniques. Cosmetic techniques have two functions: to prepare the model for make-up application and to enhance the completed make-up.

Aim and objectives

Aim of this chapter: to provide the underpinning knowledge and skills of basic cosmetic techniques required by the make-up artist.

You should achieve the following **objectives:**

* List and describe a range of skin types
* Discuss skin care and advise your clients on suitable products and routines
* Carry out a cleanse, tone and moisturise routine
* Pluck the eyebrows, giving full consideration to the final shape
* Tint or bleach the eyebrows
* Tint the eyelashes
* Apply individual and strip false lashes
* Curl the natural lashes
* Shape and paint the nails.

In order to help you proceed through this chapter, re-read the sections from Chapter 4 'Anatomy and physiology for the make-up artist' on the following:

* The structure of the skin (page 52)
* Acid mantle (page 56)
* Skin diseases and disorders (page 58)
* The skin and the ageing process (page 56).

Re-read also from Chapter 3 'Establishing positive consultation with relationships' the section on the model (page 39).

> **KEY NOTE**
>
> Ensure you are familiar with the COSHH regulations for the products described in this chapter.

Skin types and conditions

Skin types

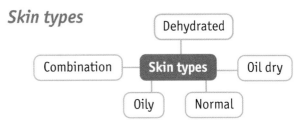

Normal skin

* Appears in good condition.
* Has a sufficient supply of sebum and moisture.
* Is free of blemishes.
* Will benefit from maintenance treatments to keep it healthy and attractive.

When caring for a normal skin, the main objectives of the make-up artist are to cleanse the skin so that dead cells are removed from the surface, impurities are removed from the pores and the skin is free from grease and make-up.

Oil dry skin

* Sebaceous glands are sluggish and fail to produce enough sebum.
* Is prone to milia.

* Feels rough to the touch.
* Has small pores.
* Appears matt.
* Feels 'tight'.

Skin can be dry due to inactivity of the sebaceous glands that produce sebum (oil). The condition may be caused by too much sun or wind, the use of harsh products, poor diet, ageing or medication. Facial treatments and home maintenance will help stimulate the sebaceous glands and normalise the production of sebum. The make-up artist must ensure the skin is conditioned after make-up removal with a rich moisturiser.

Dehydrated skin

* Is lacking in moisture.
* Is prone to fine lines and wrinkles that disappear when the skin is gently stretched (compare with the skin of a dried-out apple or peach).
* Appears to be thin.
* Feels coarse to the touch.
* Feels taut.

A dehydrated skin may have a normal amount of sebum but may still be flaky and feel taut and dry. This condition is due to lack of surface moisture. Dehydration of the skin may be a temporary condition and may be caused by the weather or environmental factors. A good homecare routine will help to improve the general health of the skin and will help it to retain moisture. Clients with this skin type should be encouraged to drink plenty of water. Dry, flaky skin can be exfoliated prior to make-up application to ensure a smooth application. The make-up artist should also ensure the skin is well moisturised after make-up removal.

Oily skin

* The surface texture resembles the skin of an orange.
* Is characterised by an over-production of sebum (oil).

* Feels thicker than dry or normal skins.
* Has enlarged pores.
* Has comedones (also called blackheads).
* Is prone to blemishes.
* Has a sallow appearance.

Oily skin can be caused by a number of factors. For example, during adolescence there may be an imbalance of hormones or a change in hormonal levels that result in an increase in the production of sebum. A diet rich in fats and oils may contribute to the oily condition of the skin and a hot, humid climate may also stimulate the sebaceous glands to produce more sebum. The make-up artist must ensure the skin's surface is completely free from any residue oil prior to make-up application, otherwise the make-up may look patchy. A mattifying lotion can be applied to prevent oily patches breaking through the make-up.

Combination skin

The combination skin is characterised by the existence of two or more different conditions. For example, the skin may be oily around the nose, forehead and chin, but dry on the rest of the face. When treating a combination skin, each area is treated for its particular condition. There are a number of product ranges available which can help to balance and normalise the conditions.

Skin conditions

The following are classified as skin conditions.

Acne vulgaris

Acne vulgaris is often accompanied by oily skin characteristics, but the skin has become infected. It is especially common during adolescence when it can affect the face, shoulders and back. Acne has a demoralising effect on a person and, if neglected, can cause scarring. Acne vulgaris can be treated to keep the condition under control and the make-up artist should not hesitate to recommend that a client see a GP for treatment. Clients should also be advised to avoid using harsh cleansing lotions,

which can exacerbate the problem. This skin condition will often display skin sensitivity and should be treated with great care.

Mature or ageing skin

As the body ages, its processes slow down and cells are not replaced as rapidly as they once were. Ageing skin is recognised by the appearance of deep wrinkles, loss of elasticity and sagging muscle tone (due to loss of collagen and elastin). There may also be certain skin blemishes present that are associated with the ageing process, for example lentigo. The make-up artist should avoid stretching the skin of a mature client. It is unlikely that you will cause any damage but clients will not appreciate it.

Sensitive skin

Clinically sensitive skin reacts on a predictable basis to an element or ingredient. Approximately 15 per cent of the population is estimated to have clinically sensitive skin, with 2 per cent of skin sensitivity reactions being attributed to cosmetic ingredients. In normal skin the cells of the stratum corneum form a protective barrier, regulating water loss and protecting against environmental aggression. In sensitive skin the basket weave appearance of the stratum corneum is not so dense and well formed, thus allowing easier penetration of external skin irritants.

Sensitive skin is often characterised by superficial flaking, dryness, a translucent appearance and redness in the cheeks due to dilated arterioles (broken veins). The make-up artist should treat a sensitive skin condition with extra care, avoiding known skin irritants wherever possible and ensuring all allergy tests are carried out and recorded. Barrier cream should be applied to the skin to provide extra protection.

Skin analysis

The make-up artist needs to carry out a skin analysis for the following reasons:

* to check the skin for contra-indications
* to identify the client's skin type
* to identify the correct products for use on the client
* to advise the client on homecare routines and products
* to record any areas requiring special attention or treatment.

There are three methods for carrying out the analysis:

* visual examination
* questioning the client
* manual examination.

Visual examination

Begin by assessing the skin before carrying out any procedure, including cleansing. During this initial examination, you are checking for contra-indications. You are also assessing the superficial condition of the skin – are there any oily patches breaking through the make-up, or does the skin look matt? This will allow you to choose an appropriate cleanser for a more thorough visual and manual examination. Once cleansed, a more detailed examination can take place. Pay particular attention to:

* skin colour
* pore size
* pigmentation changes
* skin blemishes
* surface condition – is it matt or shiny, flaky or smooth?
* lines and wrinkles.

Questioning the client

Initial questions can be asked during the cleansing procedure. This is a chance to discuss the client's current homecare routine and any problem areas. Once the thorough visual and manual examination begins, you can continue to question the client about your findings and try to establish factors that

may be contributing to the condition of the skin. Questioning of the client must be carried out in a tactful manner.

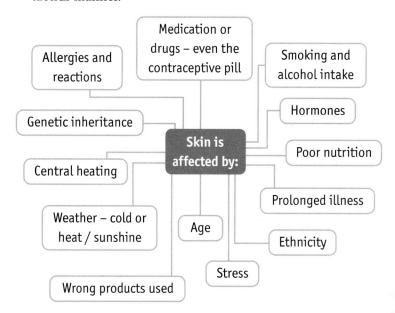

Manual examination

The manual examination should follow a logical sequence and be used in conjunction with a visual examination. Begin by assessing the skin in the following order:

* forehead
* eye area
* nose
* cheeks and sides of face
* chin and jaw line
* lips
* neck.

The manual examination should be carried out gently and particular attention should be paid to assessing the skin's texture, its elasticity (by gently pinching the skin and watching how quickly it retains its original shape) and the tone (by gently lifting the skin upwards and seeing how quickly it springs back).

Once the skin analysis has been carried out, your findings can be recorded on a facial analysis sheet.

Skin analysis

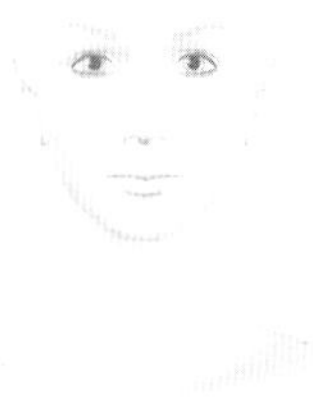

Problem areas / abnormalities noted	Area	Colour	Texture	Type	Sensitivity
	Forehead				
	Eye area				
	Cheeks and sides of face				
	Chin and jaw line				
	Neck				
	General elasticity: Firm ☐ Loose ☐				
	General colour				
Overall skin type	Treatment recommendations / adaptions				

Products used

	By make-up artist	At home
Cleanser		
Toner		
Moisturiser		
Mask		
Night cream		
Eye cream		
Specialist products		

Analysis conclusion

Product recommendations / homecare

Signed:	Date:

Facial analysis sheet

Cleansing, toning and moisturising

Knowing how to prepare the skin for make-up application and to return the skin to its original condition is essential for the make-up artist. It is also important to be able to advise your clients on suitable skin care routines to keep their skin in good condition.

The skin should be clean and free from existing make-up products and any oily residues before make-up is applied. If the skin is not perfectly clean prior to application, the make-up may look patchy and will wear off more quickly. Skin irritation may also occur.

Cleansing the skin

The skin becomes contaminated with:

* dead skin scales that are trapped on the surface of the skin
* pollution, including dust and carbon from the environment
* sweat, leaving salt and urea on the skin
* bacteria
* residue pigments, powder and oils if make-up has been previously used.

These particles are 'stuck' to the skin's surface by sebum (the oily secretion from the sebaceous gland in the dermis). Before the solid particles can be cleaned away, this excess sebum must be removed by:

* emulsifying it with a detergent – cleansing milks, bars and washes contain detergents

* dissolving it with more oil – cleansing creams remove sebum by dissolving it in oil.

When most of the excess sebum has been removed, the particles become loosened and can then be rinsed away. Cleansing twice is usually necessary as particles which have settled in the pores of the hair follicles and sweat glands are sometimes difficult to remove with the first cleanse. Cleansing preparations should:

* remove make-up and surface debris

* be pH balanced to the skin (4.5-6pH) – this will avoid disturbing the protective acid mantle

* be suitable for the client's skin type

* look, feel and smell pleasant.

Below we will look at various categories of cleansers in more detail.

Cleansing milks

Most cleansing milks have an 'oil in water' content, with a higher proportion of water to oil. As a result they often have a runny appearance. They are particularly suitable for those clients with a normal to oily skin type, who will often prefer a light, non-greasy product. They contain a detergent element and this can have a drying effect on a dry, mature or sensitive skin type.

Cleansing creams

These are usually creams with high oil content, often described as 'water in oil' preparations. They are available in a wide range of textures and consistencies, including 'mousse' preparations. Cleansing creams are very popular and are suitable for normal to dry and mature skin types or when removing heavy make-up application. The oil in the preparation mixes with, and dissolves, the sebum on the skin, removing surface particles and excess oil when the cream is wiped away.

Cleansing bars

These can be used on various skin types depending on the manufacturer's guidelines. These products look like traditional bars of soap, but do not leave the skin taut or alter the pH level as normal soap will. Facial bars should not be used with washing flannels, as these are not always sterile. Apply the soap to the face using clean dampened hands, massage in thoroughly and rinse with lots of lukewarm water.

Cleansing lotions, washes and gels

These are solutions of detergents in water and are generally recommended for normal to oily skin types. They are used on a dampened face, lathered up and rinsed off with tepid water (water too hot or too cold can damage the skin). Therefore in addition to the usual ingredients found in cleansing preparations, cleansing lotions also contain a foaming agent. Some lotions contain an anti-bacterial agent and are particularly suitable for blemished skin types.

KEY NOTE

Medicated lotions

These are generally used on oily or blemished skin types. They have a harsh, degreasing action on the skin, leaving the skin with a 'stripped, tight feeling' after use. This 'stripping' of the skin's sebaceous secretions will in turn cause over-stimulation of the sebaceous glands, which produces more sebum to compensate for this degreasing effect, so increasing the supply of sebum and worsening the original problem. The marketing of these products is aimed particularly at young people who wrongly believe the tight, oil-free feeling these cleansers leave them with will reduce the problem of blocked pores and pustules.

Typical ingredients found in cleansing preparations

The following ingredients are found in most cleansing preparations:

* water
* oils, usually mineral
* detergent, for example sodium lauryl sulphate (emulsifying)
* waxes, for example beeswax, Lanbritol Wax N21 (emulsifying)
* glycerol (moisturising)
* colouring (to make the product attractive)
* preservative (to prolong shelf life)
* perfume (to make the product appealing and pleasant to use).

Cleansing preparations may also include:

* foaming agent, for example Saponaria
* anti-bacterial agent.

Cleansing preparations will contain most of the above ingredients in varying proportions. Even products claiming to be 'natural' will include these ingredients, which will be from a 'natural source'. Recent legislation in the United Kingdom states that **all** ingredients must be listed on the product packaging.

Skin toning

Skin toning ensures the thorough removal of any residue remaining on the skin after the cleansing routine. It also leaves the skin feeling refreshed and refined. The skin may be toned using damp cotton wool pads saturated with toner that are wiped over the skin, or the toner may be sprayed onto the face. Excess toner may be blotted with a tissue.

Toners have the following features.

* Toners remove any remaining traces of grease, creams, etc.
* Toners have a bracing action and help to refine and tighten relaxed pores.

* Astringents are mildly antiseptic.
* Fresheners are soothing and calming on the skin.
* Some stimulate the circulation, improving the tone and colour of the skin.

There are various skin toners available and cosmetic houses manufacture one for every skin type. Toners can be classified as follows.

Fresheners

These contain no alcohol. They consist of mineral or distilled water and may also contain herbs or aromatherapy oils. These can be selected for the appropriateness of their properties on a particular skin type, for example lavender or camomile for a sensitive skin type, tea tree for a blemished skin type.

Skin tonics

Skin tonics contain between 1 and 25 per cent alcohol and can be used on any skin type. They have a mild and gentle effect on the skin. Some can be slightly stimulating. They are usually based on natural ingredients, for example rose water. A wide range is available to suit different skin conditions.

Astringents

Skin astringents contain between 25 and 60 per cent alcohol and should only be used on oily skin types as they have a drying and stimulating action.

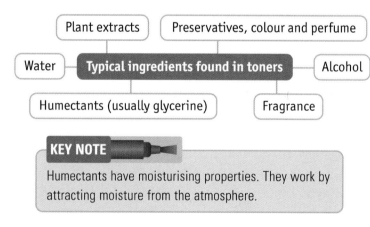

KEY NOTE

Humectants have moisturising properties. They work by attracting moisture from the atmosphere.

Skin moisturising

Moisturising creams are basically emulsions of water in an oil base; moisturising lotions are oil in a water base. Moisturisers have varying properties depending on the ingredients they contain and the skin type they have been designed for. They should be applied thinly to the whole of the face and neck. Generally a moisturiser should have the following features and benefits.

Feature	Benefit
Contains oils and waxes providing an occlusive barrier.	Prevents loss of moisture from the skin.
Contains humectants that attract moisture from the air.	This will moisturise and soften the stratum corneum.
Contains water.	Re-hydrates the skin, providing a smooth base for make-up.
Contains **S**un **P**rotection **F**actor.	Helps to prevent damage caused by harmful effects of UV rays.
May contain antioxidants – the most important are vitamins A, C and E.	The formation of 'free radicals' is part of the ageing process. These are unstable molecules that cause damage to cells, resulting in poor skin tone and elasticity. As we age, we become less able to counteract free radicals, but antioxidants help to neutralise their effects, promoting natural skin repair and slowing down ageing of the skin by providing skin cells with beneficial, nutrient vitamins.
May contain alpha hydroxy acids (AHAs).	These are naturally occurring substances that have been used for centuries (perhaps back to the Egyptians) to refine the texture of the skin. They work by accelerating the natural process of desquamation.
May contain collagen and elastin fibres.	Many moisturisers claim to be 'anti-ageing' and contain ingredients to help strengthen a mature skin type.

Night creams

These are moisturisers that are specifically designed for use in the evening. They are usually richer in texture than a day moisturiser and will not contain an SPF. The skin naturally repairs itself whilst we sleep and is thought to be more receptive to the benefits of various ingredients at this time.

Eye make-up removers

These are very gentle cleansing lotions especially formulated for the delicate eye area.

Exfoliators

Exfoliators remove dead cells from the skin's surface. They will improve the skin's texture and stimulate the circulation. Dry skin types need more frequent use of exfoliators than oily skin types. Exfoliators can take the form of grainy creams, thin creams that you slough off or 'peels' containing fruit acids.

Face masks

Face masks are usually recommended on a weekly basis. Benefits will depend on the individual properties of the mask but can range from deep cleansing to nourishing.

Eye gels and balms

These products are especially designed to condition the delicate eye area. Gels tend to reduce puffiness and have refreshing, soothing properties, whereas balms tend to smooth and improve the texture of the skin.

REMEMBER

Remove products from containers using a spatula rather than your fingers. Otherwise you will contaminate the product, reduce its shelf life and risk cross-contamination.

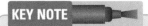
KEY NOTE

As a make-up artist you should ensure you are up to date with new skin care products on the market. Try out products from the vast number of ranges available until you find a selection that you would like to include in your kit. It may be impractical to carry a number of products for each of the individual skin types; you may prefer to choose products that are suitable for use on a range of skin types.

Skin care routines

Skin type	Morning	Evening	Weekly
Normal	Light cleansing cream, milk or wash Skin tonic Light moisturiser	Light cleansing cream, milk or wash Skin tonic Light night cream Eye balm	Face mask – deep cleansing, hydrating or soothing Exfoliate
Oil dry	Cleansing cream Skin freshener Rich moisturiser	Cleansing cream Skin freshener Night cream Eye balm	Face mask – nourishing Exfoliate up to twice a week
Dehydrated	Cleansing milk or cream Skin freshener Hydrating moisturiser	Cleansing milk or cream Skin freshener Hydrating night cream Eye balm	Face mask – hydrating Exfoliate
Oily	Cleansing bar or wash Astringent toner Oil-free or mattifying moisturising lotion	Cleansing bar or wash Astringent toner Light, oil-free moisturiser on any dehydrated patches Eye gel	Face mask – deep cleansing Exfoliate – provided skin is not blemished
Combination	Cleansing milk, cream or wash depending on client's preference Skin tonic Balancing moisturiser	Cleansing milk, cream or wash depending on client's preference Skin tonic Balancing night cream Eye gel or balm	Face mask – balancing Exfoliate
Sensitive	Hypo-allergenic cleansing milk or cream Skin freshener Hypo-allergenic, soothing moisturiser	Hypo-allergenic cleansing milk or cream Skin freshener Hypo-allergenic, soothing night cream Eye gel or balm for sensitive eyes	Face mask – calming and soothing Exfoliating should be avoided on irritated skin
Mature	Cleansing cream Skin tonic or freshener Moisturiser with anti-ageing properties	Cleansing cream Skin tonic or freshener Night cream with anti-ageing properties Eye balm Neck cream	Face mask – anti-ageing Exfoliate

STEP-BY-STEP Facial cleanse

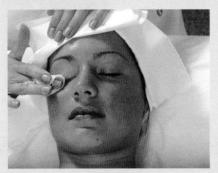

Using damp cotton wool apply eye make-up remover, working around the eye, over lid, underneath and over lashes. Work from inner to outer area. Remove with damp cotton wool.

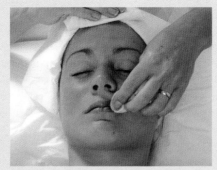

Apply a small amount of cleanser using damp cotton wool. Remove any lipstick using small circular motions.

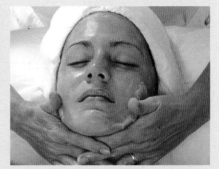

Apply dots of cleanser over the entire face. Working from the neck upwards use upward movements towards the jawline.

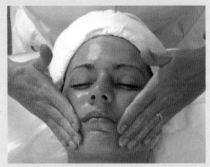

Work from the jaw line; use alternate hand movements to cover the entire cheek area.

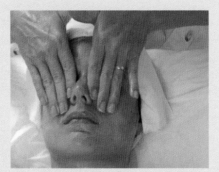

Using the index fingers, work into the nose, with small circular motions, without blocking the nostrils in! Use light pressure only.

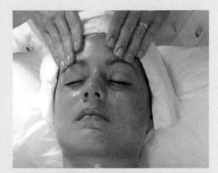

Travel over the bridge of the nose, onto the forehead working out towards the temple areas. Using index fingers, apply a little pressure to the temples.

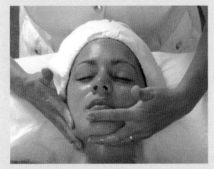

Sweep back down to the chin, working over the jaw line with alternate hand movements, to finish the cleanse routine.

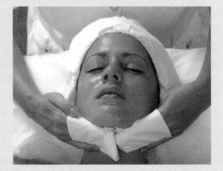

Remove cleanser, following the same routine direction as for the application of cleanser, with tissues, damp cotton wool or sponges.

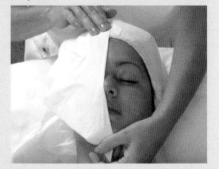

Blot the face with the tissue folded in a triangle. Pat gently with the hand, turn tissue over and repeat on the other side of the face.

For a deeper cleanse, repeat the procedure (useful if model arrives wearing make-up). Follow the routine by toning the skin and applying a thin layer of moisturiser to the face and neck.

Cleansing routine

Prepare the model for the cleansing routine by securing hair away from the face with a headband or sectioning clips. You should ensure you do not get any product in the hair. Jewellery from the neck and ears should also be removed. Clients with hard contact lenses may prefer to remove them. Remember to protect the client's clothes.

It is important your 'touch' feels confident and professional to the model. Try to ensure your hands flow smoothly over the skin and mould to the face beneath them.

Maintaining the appearance of eyebrows and lashes

The functions of eyebrows and lashes are to:

* collect perspiration
* prevent particles from falling into the eyes; lashes also protect the eyes from strong light sources
* give definition – frame the eye
* display expression – anger, surprise, disapproval, fear, etc.

The following are contra-indications to all eyebrow and lash treatments:

* cuts and abrasions to the area
* skin infection
* new scar tissue (under six months)
* bruising to the area
* swelling around the area
* eye disorders – conjunctivitis, stye, blepharitis
* prior to an eyebrow tint
* watery eyes
* positive reaction to allergy tests
* very nervous clients
* contact lenses (best removed for eyelash tinting).

(Refer to 'Skin diseases and disorders' section in Chapter 2, page 58, for further information.)

Eyebrow shaping

Eyebrow shaping is carried out to:

* remove superfluous (unwanted hair) hair from the brow area
* accentuate the natural brow shape
* accentuate the eyes
* enhance the application of make-up
* add definition to models with light or sparse eyebrows
* create a specific high fashion look.

KEY NOTE

Always check for permission from the model or artiste before you start plucking or changing the natural shape.

The make-up artist should consider the following points prior to plucking:

* the model's facial proportions
* the spacing of the eyes
* the state of the existing eyebrows
* the age of the model
* the desired final effect
* fashion.

Plucking is a suitable form of hair removal from the eyebrow area as it removes the complete hair shaft and root, delaying re-growth. It is a temporary method of hair removal, so the eyebrow shape may be changed again at a later date. It does not irritate the skin beyond a temporary erythema (reddening) and is a quick, painless procedure when carried out properly.

The correct eyebrow width and height is determined as follows:

1 Rest an orange stick against the widest part of the nose and the inner corner of the eye. The eyebrow should not extend beyond this line.

2 Move the orange stick so that it makes a diagonal line from the nose across the outer corner of the eye and up to the eyebrow. The eyebrow should not extend past this point.

3　To find where the highest point of the eyebrow should be, hold the orange stick vertically so it passes the outside edge of the iris of the eye. The point where the orange stick passes through the brow indicates the highest point.

4　The horizontal position of the eyebrow is determined by the depth of the eye, from the upper lash line to the lower lash line. The eyebrow begins one eye depth above the top lash line. The top of the eyebrow (at the arch) is another full eye width from the base of the eyebrow.

The eyebrow shape should be determined according to the facial proportions of the model.

* If the model has a high forehead, the eyebrows should have a high arch to give the illusion of reducing the depth of the forehead.

* If the model has a low forehead, the eyebrows should appear straight (low arch) to give the illusion of increasing the depth of the forehead.

* If the model has wide set eyes, extra length on the inner corner of the eyebrow (by leaving extra hairs here) can give the illusion of reducing the distance between the eyes.

* If the model has close set eyes, a few extra hairs can be removed from the inner corner of the eyebrows giving the illusion of increasing the distance between the eyes.

* If the model has a round face shape, eyebrows should be straight or angular.

* If the model has a square face shape, eyebrows should be gently rounded in shape.

* If the model has a prominent nose, eyebrows should be arched to help balance large features.

Some shapes should be avoided.

* Never pluck above the natural eyebrow line or you will end up with a hard, unnatural looking shape.

* Do not over-pluck the brow – thin brows look dated and can give a surprised expression to the wearer. Teenagers are particularly guilty of over-plucking – encourage them to visit a professional for their first brow shape. Clients who have previously over-plucked their brows should be encouraged to grow back a more natural, flattering shape. You can use an eyebrow pencil or powder to fill in the over-plucked areas. This will help the client visualise

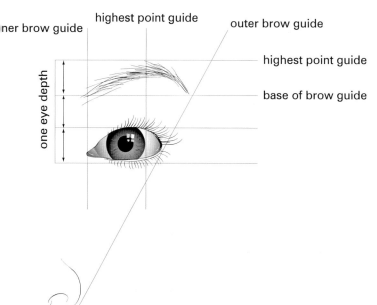

How to determine eyebrow shape

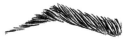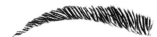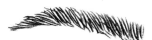

Different eyebrow shapes

a new shape to work towards. Stray hairs outside the pencilled-in area can be removed to prevent the eyebrow area becoming untidy during the period of re-growth.

* Do not shape the brow so it has a thicker 'clump' at the inner corner that suddenly becomes very thin – this doesn't suit anyone.

KEY NOTE

Clients may sometimes come to you with **unrealistic expectations**. You can only work with the eyebrow's natural shape and you may need to tactfully explain this to your client.

You can help clients visualise the shape you are proposing by using a white eye pencil to mark the hairs you intend to remove and then asking the client to look in a mirror. The whitened hairs will 'disappear', leaving the suggested brow shape for the client to view.

KEY NOTE

Make sure you have a good light source before attempting an eyebrow shape – fine, blond hairs are easily missed.

STEP-BY-STEP **Shaping eyebrows**

Equipment required

* Steriliser
* Eyebrow brush
* Tweezers
* Damp cotton wool pads
* Orange stick
* Medicated alcohol wipe
* Soothing lotion
* Tissues
* Lined bin with lid
* Mirror

1 Ensure the tweezers are sterilised prior to use. Suitable methods of sterilisation are an autoclave or sterilising solution. Refer to Chapter 2 (page 23) for further information.

2 Ensure the model is comfortable, and that her neck and head are well supported. Check for any contra-indications and secure her hair away from the face. Always try to work quickly – a complete eyebrow re-shape may take up to 30 minutes; a simple eyebrow tidy should take no longer than 15 minutes.

3 Cleanse the area (an alcoholic skin wipe is useful for this) and ensure all grease is removed from the brows.

4 Brush the brows and consult the client regarding the appropriate shape and desired effect.

5 Establish the correct position and height of the brows and apply warm cotton wool pads to the area (this will relax the pores and reduce sensation for the client).

6 Place a clean tissue on the client's forehead.

7 Use sterile tweezers and commence treatment at the bridge of the nose. Stretching the skin of the area you are working on will enable swift, painless hair removal and avoid pinching the skin. Hairs should be removed in the direction of hair growth.

8 Place removed hairs on the tissue for appropriate disposal later.

9 Continue by removing hair from beneath the brows. Treat the brows alternately and occasionally wipe them over with a soothing lotion to relieve sensation and reduce redness.

10 Check the shaping is correct and that both brows are even. Confirm client approval by showing her the result in a mirror.

11 Apply soothing lotion to cool down the area.

12 Dispose of waste in accordance with health and safety legislation.

Possible contra-actions

The following contra-actions may occur:

* erythema to the area
* blood spots (more common when removing very coarse hair)
* swelling.

Aftercare advice for eyebrow shaping

It is important to give the client aftercare advice following an eyebrow shape to avoid contra-actions and maintain the effect.

* Applying a soothing lotion such as witch hazel will help to reduce any erythema and swelling.
* Make-up should not be applied to the area for twelve hours after treatment.

* An eyebrow tidy should be carried out every four to six weeks to remove re-growth.

> **KEY NOTE**
>
> Two types of tweezers are available:
> * manual tweezers: ideal for tidying the brow and fine shaping; available with slanted or straight edges
> * automatic tweezers: ideal for removing the 'bulk' of hair quickly.

Eyebrow and eyelash tinting

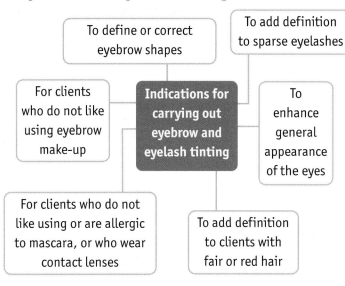

To define or correct eyebrow shapes

To add definition to sparse eyelashes

For clients who do not like using eyebrow make-up

Indications for carrying out eyebrow and eyelash tinting

To enhance general appearance of the eyes

For clients who do not like using or are allergic to mascara, or who wear contact lenses

To add definition to clients with fair or red hair

Allergy patch test

An allergy patch test should be done at least 24 hours before the treatment is performed to determine whether or not the client is hypersensitive to the tinting products. Although modern tints are mainly of vegetable origin, they are still activated by a peroxide solution and for that reason can cause irritation. Even patch testing does not completely rule out the possibility of contra-actions. Certain procedures can be followed to reduce the risk:

* carefully applying the tint
* adequately protecting the surrounding skin
* removing the tint thoroughly.

If a reaction does occur during the allergy test, no matter how minor, the treatment should not be carried out. Allergy patch tests should be carried out every six months, even on regular clients, as sensitivities and allergies can develop over a period of time. Even if a new client insists they are not allergic to tint, **never** undertake this treatment without performing a patch test first, as previous treatments may have been carried out using a different product range.

Positive reaction

The skin will become red in the area of the patch test and there will be severe itchiness and in some cases swelling of the tissue. The treatment is therefore contra-indicated.

Negative reaction

If the client experiences no discomfort or irritation then the treatment may proceed. However, should the client experience irritation or discomfort during the treatment, it should be halted and the tint removed immediately.

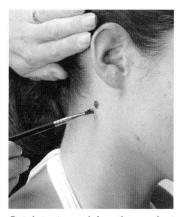

Patch test: applying the product

> **STEP-BY-STEP** **The allergy patch test**
>
> 1 Choose the area to be tested, usually behind the ear.
> 2 Cleanse the area with an alcohol skin wipe.
> 3 Mix a small quantity of tint (about 1 cm) with 3–4 drops of 10% hydrogen peroxide.
> 4 Paint the size of a one pence piece onto the area – not too thickly or it will not dry.
>
> 5 Inform the client that the tint should be left on for 24 hours unless a positive reaction occurs, in which case the tint should be removed and a soothing lotion applied to the area. If no positive reaction occurs, the tint can be washed off after 24 hours and the treatment performed.
> 6 Enter all the details onto a record card for future reference.

ALLERGY PATCH TEST – RECORD CARD

Name of model: ....

Address: ....

....

Contact tel no: ....

Date patch test given: .... /........ /........

Products used: ....

Reaction: negative / positive

Model's signature: .... Date: .... /........ /........

Make-up artist's signature: .... Date: .... /........ /........

Allergy patch test record card

The chemical reaction

A chemical reaction is responsible for the tinting process. The process begins when the tint is mixed with the hydrogen peroxide (10 per cent volume) so the mixing must not be done until the tint is required for application. The higher the percentage, the stronger the peroxide: 20 per cent volume is twice as strong as 10 per cent volume. The weakest solution is used for the eyes (10 per cent); hairdressers use up to 60 per cent volume.

STEP-BY-STEP **Tinting eyebrows**

Eyebrows take the tint colour very quickly so it should never be left on for longer than one to two minutes at any one time. It is best to layer the colour by re-applying the tint if a stronger effect is desired. Eyebrow tinting should not be carried out directly following an eyebrow shape as the skin will already be irritated and prone to further contra-actions. It is important not to leave the client during this procedure.

Equipment required

* Eye make-up remover
* Selection of tint colours
* 10 per cent volume hydrogen peroxide
* Mixing pot (non-metal)
* Spatula
* Petroleum jelly (or other suitable barrier cream)
* Orange stick or small brush for application
* Eyebrow brush
* Damp cotton wool pads
* Damp cotton buds
* Mirror

1 Ensure the model is comfortable and that the neck and head are well supported. Check for any contra-indications and secure the hair away from the face. Check an allergy patch test has been carried out.
2 Select the tint colour.
3 Thoroughly cleanse the eyebrow area, removing all traces of grease (this could act as a barrier to the tint).
4 Apply petroleum jelly around the eyebrow to protect the skin using a brush or an orange stick tipped with cotton wool.
5 Discuss, select and mix approximately 1cm of tint with three to four drops of hydrogen peroxide.
6 Brush the first eyebrow upwards and apply the tint using the tip of a clean orange stick or fine brush. Brush the tint and hair down into a natural shape. Care must be taken not to touch the skin with the tint, but you must ensure the entire hair shaft is covered.

7 Repeat on the other eyebrow.
8 Immediately after the tint has been applied to the second eyebrow, return to the first eyebrow and remove the tint with dampened cotton pads.
9 Reapply the tint if a darker colour is required.
10 Remove the tint from the second eyebrow as above. Reapply the tint if required.

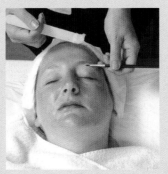

Decant barrier cream onto a spatula and paint onto the skin surrounding the eyebrow to prevent accidental staining

Hydrogen peroxide, the liquid that is added to the tint, carries an extra atom of oxygen. When it is mixed with the tint it begins to release this extra atom. This atom attaches itself to the colour molecule in the tint, which in turn swells, beginning the process known as oxidisation. It is this growth in the molecule size that allows the colour molecule to become trapped within the hair shaft, making the tint semi-permanent.

STEP-BY-STEP | Tinting eyelashes (open eye method)

Equipment required

* Eye make-up remover
* Selection of tint colours
* 10 per cent volume hydrogen peroxide
* Mixing pot (non-metal)
* Spatula
* Petroleum jelly (or other suitable barrier cream)
* Orange stick or small brush for application
* Eyebrow brush
* Damp cotton wool pads
* Damp cotton buds
* Mirror

It is important not to leave the client during this procedure.

1 Ensure the model is comfortable and that the neck and head are well supported. Check for any contra-indications and secure the hair away from the face. Check an allergy patch test has been carried out.

2 Thoroughly cleanse the eye area, removing all traces of grease (this could act as a barrier).

3 Explain the application process to the model to relieve anxiety.

4 Apply petroleum jelly around the eye area to protect the skin using an orange stick tipped with cotton wool. Make sure you take the barrier cream up to the lash roots at the top and bottom, but do not get any on the lashes themselves.

5 Shape dampened cotton pads for 'under eye' protection. Place into position under the lower lashes.

6 Discuss, select and mix 1 cm of tint with three to four drops of peroxide 10 per cent volume.

7 Instruct your client to keep the eyes open and look upwards (not directly at a light) whilst you apply the tint to the lower lashes using an orange stick or fine brush. If the client is nervous, you may prefer to omit this step (closed-eye method).

8 Ask the client to close the eyes and keep them closed from this stage onwards until instructed to open them again (otherwise the tint will seep into the eyes).

9 Apply the tint evenly over the lashes ensuring you take the tint to the roots. Make sure you do not miss the shorter hairs at each corner of the eye.

10 Cover the lashes with slightly dampened cotton pads to prevent the client from opening the eyes.

11 Leave for approximately 10-15 minutes, checking the tint development every five minutes. If the client complains of severe itching or burning, remove the tint immediately.

12 Gently remove excess tint whilst holding the eye pads (on top and under the eye) together. Remind the client to keep the eyes closed.

13 Using cotton buds, remove any remaining tint, working from the roots to the tips. Continue by sweeping a cotton bud under the lower lashes whilst the client's eyes remain closed.

14 When most of the tint has been removed ask the client to blink a few times before opening the eyes fully. Work quickly, removing any remaining tint from the lower lashes. Ensure all traces of tint are removed.

15 Give the client a fresh damp cotton pad for each eye and ask the client to gently rub the eyes – nothing will feel better!

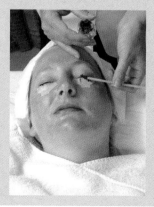

Ask client to close her eyes, and apply tint to the top lashes. Cover the eyes

Once oxidisation begins it cannot be stopped, and once it has stopped it cannot be restarted. Since the oxidisation process only lasts for approximately 15 minutes, if you were to mix a tint too soon, by the time you were ready to use it the oxidisation process would be partially complete and the tinting procedure would produce poor results.

Choosing a tint colour

You must only use tints that are specially formulated for use on the lash and brow areas. These tints are available in a small range of colours, usually, blue-black (the darkest), black, brown and grey. They can be mixed together to get further variations of tinting colour. When deciding on which colours to use the following should be considered:

* the client's natural colouring
* the colour of make-up usually worn.

Natural effects can be achieved from brown and grey colours and more dramatic results from black and blue-black. Adding a touch of black to a brown tint can give a lovely dark-brown shade that suits most people. Using brown on its own can sometimes result in a red-brown colour that does not give the same depth of colour. Mature clients tend to suit soft, natural shades. Mixing grey and brown gives a lovely shade suiting clients with white or grey hair. For a colour with more depth, a touch of black can be added to the mix. Clients with naturally dark lashes can still benefit from a lash tint as you will often find the tips of the lashes are lighter in colour – by tinting them with black or blue-black, the natural lash will appear longer in length.

Evaluation

Common problem	Troubleshooting
Roots not coloured	Take extra care to ensure the tint is applied right up to the roots of the lashes. Make sure the barrier cream has not spread onto the lashes themselves.
Corner lashes not coloured	Take extra care to ensure you 'catch' the shorter lashes at the corners of the eye.
Tint has not taken or colour is weak	Check the hydrogen peroxide and tints have not exceeded their shelf life. The tint and peroxide may have been mixed incorrectly or too soon. Check there is no grease, make-up or barrier cream on the lashes.

REMEMBER

First aid procedure should tint seep into the eye:
* Remove excess tint with dampened cotton wool
* Calm and reassure the model
* Run cool water through the eye
* Give an eye bath.

KEY NOTE

Some natural hair colours require a slightly longer development time. Red and grey hairs are resistant to the oxidisation process. In these cases, the tint needs to be left on for longer.

Possible contra-actions for tinting

The following contra-actions may occur:

* erythema
* stinging
* watery eyes
* itchy eyes
* swelling.

Aftercare and advice for tinting

Once treatment has been completed the client must be shown the results, which should of course match the client's expectations. It is also necessary to advise the client of the following.

* As a general rule, eyelash colour will last four to six weeks and eyebrow colour two to four weeks. Much depends on the colour chosen and the depth of colour achieved. Strong sunlight will fade the colour faster.

* If there is any sensitivity after the treatment then make-up and any other form of eye treatment should be avoided.

* Any client suffering any long-term discomfort, i.e. for more than a couple of hours, should see a GP and avoid similar treatments in the future.

Bleaching the brows

In most cases, the brows should be one to two shades lighter than the hair. If a client is very blond or grey, the opposite is true. If brows need lightening, you can bleach them using kits specially designed for lightening facial hair. Lightening the brows will give a soft effect and is useful when the brows dominate the face and distract from the features. They can also be bleached as a fashion statement.

Bleaching the brows is a straightforward process, but you should proceed with caution. Overusing the bleach can seriously weaken the hair, so it is best to test the effect of the bleach (and check the colour change) by removing a bit of the bleach and testing the colour and texture underneath at regular intervals during the process. When bleaching the brows, the bleach should be left on the hairs for **no** longer than **half** the time on the package recommended for other facial hair.

Because of the strong ingredients within bleach it is necessary to carry out a patch test, following the manufacturer's instructions, before proceeding with the treatment.

Aftercare and advice

Once treatment has been completed the client must be shown the results, which should of course match the client's expectations. It is also necessary to advise the model of the following.

* How long the treatment will last will depend on the area treated. As a general rule eyebrow bleaching will last two to four weeks.

* Should the model suffer any sensitivity after the treatment then make-up and any other form of eye treatment should be avoided.

* Any client suffering any long-term discomfort, i.e. for more than a couple of hours, should see a GP and avoid similar treatments in the future.

Curling the natural lash

Curling the lashes opens up the eye area, making them look larger. Some clients have naturally curly lashes and all that is needed is to sweep the lashes upwards from underneath with the mascara

---

STEP-BY-STEP **Bleaching eyebrows**

Equipment required

* Spatula
* Palette
* Facial bleach
* Damp cotton buds
* Toner
* Moisturiser

It is important not to leave the client during this procedure.

1 Check for contra-indications. Ensure a patch test has been carried out.
2 Clean the area.
3 Mix the bleach following the manufacturer's instructions carefully.
4 Apply the bleach to both brows, working quickly and carefully. Do not forget to bleach the finer hairs around the eyebrows or these will end up looking more obvious.
5 Every few moments check the effect of the bleach and colour change.
6 When the desired effect is attained, remove the bleach thoroughly using damp cotton pads.
7 Apply a mild toner and moisturiser (this will help re-condition the hair).

applicator to emphasise and lift the curl. Some mascaras also claim to have their own 'curling' properties.

When models have long but straight lashes, these may be curled with eyelash curlers or permanently curled with a chemical process called 'eyelash perming'.

Using eyelash curlers

* The client is asked to look straight ahead.
* The eyelash curlers are opened and the rubber-covered blades placed over the lashes. The curlers are squeezed together and held for three to five seconds. Heated eyelash curlers are also available – follow the manufacturer's instructions if these are your choice.
* Care must be taken not to pinch the skin.
* Use mascara **afterwards** to 'set in' the curl. Do not use mascara before curling the eyelashes or you may cause the lashes to break off.

False lashes

There are two types of false lashes to choose from – strip and individual (also known as semi-permanent). Each creates a different look. Strip lashes add immediate density to the whole lash area. Individual lashes are best when you want to fill in sparse areas and for creating a more natural look.

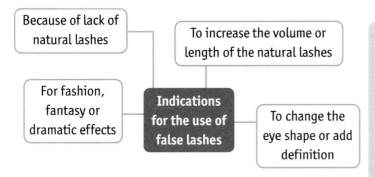

The make-up artist should consider the following points when applying false lashes:

* colour of lashes
* length of lashes
* density of lashes.

These all depend on the desired effect. In addition, the make-up artist should consider:

* the time available for application (strip lashes take approximately ten minutes to apply; individual lashes take up to 30 minutes depending on how many are applied).
* maintenance (strip lashes need to be applied daily; individual lashes can last a couple of weeks if aftercare advice is followed).

Eye shape	False lash application
Close set eyes	Feathery lashes, longer at the top and bottom outer corners.
Downward slanting eyes	Medium length lashes on upper lids, longer and curled upwards at the outer corners, none on the lower lash.
Wide set eyes	Natural medium lashes uneven in length.
Deep set eyes	Extra fine lashes with upturned tips. Lower lashes should also be added.
Small eyes	Longer, individual lashes at outer corners.

Correct false lash application for eye shapes

Allergy patch test for adhesive

This should be done at least 24 hours before the treatment is performed to determine whether or not the client is hypersensitive to the adhesive. Follow the same procedure as allergy patch testing for tinting products (see page 137).

STEP-BY-STEP **Applying strip lashes**

Strip lashes are synthetic fibres attached to a fine strip that runs the full length of the eye. They are attached to the base of the eyelid with special adhesive (usually latex-based). Available in a wide range of styles, strip lashes are suitable for a number of uses from enhancing the eye to dramatic, fantasy effects. Strip lashes are usually applied **after** make-up and will only last a day.

Equipment required

* Tweezers
* Tissues
* Adhesive
* Orange stick
* Cotton wool
* Palette
* False lashes
* Eyelash brush

1 Check the length of the false lashes against the client's eyelid. If the strip is too long it should be trimmed from the outside corner (usually lashes are longer in length here).

2 Soak the lashes in warm water for three to four minutes to remove the sizing that makes them stiff (optional).

3 Flex the base lightly to shape the lash to the contour of the client's eye.

4 Place a small amount of adhesive on the palette.

5 Apply the adhesive in a fine strip to the base of the false lashes with an orange stick. Leave for a minute to go tacky.

6 Ask the client to keep the eyes in a semi-closed position. Do not allow the client to close the eyes completely or the upper lid may become stuck to the lower lid.

7 Hold the false lashes firmly with tweezers. Place them gently in position on the eyelid immediately against the roots of the natural lashes in the centre of the eye.

8 Press gently but firmly against the width of the eye making sure the lashes are firmly fixed at the corners.

9 Allow the lashes to 'set' for five minutes. Any visible adhesive will dry clear.

10 Gently curl both natural and false lashes together and apply eyeliner to disguise any visible edges.

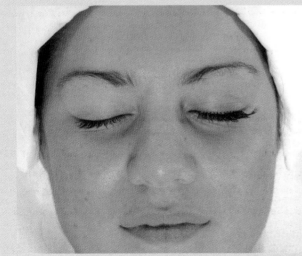

Strip false lashes applied to the eye on the right

KEY NOTE

If you need to trim the lashes, use a small pair of scissors to cut irregularly at the tips. This will create a more natural look than cutting in a straight line.

Removal of strip lashes

Special adhesive removers or solvents are used to dissolve the glue, freeing the lash from the skin. Alternatively, an oily eye make-up remover will also remove false lashes.

1 With the client in an upright position with the eyes closed, apply the solvent to the strip of the lash using a cotton bud in a rolling action.

2 The eyelid must be supported when removing the lashes to prevent stretching the skin.

3 Wait a few moments then gently peel back the lash from the outer corner to the inner corner.

4 Any adhesive left on the lashes can be gently lifted off.

5 Wash the lashes in clear warm water or with a gentle eye make-up remover.

Maintenance of strip lashes

Strip lashes can only be re-used on the same client. If they are to be re-used you will need to maintain the lashes between applications. Once they have been removed from the client, they will need cleaning in warm, soapy water. Any remaining glue can be peeled away from the strip. When the lashes are clean, you will need to re-curl them.

1 Wrap a tissue once around an even barrelled object such as a pencil.

2 Place the clean false lashes side by side on a tissue ensuring the bases of the lashes are straight.

3 Roll the object onto and across the tissue so that the lashes are evenly curled.

4 Secure the lashes with cotton or an elastic band and leave them to dry.

5 Once dry, you can store the lashes in the original container. It may be useful to mark this with the client's name.

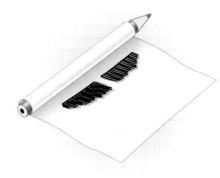

A simple way to restore the shape of strip lashes

STEP-BY-STEP Applying individual lashes

Also called semi-permanent lashes, these lashes are applied to the base of the client's own eyelashes rather than to the skin. Individual lashes come in three lengths: short, medium and long. The most natural looking effect is achieved by using a combination of two to three lengths. It is advisable to use the short lengths at the inner corner of the eye to achieve a more natural result. When applied correctly the lashes will stay on for a couple of weeks (a stronger type of glue is used than for strip lashes). They are usually applied prior to make-up. A full set of lashes across the top lash line will take between seven and eleven lashes. It is best to start from the outer corner and work inwards.

Applying individual false lashes

Equipment required

* Tweezers
* Tissues
* Adhesive
* Orange stick
* Cotton wool
* Palette
* False lashes
* Eyelash brush

1 With a clean eyelash brush, brush the upper lashes to separate them.
2 When applying lashes to the upper lid, work from behind the model, asking her or him to look slightly downwards. When applying lashes to the lower lid, work from the front of the client.
3 Place a small amount of adhesive on to the palette.
4 Pick up an individual lash with tweezers about half way down its length and dip it into the adhesive, so a small amount is on the root.
5 Using tweezers, place this on top of the root of the natural lash as close to the lid as possible and hold for a second. On the top lash line, lashes should curl upwards; on the bottom lash line, lashes should curl downwards. Work across the lid, ensuring the tips of the lashes overlap slightly.
6 After completing both eyes, check to see if they match.

Removal of individual lashes

1 With the client sitting upright, place a tissue under the lower lashes. The eyes must be closed.
2 Using an eyeliner brush, brush adhesive solvent over the base of the false lashes.
3 Wait a few seconds and the lash should easily come free.
4 Repeat if necessary.
5 Never attempt to pull the lashes off, as the natural lashes will be removed as well.

If adhesive solvent enters the eye, do not panic, but rinse immediately with cool water and follow with an eye bath.

Aftercare and advice for false lash application

You should instruct the client:

* not to rub the eyes
* not to pull at the lashes
* not to use oil-based cleanser or eye make-up remover as this will dissolve the glue
* not to use mascara on false lashes

Advise the client of the procedure to follow when the lashes need to be removed.

Maintaining the appearance of the hands

As a make-up artist you may occasionally be asked to tidy up the nails of a model and apply colour. In general, though, a manicurist will be employed if anything more than a quick tidy up is required. The basic manicure skills of shaping the nails and applying polish are useful, and these are covered briefly in the next section. Remember to check for any contra-indications.

KEY NOTE

Do not use a sawing action when filing as it can cause the nail to split. The nail plate is made up of several layers. Bevelling the nail edge 'holds' these layers together, prevents splitting and gives the nail a smooth edge.

Tips for nail painting

* Hold the polish in the palm of the non-working hand. With the same hand, use your thumb and index finger to hold the sides of the nail being painted, gently pulling the skin away from the nail plate.

* With your working hand, load one side of the brush with polish and apply to the nail bed. Begin each stroke just short of the cuticle, and re-load your brush at the end of each stroke.

STEP-BY-STEP | **Shaping the nails**

Equipment required

* Sterilised nail scissors or clippers   * Emery board

Discuss with your model the desired nail shape.

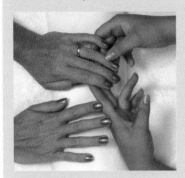

1 During the consultation discuss your client's needs, preferred shape of nails, and type of polish required. Providing there are no contra-indications present you are ready to begin.

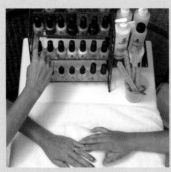

2 As your nail bar has all equipment and stock ready to begin treatment, ask the client to pick her choice of varnish – dark, plain, frosted or French manicure.

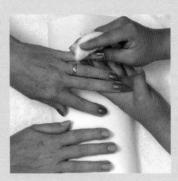

3 Remove the old varnish and check the nails for ridges and possible problems as you go.

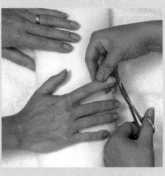

4 Cut the nails into shape if required, using sterilised scissors. Nail clippings need to be caught in a tissue and disposed of.

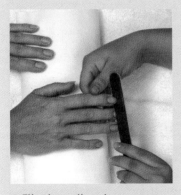

5 File the nails using an emery board working outside in, one way, one side then the other – avoid using a 'sawing' action. (There are different thicknesses of emery board.)

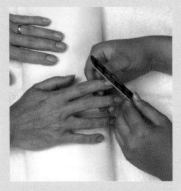

6 Bevelling seals the free edge layers to prevent water loss and mechanical damage.

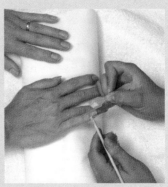

7 Using an orange stick, decant and apply cuticle cream around the cuticles.

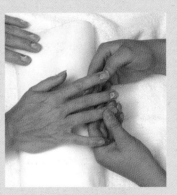

8 Gently massage the cream into the cuticles.

* Try to avoid flooding the sides and cuticles.

* Mistakes can be tidied up by dipping a clean orange stick into some nail polish remover and rubbing over areas you wish to remove. Do not use cotton buds as the fibres will stick to the damp polish and ruin the final effect.

* The nails can be allowed to dry naturally or a 'quick drying' product can be applied over the top coat to speed up the process.

KEY NOTE

It is a good idea to practise painting nails with red polish – this will show any mistakes and encourage you to paint meticulously.

French polish

A French polish comprises a white and transparent pink or beige polish and gives a very natural finish. French polish can be applied in a number of different ways. The following is one suggestion.

1 Apply a base coat.
2 Apply white polish to the tip of the nails.
3 Apply pink or beige polish over the entire nail.
4 Repeat the above if required.
5 Apply a clear top coat.

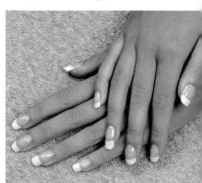

The finished results of a French polish

Knowledge Check

1 What are the reasons for cleansing, toning and moisturising?

2 What type of cleanser would you choose for the following skin types: oily, mature, oil dry, sensitive?

3 What toner would you choose for an oily skin type?

4 When would it be appropriate to use barrier cream in a make-up session?

5 How would you decide on how to reshape the eyebrows of a model?

6 What would you do to prepare the brows for treatment?

7 What contra-actions may occur during or following shaping the brow?

8 How can you avoid pinching the skin?

9 What can you apply as aftercare to an eyebrow shape and why is it advised?

10 What is the chemical reaction called that takes place during the tinting process?

11 Briefly describe how to carry out an allergy patch test.

12 What colour eyebrow tint would you use on a mature client with white hair?

13 Approximately how many individual lashes would it take to cover the entire upper lid?

14 What are individual lashes also called?

15 What are the lashes that are attached to the skin of the eyelid called?

16 What type of cleanser or eye make-up remover will dissolve eyelash glue?

17 What should be applied to the eyelashes to remove individual eyelashes?

18 What type of false lashes can be used again on the same client?

19 Should eye make-up be applied before or after the application of strip lashes?

20 Why is it best to bevel the nail plate when filing?

Designing and creating fashion and photographic images

Contemporary fashion photography is more than simply presenting clothes, but is also a platform from which personal styling can be contextualised within current cultural and social themes. To be an image-maker in this environment, the make-up artist not only requires excellent application skills but also a clear understanding of contemporary lifestyles.

Aim and objectives

Aim of this chapter: to provide you with an understanding of the requirements of fashion, photographic and straight beauty make-up for screen work.

You should achieve the following **objectives:**

* Evaluate the concepts of beauty and fashion
* Discuss the function of pre-bases and foundations
* List the types of foundation available and evaluate how to choose the most appropriate type
* Explain why make-up needs to settle on the skin and why it occasionally changes colour
* List the colour correction products for different skin problems
* List the types and function of powder available and discuss the problems associated with 'ghosting' or 'flash back'
* Discuss the principles of facial proportion and carry out contouring techniques to achieve balance in the face
* List the types and function of blushers and discuss the different effects produced by varying their placement on the face

* Apply make-up to the eyebrow
* List the types of eye make-up available, including textures and finishes, and contour various eye shapes
* List types of lip colour, including textures and finishes, and contour various lip shapes
* Carry out a full make-up application using pre-bases, foundations, concealers, contouring techniques, powder, blushers, eyebrow and eye make-up, lipsticks
* Create various make-up designs
* Carry out a straight, corrective make-up on a male model
* Discuss basic design principles, and develop and create a design for a photographic shoot
* Evaluate your work.

What is beauty and fashion?

Images of beauty and fashion are everywhere. In the developed world, the preoccupation with the notion of beauty is especially prevalent and the beauty and fashion business, despite three decades of feminism, is a multi-million pound a year business. It is hard these days to escape from images of beautiful women and handsome men: they grace the pages of glossy magazines, television, advertisements and the internet. However, the ideal notion of beauty changes over time and continents and is therefore far from fixed.

HANDS ON

Botticelli's Venus is perhaps one of the earliest representations of the ideal female form (1490). Leonardo da Vinci's *Mona Lisa*, painted in the sixteenth century, displays the characteristics associated with beauty at this time – but how would she fare by today's standards?

A Mangbettu woman's head is artificially moulded to a cone shape – babies have their heads tightly bandaged to produce this head shape in adulthood.

Do Pamela Anderson Lee and Jordan represent the Western notion of beauty in the early twenty-first century?

Use magazines, the internet and other reference sources to compile images of beauty from different periods in history and different cultures. Do they have anything in common? Are you surprised by anything you've discovered?

This changing view of the notion of ideal beauty is what can be defined as 'fashion'. Fashion can be thought of as communicating personal taste, along with cultural and social ideas, by using the appearance of the body. We use it to communicate messages about social status, sexual attractiveness and cultural aspirations to others, and are often willing to endure personal suffering to achieve the ultimate goal of beauty. A detailed historical overview of fashion is given in Chapter 15.

Despite the ever-changing concept of fashion, reflecting personal taste and cultural influences, there are underlying principles that affect our perception of beauty. These principles transcend time, gender and racial differences. It has been proved that our judgement of beauty is affected by:

* evolutionary biological responses, for example health, procreation, protection
* symmetry and proportion.

Faces are generally considered more beautiful by both men and other women if they possess the following qualities.

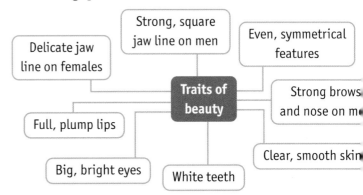

Evolutionary biology factors are related to our perception of beauty.

* Scientists have suggested that symmetrical bodies are an indication of healthy genes and therefore our attraction to symmetrical faces is an instinctive response to finding a healthy mate to procreate with, increasing our chances of having healthy offspring.

* Clear eyes and unblemished skin are indications of health and increase our attractiveness to others.

* Babies' features are designed to bring out a nurturing and protecting instinct in us, ensuring the survival of the human race. Big eyes, round cheeks, high forehead, small nose and rosebud lips are typical characteristics of a baby. When the female adult face retains an essence of these traits into adulthood, psychologists have suggested that it will evoke a similar response from the male.

Using make-up to enhance a person's appearance

The classical ideals of symmetry and proportion were discussed on page 80; proportion and symmetry in contouring make-up are covered on page 157.

It is important that the make-up artist understands the theory of what makes a face appear beautiful. Armed with this knowledge the make-up artist can help to exaggerate or add the features and traits that will make an individual be perceived as more attractive using make-up application techniques:

* foundation provides a clear, unblemished skin
* eyeliner, eye shadow and mascara help to make the eyes look larger
* gloss and lipstick create fuller looking lips.

This is sometimes taken to extremes, particularly in the glamour industry where models are transformed with cosmetics techniques (often using surgery along with make-up application) that overtly exaggerate the features associated with sexuality: look at images of Pamela Lee Anderson and Jordan for examples of this.

Cosmetic and fashion make-up application may be applied for a number of reasons:

* to portray an image
* to increase personal confidence
* to improve appearance
* to make a statement.

There is no better example of how make-up and hairstyling can be used to successfully change a person's image than Madonna. She has become an expert in using her appearance to maintain her iconic position throughout her career. Her various personas have included a Marilyn Monroe look-alike, a dominatrix, a geisha and a spiritual earth mother. Perhaps these frequent changes have helped maintain Madonna's longevity in show business by enhancing her visual appeal and preventing public boredom.

It is generally the role of the cosmetic, fashion or photographic make-up artist to employ make-up design and application techniques to improve a person's appearance with the aim of making them look as beautiful as possible. However, for high fashion photographs or shows, the portrayal of a particular image or cultural statement may be more important than achieving a picture of 'idealised beauty'. We will now look at the various stages of a cosmetic, fashion or photographic make-up. The following application techniques also apply to straight beauty make-ups for television and film.

Pre-base and under-base products

These products are applied to a cleansed skin prior to the application of foundation. Some brands can be used in conjunction with moisturiser, particularly on a drier skin type, whilst others are recommended for use directly on a 'naked' skin. In general, they will have one or more of the following functions:

Provide a base on which the rest of the make-up can be built

Provide protection from UVA and UVB rays

Some are iridescent giving the skin a shimmery, light-reflecting surface

Functions of pre-base products

Pre-bases can be mixed with the foundation to create a sheer finish

Brighten and smooth the skin tone

Mattify the skin and prevent oily breakthroughs

Increase the longevity of the make-up application

Temporarily 'lift and tighten' a mature skin

Tinted pre-base products colour-correct skin tones

Foundations

A smooth, healthy-looking and even-toned skin is the essential canvas required for fashion and photographic make-up. Foundations are applied to achieve this whilst providing protection for the skin from the environment. Numerous types of foundation are available on the market. When choosing a foundation the following considerations should be taken into account:

* colour
* texture
* coverage.

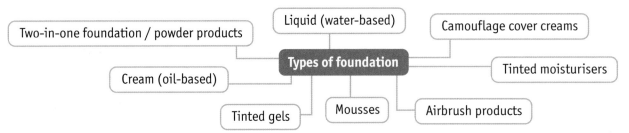

Foundation type	Skin type	Texture and coverage	Ingredients	Notes
Liquid (oil in water)	Suitable for normal and combination skins. Oil-free, medicated or matt foundations are available for oily or greasy skins.	Light, fine coverage, normally with a semi-matt finish, providing excellent 'flesh impact' (skin looks natural and healthy in pictures or on the screen).	Mineral oil, ceresin wax, pigment, titanium dioxide.	Shorter working time on skin than cream foundations.
Cream (water in oil)	Suitable for most skin types, but give dry skins extra moisture and nourishment.	Medium coverage. Thick with a glossy texture, providing good 'flesh impact'.	Same as liquid but has a higher oil content.	Available in 'stick' or 'compact' form. Long working time on the skin, excellent colour stability and very durable when applied and set properly.
Two-in-one foundation and powder products	Particularly suitable for oily skins because of the high powder content. Also a good choice for very dark skin tones.	Medium to heavy coverage with a drier texture, providing a matt finish.	Small amount of mineral oil, high content of powder products, e.g. talc and kaolin, pigments.	Essentially a form of traditional cake make-up. Very durable on the skin.
Tinted gels	Gels are transparent and are particularly suitable for young unblemished skins or men, which need only the lightest cover. Gels can cause dryness on sensitive skins.	Provides very light, sheer cover.	Pigments in a water-based gel.	Useful for adding enhancement and gleam to a tanned skin. Short working time, and therefore care should be taken to avoid a streaky application.

Foundation type	Skin type	Texture and coverage	Ingredients	Notes
Tinted moisturisers	Suitable for all skin types, but particularly those that require very little coverage, e.g. unblemished, clear skin.	Light coverage providing a very sheer, natural finish.	Same as moisturisers (oil and water; humectants, etc.) with added pigments.	Particularly useful for men and children when a very natural effect is required.
Mousses	Suitable for all skin types, but particularly those that require little coverage.	Light coverage providing a very sheer, natural finish.	Either oil or water based, with same ingredients as cream or liquid foundations.	Supplied in an aerosol can, allowing the product to be dispensed as a fine foam, which is easily blended onto the skin.
Airbrush products	Suitable for all skin types.	Coverage depends on application technique, but can be sheer or applied to provide more coverage. Available in a variety of finishes.	Pigments dispersed in either water, alcohol or polymers (plastics). For beauty make-ups, water-based products are usually preferred.	Very liquid so products can be applied with an airbrush.
Camouflage cover creams	Suitable for all skin types, but particularly those that require heavy coverage.	Provide excellent, opaque coverage, without the look of a heavy application.	High pigment content.	Water-resistant when set properly. Excellent for use on transvestites when beard-shadow cover is required.

KEY NOTE

Finishes of foundations range from matt, semi-matt, dewy to shimmery. New technology includes the use of light-reflecting ingredients, which claim to create a smooth, vibrant surface. Although they can look very attractive to the eye, shimmery finishes can create problems with lighting on screen and photographs, so should be avoided.

Application of foundation

Choosing a colour

For street make-ups, still photos and most naturally lit screen make-ups it is best to match the foundation to the model's natural skin tone. All skin tones tend to be enhanced by the application of a yellow rather than pink-toned foundation colour (see basic colour theory in Chapter 5, page 70). There are three basic skin colours, made up from tints and shades of quaternary colour mixes. These tints and shades make up various skin tones ranging from the lightest to the darkest.

Most cosmetic companies produce a wide variety of colours within their foundation ranges, meeting the needs of most skin tones. However, as professional make-up artists will not be able to carry the full

Quaternary colour mix	Basic skin colour	Tints	Shades
Orange and violet	russet brown (red toned)	ruddy complexions, rose	russet, red-brown, cinnamon
Orange and green	sallow brown (yellow toned)	ivory, alabaster, cream	golden, bronze, honey, sand
Green and violet	olive brown (blue toned)	olive, beige	the darkest skin tones

colour range in their kit, they will often select a number of key foundation colours that when mixed will cover the full spectrum of skin tones.

Choosing the wrong colour can be disastrous, leaving the skin looking unnatural. Light skin tones may look washed out or exhibit the classic 'tide-mark' if a shade is chosen that is too dark. Darker skin tones may look grey and dull.

KEY NOTE

Occasionally in television and film, the correct shade of foundation is chosen not for an exact skin tone match but to balance or correct the skin colour on camera according to screen requirements. However, the make-up artist must ensure the finished effect still appears natural to the audience. In these cases, the foundation must be carried to slightly below the costume line at the neckline or décolletage and should include the shoulders, arms and hands if on show.

Applying foundation

When choosing a foundation colour, the natural skin tones should be viewed after **a cleanse** when the model has no make-up on the face. This will allow you to make an accurate assessment of the natural colouring.

↓

An easy way to select foundation colour is to hold a few shades (in their containers) near the skin and select the one that is closest in colour to the model's skin. Test the foundation colour on the model's jaw line. If colour is correct, once lightly blended the foundation should become invisible to the eye.

↓

It is sometimes necessary to mix two or more foundations together to get the correct shade. For example, if one shade is too light and another too dark, then two shades can be blended together to achieve the desired shade. If the shade is too warm a cooler tone can be added, etc.

↓

Many make-up artists will use the back of their hand to mix colours. However, it is more hygienic to blend the foundation on a small clean palette with a spatula. This custom-blended foundation should be kept until the make-up is completed in case additional foundation is required during the rest of the make-up application or for maintenance during the shoot.

↓

To apply foundation, you will use a slightly damp, disposable, synthetic or natural sponge (wet a sponge and wring it out in a tissue to remove excess moisture), a foundation brush or sanitised fingers (with the model's permission).

↓

Apply carefully, with one stroke overlapping the other to produce a smooth, even application. Blend the foundation towards the edges of the face and under the jaw line (not forgetting under the chin), continuing down the neck if required. Using a brush will allow easier access to small areas, e.g. around the eye socket and nostrils. Blend gently and carefully, especially around the hairline, eyes, nose and mouth. Do not drag or rub at the skin. Always work to the same routine, e.g. centre, forehead, sides and neck, finishing with a downward stroke over areas covered with fine, downy hair. Do not forget to cover the ears (which often look red on camera), eyelids and the outer edge of the lips, as this will help to keep eye shadow and lipstick in place.

↓

On mature skins where wrinkles are present, it is useful to use your sanitised fingertips in a tapping motion over the foundation application. This helps to prevent the make-up from settling in the wrinkles and accentuating them. It is important to ask the model for permission before touching the skin with your fingertips – some models may object.

↓

If any minor imperfections or discolouration show through, apply another light covering of foundation to these areas (a brush and finger-tapping motion is useful for this). The finished application should always be light, even and perfectly blended. Never apply a thick layer of foundation to cover up skin problems, but use the corrective techniques discussed in the next section.

Foundation does not have to be applied over the entire face, but can be applied only to the areas that require coverage, leaving the rest of the skin with a simple application of moisturiser or pre-base product.

Allowing the make-up to settle

Make-up should be left to settle on the skin for at least 20 before it is photographed. This allows the application to 'become one' with the skin, improving 'flesh impact' on camera. During this time, the oils in the make-up will warm and merge with the oils of the skin, softening and further blending the application, and optimising the final effect.

Colour change

Sometimes you may notice that as you allow the colour to settle, it actually changes colour. The oils in the make-up react to the skin's acidity causing this reaction. It is most common in models with an oily skin type. These days most products are likely to be colour stable, as any colour shift will have already taken place during its manufacture. However, anything that affects the skin by increasing its acidity, such as drinking alcohol, perspiring and applying medicated skin products, will increase the likelihood of a colour change.

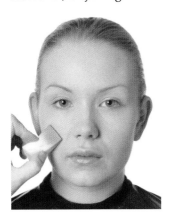

Application of foundation

Concealers

Sometimes foundation is enough to cover minor under-eye circles and other skin imperfections. However, if the circles are dark and the imperfections more apparent, because foundation tends to be semi-translucent it provides insufficient coverage. This is where concealers will give better results.

Concealers are solid, thick preparations giving excellent coverage, and are available in pencil, stick or compact form. They can be applied before or after foundation to cover blemishes, scars, uneven pigmentation and shadows. Various shades are available and they should be used with discretion as a little goes a long way. Concealer should not feel greasy (which would tend to slide over the skin) or have a chalky consistency (which would cause the make-up to 'cake' on the skin), but should be smooth to the touch. Many formulations now contain light-reflecting ingredients that enhance their effect on the skin. Many make-up artists prefer to use camouflage cover creams, such as Dermacolour or Veil, to conceal with. These possess excellent coverage qualities being almost opaque, and are available in a wide colour range.

Two shades of concealer are useful for general make-up application.

Shade 1

A shade should be chosen that matches the colour of the foundation and is used to conceal general skin imperfections.

Shade 2 – Light skin tones

A shade slightly lighter (one to two shades) than the foundation can be used to hide unwanted shadows. This is useful for hiding dark shadows around the eye, at the corners of the mouth, around the nostrils, etc. This lighter shade of concealer should not contain too much white as this can unattractively 'bloom' on film or screen. Yellow-toned concealers counteract purplish or bluish areas of shadow.

Shade 2 – Dark skin tones

For dark skin tones, use an orange-toned concealer to lift and disguise natural areas of dark shadow or hyper-pigmentation. The darker the skin tone, the more orange the concealer can appear. For lighter shades of dark skin tones, a more subtle effect can be created by mixing an orange concealer with Shade 1 (in a ratio of approximately 50/50).

Use of colour corrective concealers and bases

In addition to the standard two shades of concealers that you will require for a corrective make-up, you may also need to use colour corrective products to correct discolouration in the skin tone. These products are available in stick, compact or fluid form, but should be used with caution – using too much can make your client look ill. They can be used on their own, under the foundation, or mixed with the foundation or standard concealer shade for a more subtle effect.

Problem	Colour corrective concealer
Redness in the skin tone, blotches	Green
A dull, sallow complexion	Lilac
Blue discolouration, e.g. heavy beardline, shadows on a dark skin tone	Orange

KEY NOTE

Colour correction is based on complementary colour theory (refer back to Chapter 5, page 70). When complementary colours are overlaid, they neutralise each other.

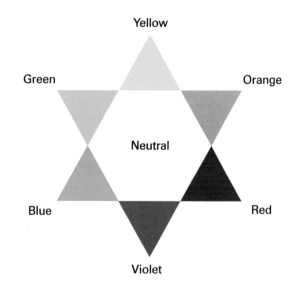

The colour star

Applying concealers

It is important to study the model with a critical eye, using your mirror to help you. Try to 'remove' anything that looks unattractive or detracts from the perfect canvas on which you will create your make-up. Using the foundation on the palette as your colour guide, mix concealing Shade 1. As with foundations, you may have to mix more than one colour to achieve the desired result. Once you are happy you have created an exact match to the foundation, use half the mixture to create Shade 2, adding further colour (avoid white) to lighten the mixture (by one to two shades) for light skins, or adding an orange tone for darker skins.

Concealers are generally applied using a small brush that allows you accurate control over its placement. Only a small amount is required as a little goes a long way. The application is then blended with a clean brush until its edges are completely blended with the foundation. (If you prefer to apply concealer prior to foundation, the foundation can by stippled lightly over the area with a sponge to aid blending). To set the concealer, dust on a layer of powder. Keep it light if working around the eye area and brush away any excess. A touch more concealer can now be added if required for very dark circles or stubborn blemishes.

KEY NOTE

Setting the concealer with powder between applications is very important; otherwise the layers of colour will slide and merge into one thick coating.

Concealing common problems

Dark circles under the eyes

Apply concealer one to two shades lighter than the foundation (or orange-toned on darker skins) on the area with a small brush. Be careful to apply the lighter shade only to the shadowed area, otherwise you may form an eye-bag! The darkest areas on most people tend to be on and under the inner corner of the eye.

Shadows in the outside corners of the eyes

Concealing these shadows can help to 'lift' the eyes. Application is as for dark circles.

Uneven pigmentation under the lower lashes and on the eyelids

Many people have red or purple pigmentation in this area, making the eyes look tired. Using a concealer the same shade as the foundation can hide it. (Using a lighter shade would form an eye bag under the lid and make the eyelids look heavy).

Blotchy skin

Areas of the skin that are redder than normal can be toned down to a neutral colour by the careful application of green concealer or a green-tinted pre-base before the application of foundation. Alternatively, a little green concealer can be mixed with a concealer the same colour as the foundation for a more subtle effect, and applied before or after the foundation.

Small blemishes and facial marks

These can be hidden with the application of a little concealer the same colour as the foundation. Blemishes that have a red appearance can be neutralised by adding a little green to the mix.

Shadows at the corners of the mouth

These can be lightened using concealer one to two shades lighter than the foundation (or orange-toned), helping to lift a down turned mouth.

Heavy beard line on a man

Using an orange-toned concealer prior to the application of foundation can reduce a beard line.

Freckles (ephelides)

These are not generally considered a problem. If you are working on a model with freckles she or he has probably been cast because of them. However, if you are asked to minimise the appearance of freckles, you will need to opt for a foundation with a medium to heavy coverage and choose a colour that is slightly darker than the natural skin tone and slightly lighter than the freckles themselves.

> **KEY NOTE**
>
> As a make-up artist you cannot get rid of eye bags – a good photographer will achieve this with the use of clever lighting. Do not attempt to shade the eye bag, as this will simply draw more attention to it or to shadow under the eye.

Powder

Powder should feel silky to the touch and have a very light, fine consistency. Ingredients may include zinc oxide or titanium oxide, talc and pigments (if tinted). Many products now contain light-reflecting ingredients that help to minimise imperfections on the skin's surface, brightening the skin tone.

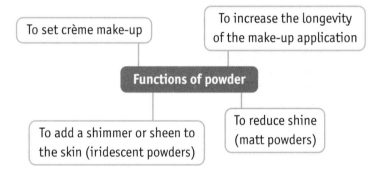

Types of powder

There are two main types of powder:

* loose (the preferred option of professional make-up artists)
* compact or pressed (useful for maintaining make-up on set, when a loose powder may be impractical).

These are available as follows.

* **Translucent powder** allows the colour of the foundation to show through. However, even translucent powders vary in colour tints and sometimes create undesirable effects to the eye and camera. A yellow-toned powder (or orange-toned for darker skin tones) is nearly always the

preferable option for photographic work. Pure yellow or orange powder can also be used directly under the eyes to help lift dark shadows.

* **Colourless powder** is truly without pigment and therefore looks white in its container, but colourless on the skin. It will therefore not create any changes to the foundation colour. It is usually the preferred option for screen work.

* **Tinted powders** should match the colour of the foundation exactly.

* **Bronzing powder** lightly used can give a healthy, sun-kissed glow to the skin. This is also useful for contouring the face.

* **Iridescent powder** creates a shimmery complexion. Use with caution as it can also accentuate unevenness in skin texture such as scarring, wrinkles and blemishes. It is useful as a highlighter when contouring the face.

Titanium dioxide and 'ghosting' or 'flash back'

Many products contain titanium dioxide and iron oxides. They are used in powders to reflect UV light and prevent photosensitive reactions. These ingredients have two disadvantages.

When photographed (particularly when using flash light), these ingredients can cause 'whitening' and a pale, white bloom may be visible on the skin in the photographic image, known in the trade as 'flash back' or 'ghosting'. If you know your work may be photographed, it is important to use products free of these ingredients.

When used on dark skin tones these ingredients can give a greyness to the area.

Application of powder

1 Place a small amount of powder into a tissue.
2 Using a clean velour powder puff or firm synthetic make-up wedge, press lightly onto the base with a rocking motion covering the entire face.

3 Remove excess powder with a powder brush using light strokes – first brush upwards to lift the hairs and remove trapped particles, then brush downwards to flatten facial hairs. Check hairline and eyebrows.
4 If the skin is mature, gently stretch the surface as you apply the powder to ensure it reaches into the creases.
5 To restore a natural sheen to the skin, lightly mist with water, using a fine spray or atomiser.
6 Blot any excess moisture with a tissue.

KEY NOTE

Powder application should be kept especially light over wrinkled areas as well as over hairier areas such as the sides of the face, upper lip, eyebrows and hairline.

Contouring make-up

Facial proportions

What is considered as the ultimate in beauty, or the perfect face, varies over time and continents. However, an oval-shaped face that is symmetrical with evenly spaced features is considered the most 'balanced' face. Contouring techniques are employed by the make-up artist to balance the model's face shape and features to enhance his or her appearance on camera.

On the next page is a list of standard facial proportions found in the 'balanced' white face. Measurements will vary in black and Asian faces (see Chapter 14, page 326).

For many years now, the professional make-up artist has referred to a number of basic face shapes as a way of categorising facial proportions. However, in reality a model's face is unlikely to 'fit' a specified face shape exactly and it is best not to take the named shapes too literally. When did you last see a person with a truly square face? It is much more appropriate to use the face shapes detailed below as a guideline whilst looking upon your model as an individual with unique proportions and contouring requirements.

Feature	Ideals found in the 'balanced' white face
Length of face	1.5 times the width
Widest part of face	Two thirds of length
Width across jaw bone	Slightly less than width across cheekbones
Width of mouth	Corners should lie between inner edges of the eyes' iris
Placement of eyes	Eyes are halfway between the top of the head and the chin
Length of nose	The bottom of the nose is halfway between the eyes and the chin
Distance between eyes	One eye width apart
Chin in profile	Taking a straight line from the tip of the nose to the chin, the lips should just touch this line

The technique of contouring

Contouring make-up means using the art of chiaroscuro (painting with light and shade) to create the illusion of reshaping and sculpting the face and features. It is based on the principle that light comes forward and shade recedes.

When applying shadows and highlights to the skin it is important to ensure there is a significant tonal difference between them and the base colour, otherwise they will be lost. You can test this by applying some of the shadow and highlight colour, blending them lightly, then stepping back and squinting at the tones (use your mirror if your workstation has one). If they fade into the base colour you will need to strengthen them; if they look very harsh you may need to reduce their strength.

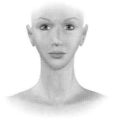

Heart face shape

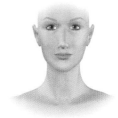

Oblong face shape

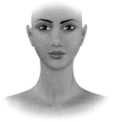

Oval face shape

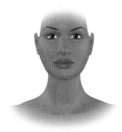

Pear face shape

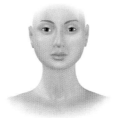

Round face shape

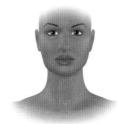

Square face shape

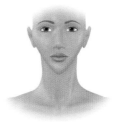

Triangular face shape

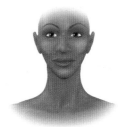

Diamond face shape

Shading

Shading is the blending of a make-up shade **darker** than the foundation or skin tone in order to **diminish** a feature. A large nose could be shaded at the sides to make it appear thinner, for instance, or a double chin could be made less obvious by shading underneath the jaw line. Shading colours should be similar in tonal value to the natural shadows of the face. Begin by looking at the inner corners of the eyes or any other area of natural shadow. This will

mediums, the application can be more dramatic. Shaders and highlighters are available as either powder or creams: cream products are applied before powdering the face; powder products are applied after general powdering. Remember that the contouring should look completely natural in the conditions under which it will be seen so careful, clean blending is always called for, whatever type of product you choose. The following will ensure a professional application.

Shadow tonal range	Colours found in dark skins	Colours found in white skins
Two to three shades darker than the base	Purple, blue, and for very dark skins a touch of black	Greyish-brown or brownish-grey, red-brown for darker areas of definition

give you a good idea of the kind of colour and tone that will look natural on the model. Generally, a correct colour selection will involve shifting two to three shades down the tonal range of the foundation or skin tone, ensuring that you remain within the correct underlying skin colour. The application of shading needs to be carefully blended. Bronzers or tinted powders can make useful shaders.

* Always use a good quality, soft brush when applying powder products, appropriately sized and shaped to the area you are working on.

* Crème products may be applied using a sponge or brush.

* Always apply the golden rule – less is more. You can build up the colour if further definition is required.

Highlight tonal range	Colours found in dark skins	Colours found in white skins
Two to three shades lighter than the base	Muted orange and yellows	Pale pink and pale yellow, cream, and for very light skins a touch of white

Highlighting

Highlighting is the blending of a make-up shade **lighter** than the foundation in order to **accentuate** a feature or facial plane. A correct colour selection will involve shifting approximately three shades up the tonal range of the foundation or skin tone, ensuring that you remain within the correct underlying skin colour. As with shading, the application will require careful blending. Iridescent powders can be useful highlighters.

Application techniques

For colour editorial and screen work, a subtle use of contouring make-up is called for. For the stage and in photographic work, particularly black and white

* Use your mirror to help you achieve balance and symmetry.

* Keep highlighter away from the under-eye socket area, otherwise you may make the eyes look puffy.

* Only contour where necessary – the final effect should enhance the model's bone structure and facial features.

KEY NOTE

Refer to Chapter 5 (page 68), for a recap on blending techniques.

Common areas for highlight application are:

* brow bone (on young models)
* centre of the eyelid
* centre of the forehead down through the bridge of the nose
* cheekbone plane
* centre of the chin
* collarbone
* top of the breast.

Common areas for shader application are:

* hollows under the cheekbone
* just below the inner corner of the eyebrow
* cleavage
* under the chin
* socket line of the eye
* hairline
* sides and tip of the nose
* temples
* hollows of the collarbone.

Contouring face shapes

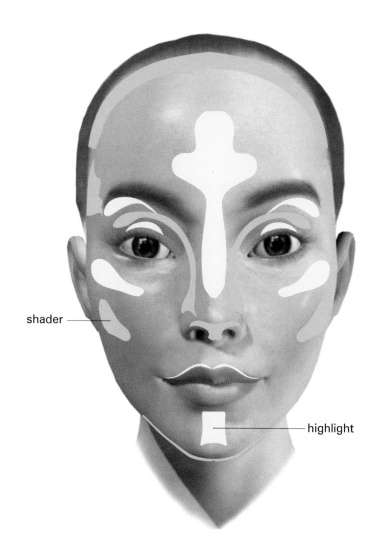

shader

highlight

Common placement of highlight and shading

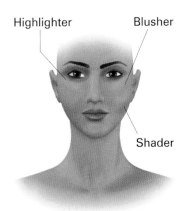

Oval

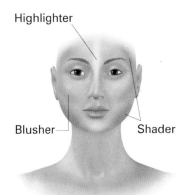

Round

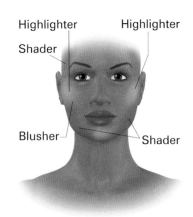

Square

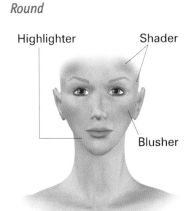

Oblong

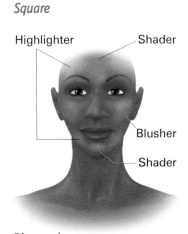

Heart

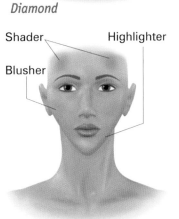

Diamond

Common placement of highlight and shading

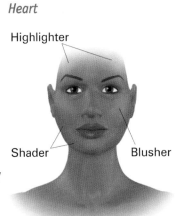

Pear

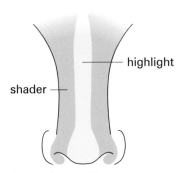

Triangular

KEY NOTE

A double chin can be reduced by using a shader on the fleshy part under the chin and a little highlighter on the chin itself.

Applying highlighter on the bony part of the chin only can bring a receding chin forward.

Shading below the hairline can reduce a high forehead.

Contouring the nose

A nose that is too wide can be narrowed by shading either side of the bridge of the nose and blending into the foundation.

shader — highlight

Contouring a wide nose

A crooked nose can be made to look straighter if the outward side of the bend is covered with shader and the inward side with a highlighter.

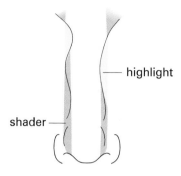

Contouring a crooked nose

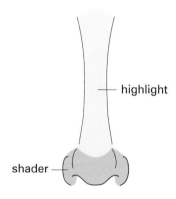

Contouring a long nose

A nose that is too long can be made shorter by shading the tip.

HANDS ON

Study the work of the late make-up artist, Kevyn Aucoin, who was a master at sculpting faces using contouring techniques.

Blushers

Blusher warms and brightens the skin complexion. It should complement the rest of the make-up, particularly the skin tone and lip colour. Placement is very important and colour should be built up in layers for a natural glow to the skin. Blusher should always be carefully blended to avoid stripes of colour.

Types of blusher

Cream blushers are good for drier skin types. They are applied with a sponge or sanitised fingertips (with the model's permission) after applying the foundation and before applying powder.

Powder blushers are similar in composition to pressed face powder and should be applied after powdering the face. Use a full soft brush with tapered edges to spread the colour evenly. They are available in matt and frosted textures.

Liquid or gel blushers are water based and give a transparent, natural glow, which looks good on highly coloured, freckled or bronzed complexions. They should be used over moisturiser or foundation. They have a short working time, so care should be taken not to streak these products on application.

Colour choice

The choice of blusher colour depends on the following.

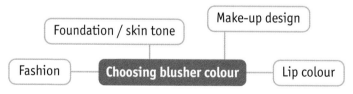

For a natural make-up the perfect blush is the colour of the cheek when it is flushed. Clear red tones are useful for creating this effect and suit most skin tones. It follows that the lighter your skin is, the lighter your blush shade should be: the darker your skin, the deeper the blush. It is a good idea to co-ordinate the lip and blusher colour for a harmonised make-up. However, for high fashion, harmony will not always be your aim and colour choice may range from the natural to strong dynamic effects. Do not be restricted by using just one colour – often overlaying a couple of shades, beginning with the lighter colour then adding the brighter colour, can create a very pleasing effect. Likewise, applying a cream, gel or liquid blusher, powdering and then adding a powder blusher over the original blush application can create a long-lasting, attractive finish.

Placement of blusher

fashion

Blusher placement is affected by:

face shape

make-up design

Blusher colour is used to enhance the model's natural features by complementing contouring techniques. Fashion has always affected the placement of blusher. If you look at fashion images from the early to mid 1980s you will notice that blusher was placed high across the cheekbone, sweeping up to the temple area, often in strong colours. However, more recent fashion trends have led to blusher being applied on the apple of the cheek in an attempt to create a flushed, natural look. The professional make-up artist will keep up to date with current trends and employ them in his or her work.

> **KEY NOTE**
>
> For high fashion, blusher need not be restricted to the cheeks. For an all-over glow, whisk gently over the forehead, temples and brow bone. However, blusher should never be used to contour the cheekbones as this would look unnatural.

Application techniques

1   All blushers that are not in powder form should be applied before the powder. Powder blushers should only be applied over a powdered base, otherwise the product will 'grab' the foundation and be very difficult to blend.

2   If using powder blush, tap off any excess from a rounded brush before applying to the face.

3   The model's pupil, when looking straight ahead, is a guide as to where to start applying the blusher. Sweep over the 'apple of the cheek' and, if appropriate, upwards across the cheekbone towards the hairline.

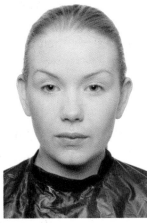

The effects of blusher vary according to the application

4   Blusher should always be blended upwards and outwards – this draws attention to the eyes and will help to 'lift' the face.

5   To soften or reduce the strength of blusher application, face powder can be applied directly over blush.

Bronzing powder and cream

To achieve a sun-kissed look, bronzing powder or cream should be applied on areas that would normally 'catch' the sun: the bridge of the nose, the cheekbones, the brow bones and temples. Shades that are too orange-toned should be avoided, as they tend to look artificial. The effect should be subtle and should enhance the foundation or skin tone.

Application of eyebrow make-up

The following section assumes knowledge of the theory of eyebrow shapes and shaping, covered in Chapter 7, page 135.

Compact powder

Types of eyebrow make-up

Eyebrow pencil

If you prefer a brow pencil, find one that is soft to avoid an artificial look. To apply powder, use a small, hard brush that is flat and angled at the tip.

Dip it into the shadow, tap off any excess and apply using a light touch. Eyebrow make-up is used to strengthen the colour of the brows and define their shape.

Application technique

1 Remove any stray hairs with tweezers.

2 Brush and smooth the brows into place.

3 Find the highest point of the brow.

4 Beginning a little in from the inside corner (this ensures the brow stays natural looking), fill in gaps until you reach the highest point, using fine, short strokes to simulate natural hair growth. This portion of the brow's shape is unchangeable without severe plucking or the use of special effect products.

5 Brows should generally taper to a fine point from the highest part to the end of the brow (use the same guidelines as for eyebrow shaping when determining the ideal length of the brow, see page 00). Unless the model has dark eyebrows, in which case the natural shape should be followed, the tapered part of the brow can often be changed to create different looks for high fashion.

6 Brush through the brows to soften any hard lines.

7 Apply a little clear mascara or hairspray to the brows, from a clean mascara wand, to hold in place.

Natural hair colour	Brow make-up colour
Blonde	Taupe
Light brown	Brown
Light red	Taupe
Auburn	Red-brown
Brunette	Dark brown
Grey	Slate (if hair is not coloured), otherwise taupe may be preferable
Black	Black-brown

Colour guidelines

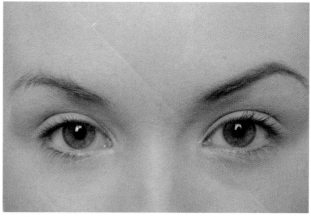

The brow before make-up application   *The brow after make-up application*

Eye make-up

Professional eye make-up is a result of meticulous application and careful build up of colour. For each look the following should be considered.

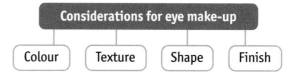

Choosing eye shadow colours

The natural skin tone, eye, hair colour and wardrobe can all act as indicators for choosing eye shadow colours.

Eye shadows need not match the eyes; in fact they often look more effective if they contrast with the eyes – try golds and coppers around blue eyes to make them look bluer; enhance brown eyes with greens, violet and gold; and try violets around green eyes to intensify their colour. There are no 'rules' when it comes to choosing eye shadow colour, but do think back to the colour theory discussed in Chapter 5 and consider how colours interact. For the more mature model, it is advisable to choose soft shades: soft greys, muted browns and peaches rather than bright, hard colours. Pastel colours or shiny products will accentuate wrinkles and skin imperfections. For screen work, matt neutral shades still remain the most reliable and favoured choice of make-up artists for straight beauty make-ups.

Types of eye shadow product

Powder-based shadows

Available in loose or compact form, powder-based shadows are made from the same ingredients as face powder. Loose powders are easier to use if they are mixed with a setting liquid or pressed into a crème base. The quality of powder-based shadows varies considerably, the best containing a high pigment content that will not lose its depth of colour as it is blended over an area.

Cream-based shadows

Cream-based shadows are available in liquid, stick or compact form. Since they contain water-in-oil they are good for dry skins and blend into the skin easily. They are applied after foundation and then set with a light film of face powder to help prevent creasing.

Eye shadow finishes

Frosted or metallic

The effect varies from a subtle shimmer to a dramatic metallic effect. They are available in liquid, crème or powder. In lighter shades they reflect light and act as highlighters. Bismuth oxychloride – found in fish scales or synthetically manufactured – is the ingredient that creates the shimmer effect.

Matt

Creating reliable results on camera, matt eye shadows remain a popular choice for make-up artists. Darker shades absorb the light and are useful for creating depth. They give the most natural finish and are an excellent choice for the more mature model.

Glossy

This look is generally used for high fashion images. It requires a lot of maintenance as after a while the gloss, and whatever is under it, tends to slide and crease. Glossy finishes should be avoided for screen work where the gloss will resemble an oily patch on the skin.

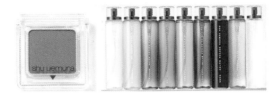

Shu Uemura coloured products

Contouring the natural eye shape

Small eyes

* Heavy or low eyebrows should be shaped to open up the eye area.
* Dark brows may benefit from being lightened by one to two shades.
* Eyelashes should be curled to open up the eye.
* A light colour should be used over the entire eyelid and blended up to the socket line.
* A medium-toned colour should then be applied on the outer corner of the eye and blended upwards and slightly outwards, into and just past the socket line.
* A darker shade, in pencil or shadow, should now be applied along the top lash line and extended slightly at the outer corner. The lower lash line can also be defined along the outer corner and extended as well.
* The brow bone should be highlighted.
* A kohl white pencil may be added on the inside rim of the eye.
* Mascara should be applied.

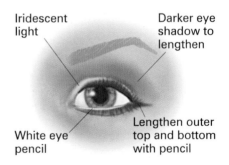

Iridescent light

Darker eye shadow to lengthen

White eye pencil

Lengthen outer top and bottom with pencil

Contouring small eyes. All contouring eye sketches by Julia Conway

Prominent or protruding eyes

* A matt colour should be used over the entire eyelid and blended up to the socket line.

* A medium-toned colour should then be applied on the outer corner of the eye and blended across the eyelid, covering about half of the original colour. Continue to blend upwards defining the socket line.

* A darker shade, in pencil or shadow, should now be applied along the top lash line. This line can be blended upwards to create a thicker, smoky line. The lower lash line can also be defined along the outer two-thirds.

* The brow bone should be highlighted.

* A dark-coloured kohl pencil may be added on the inside rim of the eye.

* Mascara should be applied.

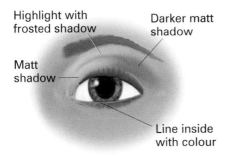

Contouring prominent eyes

Deep-set eyes

* Heavy or low eyebrows should be shaped to open up the eye area.

* Dark brows may benefit from being lightened by one to two shades.

* Apply a light colour over the entire eye area.

* Apply a medium tone slightly above the socket line and blend.

* Apply a darker tone under the outer portion of the lower lash line and soften by blending.

* Do *not* over-highlight the brow bone.

* Apply mascara, emphasising the outer portion of the lashes.

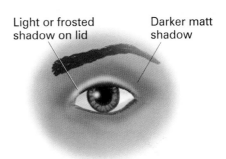

Contouring deep-set eyes

Round eyes

* Eyebrows can be shaped as angular or straight to counterbalance the round eye shape.

* Apply a light colour over the eyelid.

* Blend a medium-toned colour into the socket line to define this area and sweep outwards at the outer corner to elongate the eye.

* Apply a darker colour on the outside corner of the eye (above and under), blending upwards and outwards.

* Highlight the brow bone.

* Apply eyeliner across the top lid, extending slightly in an upward direction at the outer corner.

* Curl the lashes at the outer corner to lift the eye and apply mascara, emphasising the outer portion of the lashes.

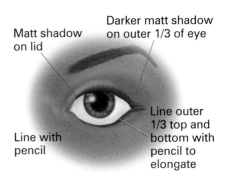

Contouring round eyes

Close-set eyes

* The inner corners of the eyebrows should be kept natural, and a few extra hairs may be removed from this area when shaping to maximise the space between the eyes.

* A light colour should be applied on the inner corners of the eye.

* Medium- and dark-toned colours should be kept to the outer portion of the eye and swept outwards to 'pull' the eyes apart.

* Highlight the brow bone.

* Apply mascara and eyeliner, emphasising the outer portion of the eye and lashes.

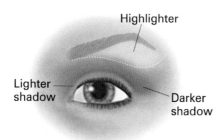

Contouring close-set eyes

Wide-set eyes

* The inner corners of the eyebrows should be emphasised a little (but not so they look heavy and unnatural), and a few extra hairs may be left in this area when shaping to minimise the space between the eyes.

* A light to medium colour should be applied on the outer corners of the eye and blended upwards into and slightly beyond the socket line, but *not* outwards.

* Medium- to dark-toned colours should be kept to the inner portion of the eye. They should be blended softly along the side of the nose into the inner corner of the brow and across to the centre of the eye, merging with the lighter shade applied earlier.

* Highlight the centre of the brow bone, but blend off before it reaches the outer corner.

* Apply eyeliner, ensuring you start from the very inner corner of the eye. This line can be blended to create a softer effect on the outer portion of the eye. Another tip is to use a lighter shade of eyeliner on the outer half of the eye.

* Apply mascara.

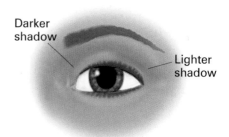

Contouring wide-set eyes

Hooded eyes

* Apply a medium colour starting at the outer corner of the eyes and shape slightly upward and across to the centre.

* Apply a dark colour over the hooded area, extending it onto the brow bone slightly. Blend well.

* Apply a light colour on the inner corner of the eyes and blend across to meet the medium colour.

* Highlight just a little directly under the brow. Do not extend the highlight down too far.

* Apply eyeliner across the top lid and outer portion of the lower lid. Soften if desired.

* Apply mascara.

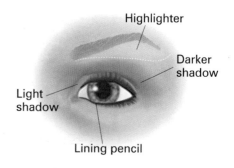

Contouring hooded eyes

The Oriental eye shape

* Groom and fill in the brow with powder or pencil. Extend the length of the brow.

* Apply a light colour over the entire eye.

* Shade and blend with a medium colour. Create a half moon, rounded shape from the lash upwards (this needs to look like a socket shadow). Start the shadow a little outside the outer corner of the eye. Blend well.

* Add a darker shadow to the outer corner of the lower lashes and blend around the lash line.

* Highlight the brow bone.

* Apply liner in a fairly thick and smoky line.

* Curl the lashes and apply mascara liberally.

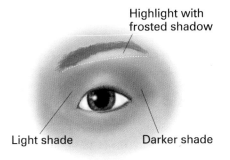

Highlight with frosted shadow

Light shade   Darker shade

Contouring the Oriental eye

Fashion eye shadow shapes

There are dozens of eye shadow shapes and each one can create a completely different effect. The following are the most useful shapes to practice.

Once you have mastered the application of eye shadow, you should be able to create any shape you like. Eye shadows can be applied with brushes (a selection of sizes is useful) or sponge tip applicators, which are useful for applying a good depth of colour quickly, for example when creating a smoky eye. Colour should be built up in layers until the required depth is achieved. Brush strokes should vary in direction to ensure the tiny creases on the eyelids are filled with colour. If you are applying dark colours, place a generous layer of face powder under the eye area to 'catch' any colour that may drop here. When the application is complete, simply dust away the powder to ensure this area is clean (you may wish to avoid this technique if the under-eye area is heavily wrinkled).

Eyeliner

Historically, lining the eyes goes back to the ancient Egyptians. Depending on the look you are trying to create, eyeliners can give a defined line of colour or a soft, smudgy look around the lash line. Eyeliner is generally available as:

* pencils (should be slightly soft to the touch)

* eye shadow used with a dampened eyeliner brush

* a block or cake used with a dampened eyeliner brush

* a liquid.

Natural or minimal
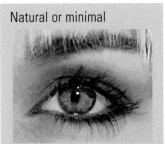

Contoured
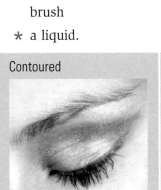

Wash
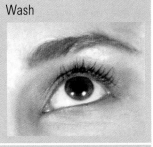

Smoky
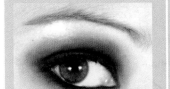

Hard-edged
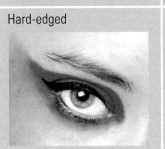

Winged
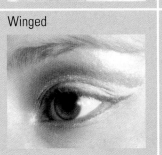

Graduated
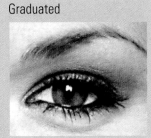
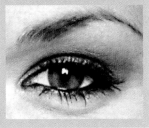

Black, brown and slate or charcoal-coloured eyeliner give the most natural finish. Strong colours are also available for a high fashion look.

Application of eyeliner

Top line

1 Whichever type of eyeliner you are using, it is important to hold the eyelid taut by lifting the brow with a clean fingertip resting on a tissue or powder puff to remove any creases in the lid.

2 The line should be kept as close to the natural lash line as possible. However, the thickness of the line can vary according to the effect you wish to create.

3 The upper lash line should be started at the inner corner of the eye as a fine line and continue, increasing in thickness, to the outer corner.

4 The thickness of the line and degree and direction of extension past the outer corner will vary according to fashion and the kind of look you wish to create. However, normally the ends of the lash line should be tapered to finish in a fine point.

5 The finished line can either be softened with a brush, cotton tip or sponge applicator, or left well defined, depending on the effect you wish to create.

Bottom line

1 The line should be kept as close to the natural lash line as possible. However, the thickness of the line can vary according to the effect you wish to create.

2 The lower lash line should be started approximately one-third along from the inner corner of the eye and continue to the outer corner.

3 The thickness of line and degree and direction of extension past the outer corner will vary according to fashion and the kind of look you wish to create.

4 The finished line can either be softened with a brush, cotton tip or sponge applicator, or left

well defined, depending on the effect you wish to create.

Kohl-rimmed eyes

This make-up technique originates from Eastern cultures. Using a finger from your free hand, gently pull the lid away from the eye. Choose a pencil with a slightly softer tip and apply a line to the inside rims. Ask the model to blink her eyes a couple of times (this will help to soften the line).

White eye pencil

Using a white eye pencil on the inside rims of the eyes can make them look bigger. To apply, gently pull the lid away from the eye and draw a line along the upper and lower inner eye rim.

> **KEY NOTE**
>
> Use kohl with caution. Stringent hygienic precautions are essential for this procedure, which is used more in fashion than screen work. Always gain permission from the model before proceeding.

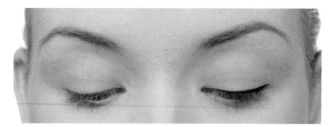

Eyeliner application

Curling the natural lash

Some models have naturally curly lashes and all that is needed is to sweep the lashes upwards from underneath with the mascara applicator and the curl will be 'set in'. Other models have long but straight lashes. These may be temporarily curled with eyelash curlers or permanently curled with a chemical process, called eyelash perming.

Using eyelash curlers

1 Ask the client to look straight ahead.

2 The eyelash curlers are opened, placed near to the base of the top lashes and squeezed together

for three to five seconds. Continue to move along the lash towards the tips, squeezing as you go.

3 Care must be taken not to pinch the skin.

4 Use mascara *afterwards* to 'set in' the curl.

Mascara

Mascara thickens and darkens the eyelashes giving emphasis to the eyes. It is better to build up layers rather than applying one thick coat.

Types of mascara

Cake

* This is the original type of mascara.
* It consists of mineral oil, waxes and pigments mixed with a soap (triethanolamine).
* It should be applied with a damp mascara wand.
* It has a longer shelf life than liquid mascara.

Liquid

* This consists of pigments mixed with water, or alcohol and water, and castor oil to soften the suspension.
* Other ingredients are often added to enhance and improve the product.
* Resins produce a waterproof mascara.
* Nylon or rayon filaments thicken the lashes.
* It is usually sold in a barrel container.
* It has a shelf life of approximately three months.

Both cake and liquid mascaras are available in a range of colours from the more traditional black, brown, aubergine and slate to the latest trend, whether that be pink, purple or gold. Navy blue mascara can help to lift tired eyes by making the whites of the eyes 'whiter'.

Application of mascara

1 Both cake and liquid mascara are applied using a disposable mascara wand.

2 Ask the model to look down. Gently lift the eyebrow at the outer corner with your free

hand. As you do this, the hairs of the lashes will separate.

3 Apply the mascara over the top of the upper lashes from the roots to the tips. When this is dry, add a second layer, this time upwards and outwards from under the upper lashes. This will help to lift the lashes.

4 Wait until the top lashes are completely dry before attempting to mascara the lower lashes, otherwise you will end up with dots of mascara across the eye make-up.

5 To apply to the lower lashes, ask the model to look upwards away from the applicator. Make sure the model is not looking directly into a strong light or the eyes may water.

6 Always protect the client's skin underneath with a tissue. Apply the mascara downwards on top of the lashes. Mascara on the bottom lashes should be used sparingly; clients with naturally dark lashes may not require it at all here.

7 Use an eyelash comb to separate the eyelashes and remove any 'lumps'.

> **KEY NOTE**
>
> When loading the mascara wand with product, do not pump the wand in and out of the barrel as this will introduce air into the product and cause it to dry out quickly.

Eye lash tinting and false lash application are covered in Chapter 7 (pages 139 and 142).

> **KEY NOTE**
>
> Contact lenses come in different types, but are either hard or soft. Hard lenses tend to trap dust, which irritates the eye. The make-up artist must be very careful not to let any debris from the make-up get into the eye. Some models are happier removing their contact lenses before make-up application; others prefer to leave them in place. Always ask the client to keep the eyes closed when applying powder products, and avoid using lash lengthening mascaras containing filaments which may irritate.

The mouth

Lip colour will enhance lips and complete the make-up by adding harmony and balance.

Types of lip colour

Lipstick

Lipstick consists of oil, wax and dyes. It comes in a variety of forms varying from the regular twist-up tubes to compacts or barrel containers complete with applicator. Moisturising, creamy textured lipsticks are good for dry lips that have a tendency to crack.

Lip glosses

Lip glosses contain more oil than lipstick. They can be used alone for a natural look, or as a final glossy coat over lipstick. Most are clear or subtly tinted. Avoid glosses that are very 'sticky'. Glosses are high-maintenance products and need to be touched up frequently.

Lip pencils

Lip pencils are available in a variety of colours and are used to define and outline the lips. They can also help to prevent lipstick 'bleeding' on a mature model.

Lip primers and sealers

Lip primers are used prior to lipstick application to help prevent lipstick 'bleeding'. Sealers are a clear liquid and are used over lipstick application to help improve its longevity.

Matt	A sophisticated finish. Look for a creamy matt texture as some matt formulas are very dry.
Sheer	Lets the natural colour show through. A transparent stain.
Glossy	Very versatile. Can look sexy or very natural, depending on colour. Can create appearance of fuller lips.
Frosted	Dramatic and three-dimensional.

Lip colour finishes

Choosing lip colour

Lip colours should complement the model's natural colouring, existing make-up and wardrobe. The following guidelines should also be taken into account.

* Matt and dark-coloured lipsticks make a mouth look smaller.

* Frosted, glossy and light-coloured lipsticks make a mouth look larger.

* Yellow-based lip colours, such as oranges, should be avoided on sallow skin.

* Warm tones such as corals, roses and peaches flatter mature models. Frosted or glossy lipsticks will emphasise any wrinkles around the mouth and will be more likely to 'bleed' into the surrounding skin.

* Redheads should avoid blue-based lip colour such as mauves and certain reds.

* Avoid orange-toned or pale pink lipsticks if the teeth are yellowed.

* The correct shade of lip pencil will either match the lipstick or match the natural lip colour (sometimes referred to as 'nude').

Application of lip pencil

1 You should have covered the edge of the lip line with a layer of foundation and powder. This will help if you wish to reshape the mouth and prevent 'bleeding' into the surrounding skin.

2 Ensure your lip pencil is sharp.

3 The desired line should be drawn on, making minor corrections to the natural lip line if required. Begin with the top lip and shape the Cupid's bow, then continue to the corners of the mouth. Aim for a clean, well-balanced, symmetrical outline. Fill in the entire lip with colour.

4 Now begin on the centre of the lower lip and continue into each corner, filling in the entire lip.

5 If you make a mistake, the wrong part of the line should be carefully wiped away using

tissue or a cotton bud. Foundation and powder should be reapplied to the wiped area, and the lip line can be re-drawn in the correct place.

Lip liner can also be applied after the lipstick application. This has a more subtle effect, but still adds definition to the lip shape.

Application of lipstick

1 Prepare the lips with Blisteze or Vaseline if they are cracked or dry.

2 Lipstick should not be applied from the stick or lip palette directly to the lips of your model. A small amount of the chosen colour should be transferred to the working palette, and this can then be liberally transferred to a lip brush.

3 Ask the model to slightly part the lips.

4 Use a lip brush to apply colour to the model's lips, but first steady your hand. You can do this on your model's face by gently resting your little finger on the chin with a powder puff. Be careful not to press – you are just making sure your hand doesn't wobble.

5 Start with the bottom lip and go to the corners. If you have enough lipstick on the brush, the colour should flow without dragging.

6 Ask the model to smudge the lips together carefully to spread colour over the top lip.

7 Using the lip brush, work carefully on the top lip, aiming to create a clean, well-balanced, symmetrical shape. Begin on the Cupid's bow. Ask the model to part the lips and fill the top corners of the lips carefully.

8 Use your mirror to assess any mistakes. At the first attempt, one side of the top lip is usually straight and the other more rounded. Even them up.

9 If required, the outline of the lips can be perfected with a touch of foundation on a clean brush.

10 Blot the lips using a tissue. Separate a two-ply tissue and use one sheet at a time.

11 Reapply the lipstick and blot again.

12 For a longer-lasting lip colour the lips can be lightly powdered after blotting each layer. If a matt finish is required or the model's lips tend to 'bleed' lipstick, powder lightly again. Alternatively a lip sealer can be applied.

13 If a shiny appearance is required, gloss can be used to finish. This should be applied sparingly.

KEY NOTE

Perfecting lipstick application is all about practice. It is a good idea to practise using a bright red lipstick as any mistakes will be obvious.

Correcting lip shapes

The basic lip shape is a fuller bottom lip and a slightly narrower top lip, but there are many variations on the basic lip shape. It is possible to correct unbalanced lip shapes when applying the lip make-up, though any changes should be kept subtle.

Thin lips

Aim to create fuller lips by increasing the curve of both the upper and lower lips slightly outside the natural lip line. Shape the Cupid's bow on the top lip and then work from the corners up to the newly shaped Cupid's bow. Working upwards, rather that down to the corners, will encourage you to create a slightly fuller, more curved shape. A highlight can be added just above the Cupid's bow to make the top lip look fuller still. Begin on the lower lip at the corners and work to the middle just outside the natural lip line. Use light lipsticks and glossy textures.

Thin upper lip or thin lower lip

Follow the procedure above but only correct either the top or bottom lip as appropriate to try to create a balance between the two lips.

Full lips

Hide the natural lip line with foundation and powder. Carefully create a new lip line just inside the natural one using a stronger colour than the fill-in shade. Dark lipsticks and matt textures should be used.

Asymmetrical lips

Aim to create a balance between the two sides of the mouth. If necessary, hide the natural lip line.

Droopy mouth

Aim to create an illusion of uplift at the corners by building them up with colour. Work on the outer corners of the upper lips, building them up with colour. Extend the corner of the lips upwards to meet the upper line and possibly outwards beyond the corner of the upper lips.

Body make-up

The make-up artist will often be required to apply straight body make-up on models; this is a standard requirement on lingerie or swimwear shoots, glamour work or any scenario where the skin of the body is exposed. There may be a number of reasons why body make-up is required.

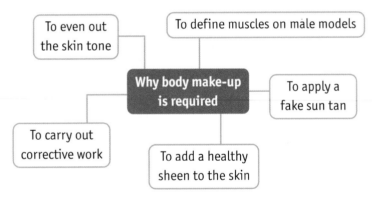

Corrective body work

Just as the face suffers from skin imperfections, so does the body. Common imperfections include blotchiness or excessive redness on the chest area and hyper-pigmentation caused by UV exposure and scars. Each problem should be dealt with using appropriate corrective make-up techniques.

Evening out the skin tone

The skin tone on the body can vary from that on the face and this is often more noticeable in

photographs. Foundation can be applied to specific areas such as the chest, shoulders and suntan marks to counteract this problem. However, when larger areas require work, it is neither practical nor economical to use conventional foundation. Instead, there are a number of formulations on the market specifically designed for body application. These are sold in larger quantities and often have long-lasting, water-resistant properties.

Fake tans

There may be occasions when the model or performer requires an all-over tan. If you are aware of this ahead of the shoot or production, you could arrange for the performer to either undertake a number of sun bed sessions or visit a beauty salon to have a fake tan applied. A fake tan usually lasts between one to three weeks, depending on the individual's skin type. However, sometimes a tan is required at short notice and again there are a number of products available on the market that give instant results. Airbrushing is an excellent method of quickly applying colour to the body.

Adding sheen or shimmer to the skin on female models

There are various types of products that add shimmer or sheen to the body: powders, liquids, oils or creams are all available. Some are tinted and give the skin a healthy glow – these look great over a tanned skin. Products that give a more subtle effect can be used all over, whereas products with more obvious finishes can be used to highlight specific areas such as the tops of the collarbones, shoulders, top of the breasts, shins, etc.

> **KEY NOTE**
>
> In an emergency, hair wax applied sparingly to the body will create sheen on the skin.

Creating muscle definition and sheen on male models

Male bodies sometimes require sheen without the shimmer associated with many of the products available. The easiest way to achieve this is to add a little glycerine to the skin's surface, though care must be taken not to dislodge any coloured base underneath. For a sporty, sweaty effect, a mixture of 50 per cent water and 50 per cent glycerine can be added to a spray bottle and applied to the skin sparingly. Muscles can be defined using conventional chiaroscuro techniques (painting with light and shade).

The make-ups that follow are typical of designs you may be asked to reproduce at any point in your career. They are, of course, just examples, and many more possibilities, bound only by the restraints of your imagination, are possible.

Minimal make-up

This is an 'un-made-up' make-up, which should enhance the model while leaving him or her looking completely natural.

1 Apply a pre-base that will add radiance to the skin (optional).

2 Apply a light, liquid foundation or tinted moisturiser where required to even out the skin tone.

3 Apply concealer to remove any blemishes and shadows.

4 Apply liquid or cream blusher to the apple of the cheeks. A touch of bronzing product can also be added to give a sun-kissed look if desired.

5 Powder lightly.

6 Brush through the eyebrows and fill in any gaps with powder or a pencil.

7 Subtly contour the eye shape by applying a soft, natural-coloured eye shadow. Blend well. Apply a little under the outer corner of the eye to add definition and blend well.

8 Curl the lashes and apply a light coat of natural-coloured mascara to the top lashes only (unless the model is blonde or red haired, in which case the lower lashes can also be covered).

9 Balance out the lip shape with a soft, nude-coloured lip line; fill in softly with a soft, natural-coloured lip stain. Alternatively, just apply a little lip balm or tinted gloss to create a sheer, healthy look to the lips.

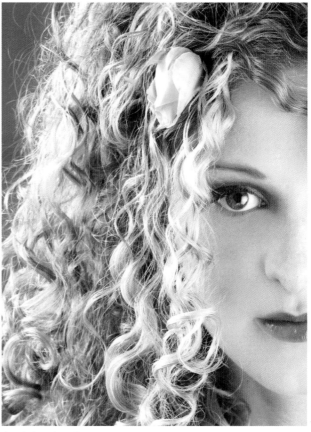

A minimal make-up

> **KEY NOTE**
>
> **A neutral make-up** is a make-up using neutral colours. Neutral colours are those that can be found in the natural colouring of the model. For example, ivory through to browns and greys on the eyes, soft pinks or apricots on the cheeks and fleshy pinky-beige tones on the lips. Colours will vary subtly according to the model's individual natural colouring. Many make-up artists confuse a neutral make-up with a minimal make-up. However, although neutral shades are often used in minimal make-ups, a neutral make-up can be quite strong depending on the intensity of application and depth of tones used.

HANDS ON

1 Try creating a minimal make-up using matt products, and then repeat it using products that create a 'dewy' or slightly shimmery finish. Compare the results and make notes for future reference.
2 Create a make-up using neutral colours only. Concentrate on creating balance in the model's face using contouring and corrective application techniques on the face shape and features. Remember to photograph your work.

Glamorous make-up with smoky eyes

1 Apply foundation, concealer and contouring products as required.

2 Powder.

3 Groom the brows and fill in any gaps with powder or pencil.

4 Apply black kohl to the inside rims of the eyes.

5 Apply black eye shadow with a sponge-tip applicator around the lashes (upper and lower), encircling the entire eye. Blend out as far as you dare, depending on the look you wish to achieve. Ensure you create the greatest depth of colour closest to the lashes.

6 Apply aubergine-coloured eye shadow to the edge of the black to soften and diffuse the edge. Loose powder can then be applied to the edge of the aubergine to soften and diffuse this edge.

7 Apply a highlighter to the brow bone and blend carefully.

8 Curl the lashes and apply black mascara.

9 Add false lashes if required.

10 Apply blush on the cheeks that is suitable for the model's colouring. Keep the colour soft – you can always add a 'pop' of brighter colour to the centre of this application at the end of the make-up if more colour is required.

11 Use natural-coloured lip pencil to outline and balance the lips.

12 Apply a red lipstick in a tone suitable for your model's colouring. If you prefer a softer mouth, blot the lipstick firmly and apply a little lip balm or gloss over the colour.

The smoky eye effect can be created in any colour, but deep dramatic shades seem to work best.

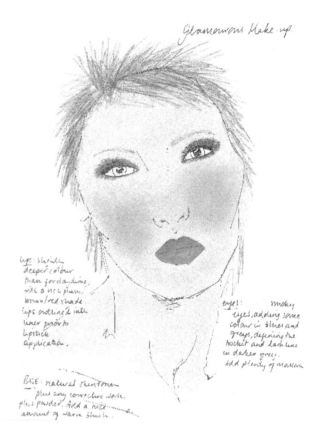

A design sheet for glamorous make-up by Louisa Morgan

Balance in make-up

The above glamorous make-up is an example of a dark-eyed, dark-mouthed design. If natural-coloured lips replaced the strong, red mouth, the mood of the final design would alter dramatically because the balance of the make-up would have changed. There are four main options when considering balance in the overall make-up design:

* dark eyes, dark mouth
* dark eyes, light mouth
* light eyes, dark mouth
* light eyes, light mouth.

There are of course many variants that exist across these options, depending on the degree of lightness and darkness you choose in each case. The different options will shift the focus between the top and lower half of the face, so it is possible to draw attention to your model's best features in this way.

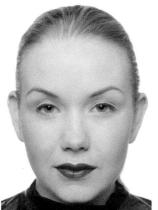 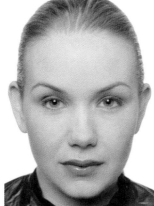

Light eyes, dark mouth   *Dark eyes, light mouth*

HANDS ON

1 Create a minimal make-up on your model. Take a photograph (light eyes, light mouth).

2 Change the above make-up by replacing the lip colour with a strong, red-toned lipstick Take a photograph (light eyes, dark mouth).

3 On the same model, create a glamorous, smoky eyed make-up, but paint the lips in a natural colour. Take a photograph (dark eyes, light mouth).

4 Change the lip colour to a strong, red-toned lipstick. Take a photograph (dark eyes, dark mouth).

5 Compare the final effect of the four make-ups. Try to evaluate your responses and make some notes for future reference.

Catwalk or runway make-up

Catwalk or runway shows are platforms for fashion designers to show their collections. They are usually spectacular performances with a distinct theatrical feel that reflects the avant-garde nature of the clothes. The styling and ideas featured at these shows are indicators of forthcoming fashion trends, which will eventually filter down to the high street.

Sometimes retailers will also put on shows to promote their collections. These shows tend to be more commercially based, i.e. taking place to promote and sell products to the mass market. Therefore the styling of these shows tends to be more conventional, reflecting current trends that the mass market is able to relate to.

KEY NOTE

An avant-garde image is a look that is ahead of current commercially acceptable styling, but often acts as an indicator of future trends. A commercial image is one that is used to promote and sell products to the mass market.

The fashion designer or client will decide the overall concept behind the show. Based on this information the make-up artist must come up with suitable make-up and sometimes hair designs that complement the styling of the clothes. The make-up can vary from the fantastical to the minimal and low key, so there are no set rules when applying catwalk make-up. However, it is worth bearing in mind the following considerations.

* Make-up for the catwalk is traditionally stronger than make-up for fashion photography as its roots are closer to the theatre than photographic work: the show is live with the audience sitting some distance from the models and the runway is lit by harsh lighting, which is sometimes coloured. Nowadays many runway shows are also televised, which means that the make-up has to look good close-up as well as from a distance. The application therefore needs to be perfect.

* The make-up should enhance the clothes, not take over from them.

* Haute-couture catwalk offers the make-up artist a chance to experiment with new ideas and display his or her creativity.

* Many designers' collections or shows are based on themes that may involve research for the make-up artist.
* Catwalk environments are frantic; the make-up artist will need to be organised, and work calmly but quickly in the midst of chaos.

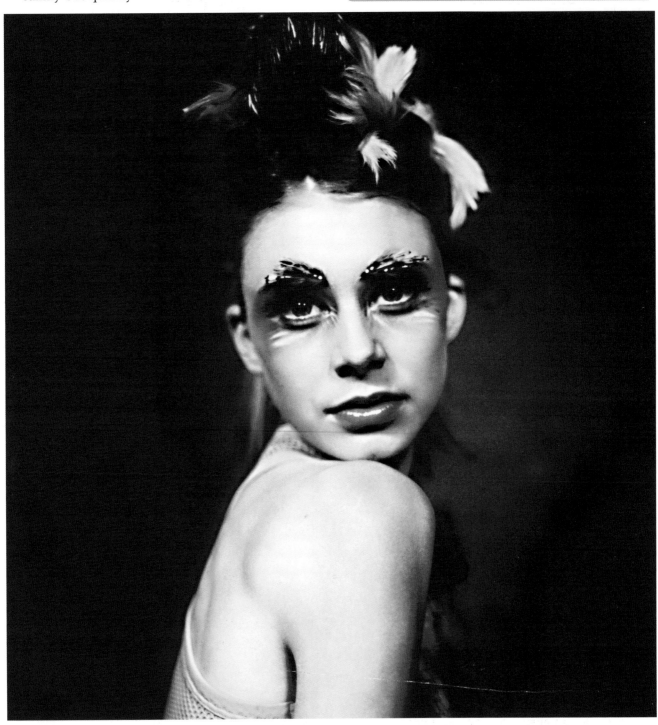

Example of avant-garde make-up and hairstyling

Bridal make-up

Many brides-to-be will employ the services of a make-up artist and hairstylist for their big day. To ensure a positive outcome, the make-up artist must establish the client's needs and requirements and ensure these are met. The best way to achieve this is by arranging a trial run. A trial run will:

* give the make-up artist a chance to collect as much information as possible

* ensure the bride is confident and happy with the make-up.

The type of considerations the make-up artist should take into account include the following.

* Is the make-up artist doing both hair and make-up or just make-up? Who will require the services? This may include the bridesmaids and bride's mother as well as the bride, so you may need to hire assistants to help you.

* How does the bride usually wear her make-up? It is generally not a good idea to dramatically change a bride's make-up for the wedding day – she will not feel comfortable and the groom may get a shock!

* How will the hair be worn – up or down, straight or curly? Will a headdress or veil be worn? This will affect the choice of hairstyle.

* What style and colour is the dress? Not all brides wear white or ivory and the style (for example romantic, classic, formal, etc.) of the dress is important when planning the overall mood of the make-up and hair design.

* What colour are the flowers, and what is the general colour scheme and style of the wedding? The make-up should be designed to complement the overall 'style' of the wedding.

* Where will the make-up and hairstyling be done? Will there be adequate space and lighting? If the wedding is not local, you will have to include your travel expenses when costing your fee.

* How will you ensure the make-up lasts throughout the day? Waterproof mascara is essential and a long-lasting lipstick is advisable. The make-up artist could also leave a few scrapings of the lipstick colour in a small sample pot for the bride to reapply herself throughout the day.

KEY NOTE

Many brides employ a make-up artist for their wedding day because they do not usually wear make-up but want to make a special effort for their big day. These brides will usually prefer a 'natural look'. Although this is by far the best option, they should be encouraged to wear enough make-up to achieve a flawless, radiant finish for the photographs. The biggest anxiety to overcome is foundations; many people feel 'over made-up' when wearing foundation, or are under the misconception that it will look obvious and unnatural. For these brides, consider the sheerer alternatives if the skin condition will allow and use the trial run to show them how foundation can enhance their appearance.

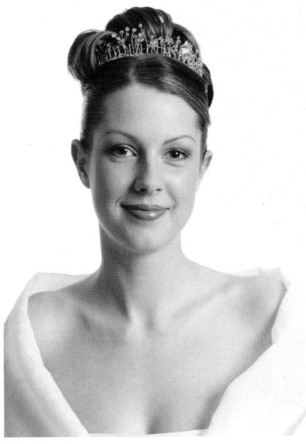

A bridal make-up

Black and white photography

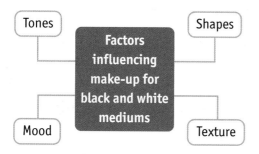

Tones — Shapes — Mood — Texture — Factors influencing make-up for black and white mediums

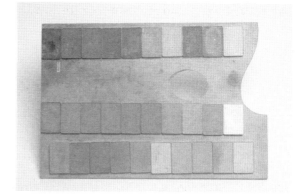

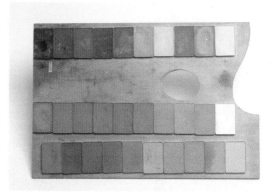

Tones are important to consider when planning make-up for black and white photos

Mood

Because colour film is widely available and used these days, if a photographer chooses to shoot in black and white, he or she is making a conscious statement about the final image. Black and white images can be very atmospheric because of the importance of texture and lighting in the absence of colour. As discussed in Chapter 6 ('Professional studies'), lighting can be high key with lots of lighter tones, or low key with lots of dark tones and shadows. The mood of the make-up can complement the lighting by the use of predominantly light or dark tones on the skin.

Tones

In black and white photography colours will register as tints and shades (tones) of grey. It is therefore advisable to:

* use neutral colours on the eyes such as browns, blacks, greys and creams as it is easy to judge their tonal value
* use shades of red and brown on the lips
* apply contouring techniques on the cheekbone instead of blusher, which is used to add colour to the face so is not required.

KEY NOTE

For a mixed shoot of colour and black and white the above colours still work well, but you may wish to add blusher. Avoid 'brick' shades as these can look like dirty marks on the skin. If you wish to experiment with other colours on the eyes, ensure you understand how they translate into tones.

Shapes

In black and white photography shapes take on new emphasis and contouring make-up techniques can be employed to take full advantage of this.

Contouring for black and white photography can be far more dramatic than for colour mediums, as the camera will translate shadows and highlights made with make-up as natural contours. Therefore contouring make-up can be up to four tones lighter or darker than the skin tone, depending on the lighting set-up. Results can be quite dramatic, with the model's face literally being re-sculpted using light and shade.

Texture

Black and white images tend to emphasise texture on the skin's surface to a greater or lesser extent depending on the photographer's lighting. It is much easier to predict the finished result when using matt products, although pearlised finishes, used sparingly, can be effective when using highlighting products. Excellent communication with the photographer is important at all times to establish the lighting arrangements so that make-up can be applied appropriately.

HANDS ON

Complete a make-up for black and white photography concentrating on using dramatic contouring techniques. Ensure you photograph the finished result using both a colour and a black and white film (or shoot in digital format and then you should be able to print the image as both). Compare and contrast the images – this will be a useful reference for the future.

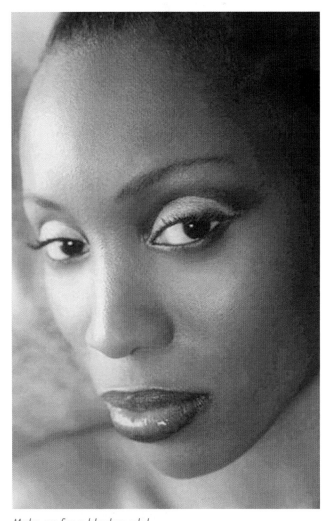

Make-up for a black model

Make-up for black skin tones

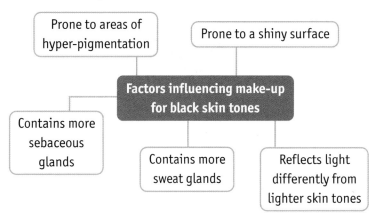

Foundation

* A mattifying pre-base can prove useful in removing excess shine from the skin. An orange-toned pre-base used sparingly can 'lift' and brighten the complexion.

* Consider using brands that specialise in colours for black skins. Avoid colours with pink undertones.

* If you are doing a photo shoot with a black model, contact her before the session and ask her to bring her own foundation along. Most black models are experts at selecting their own make-up shades. However, always take your own selection along, just in case!

* The new 'two in one' powder and foundation compacts work well on dark skins.

* To even out extensive hyper-pigmentation, first test the foundation on a lighter area of the skin, and then again on a darker patch of skin. Choose a colour foundation that is in between the lightest and darkest colouring.

Concealing

* Orange is an excellent corrective colour for lightening smaller areas of hyper-pigmentation.

Contouring

* Black models and clients will often request specific contouring techniques to be carried out for photographic work. This may include

slimming a broad nose and reducing full lips. However, for fashion work, the model will have been chosen for his or her specific look, so this specific contouring is generally not required.

Powder

* Avoid translucent powder or powders containing titanium dioxide, as this can make the model look 'grey'. Instead, choose a dark yellow or orange powder, which works well on very dark skins.

Colour products

* For a natural look, black skin suits warm-toned colours ranging from peach to reds, burgundy, bronze and browns. The darker the skin tone, the deeper the shades should be.

* Alternatively, bright colours such as lime greens, shocking pinks and electric blues on the eyes can look fantastic for high fashion effects.

* Sheer and iridescent finishes particularly suit black skin tones as they enhance the natural luminosity of the skin.

* Deep berry shades such as plums look great on lips.

Make-up for Oriental Asian skin tones

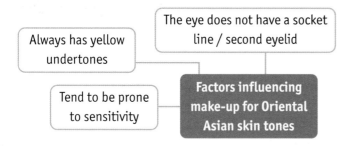

Always has yellow undertones

The eye does not have a socket line / second eyelid

Tend to be prone to sensitivity

Factors influencing make-up for Oriental Asian skin tones

Foundation and powder

* A lilac-coloured pre-base can be used to reduce extremely sallow complexions.
* Always use yellow-toned foundations and powders. Bases with pink undertones will look completely unnatural.

Contouring

* Oriental models often have a round face shape, and their features may appear flat on camera. Therefore contouring techniques for this face shape can be employed. The eye shape can either be emphasised or contoured to give the impression of a socket line, depending on the design requirements.

Blusher

* Soft colours with pink or red undertones will 'lift' a sallow skin tone.

* For added definition, apply blush high along the cheekbone, not on the 'apples' of the cheeks as this will make the face appear rounder.

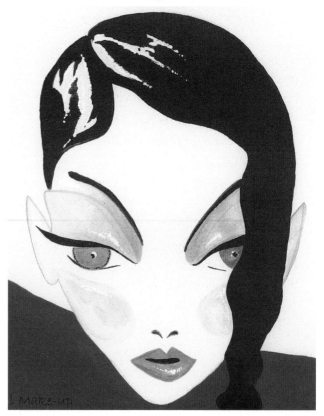

Design sheet for make-up for Oriental Asian skin tones by Julia Conway

Eyes

* Light shimmery colours with a smudgy eyeliner for definition looks great on Oriental eyes. For a more dramatic effect, a dark smoky eye works very well.

* Eyelashes that are straight and short can be curled with an eyelash curler. Sparse lashes will benefit from an application of black mascara.
* Eyebrows tend to be straight and short in length. Shaping with tweezers and extending with a pencil or shadow can define them.

Lips

* Shades from sheer pinks to deep berry colours with brown or red undertones look great.

Make-up for Indian Asian skin tones

Foundation and powder

* Once again, this type of skin tone will usually have warm, yellow undertones.
* Dark circles under the eyes are common amongst Indian Asians. Orange is an excellent corrective colour for lightening dark pigmentation patches. For lighter skin tones, mix with the skin-toned concealer.
* Yellow-toned powder is again the preferable option; darker skin tones should opt for orange tones.

Blusher

* Almond and warm coffee tones will colour the face without making it look too dark. Deeper brown-based shades with red, plum and soft berry undertones will also work well, particularly on darker skin tones.

Eyes

* Heavy eyebrows can be shaped with tweezers to open the eye area.
* All the natural tones within the warm spectrum – shades of brown, golds, bronzes, etc. – will look good. For a more dramatic effect, shades such as burgundy, black, silvers, deep blues, etc. will work well. In general, warmer, darker or brighter colours will work better than pastels.
* Black and dark brown mascara will define the eyes.

* Using kohl eyeliner can create dramatic effects.

Lips

* Shades of brown give a natural finish. Deeper berry shades are great for a more dramatic effect.

HANDS ON

Research brands that specialise in ranges for dark skin tones. Collect information from each of the suppliers and add these to your file for future reference.

Carry out a make-up on a model with dark skin. Take a before and after photo use these to evaluate your work. Ask the model for feedback as well.

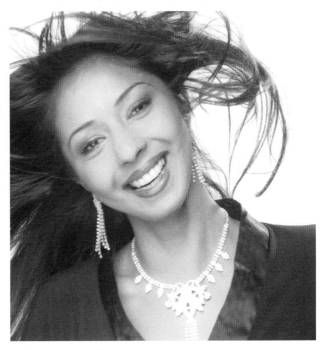

Indian Asian make-up

Make-up for mature models

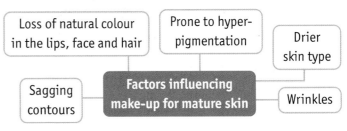

When applying make-up to mature skins it is important to be very gentle and avoid dragging the skin tissue.

Foundation and powder

* Using a pre-base product can often temporarily reduce eye bags or temporarily lift and tighten the skin. One such product is Clarins Beauty Flash Balm, which can temporarily tighten the skin's contours and smooth the skin if applied before foundation.

* Hyper-pigmentation can be concealed with a concealer one to two shades lighter than the skin tone.

* Use a cream foundation that will help to nourish a drier skin type.

* Ensure the foundation does not settle in lines and wrinkles by blending carefully and using a tapping motion over the surface.

* Keep the base matt; shimmery products can accentuate skin imperfections.

Powder

* Make sure your face powder is matt, silky, fine and light. Product technology is developing all the time.

* Apply just the lightest dusting of powder on the centre of the face (not around the eyes, where lines are all too easily emphasised).

Contouring

* Sagging jaw lines, double chins and hooded eyes can be reduced with the use of contouring make-up.

Blusher

* Cream blushers work well on dry, mature skin types. Apply cream blush over foundation and then lightly dust on face powder. A touch of powder blush can be applied on top for added definition.

* Generally, more natural colours such as peaches, corals and soft pinks are an excellent choice.

Eyes

* Grey eyebrows can be strengthened using pencil or powder in slate or taupe. Eyebrow tinting could be offered as a more permanent option.

* Matt finishes are more flattering than shimmer, which can accentuate the crepey skin texture of mature eyes.

* Subtle colours work best, but the eyes will benefit from some definition. Shades of brown (avoid red undertones), grey, khaki, soft pinks, mauves and peaches are a good choice.

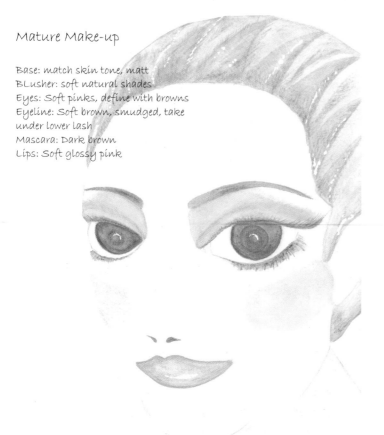

Mature Make-up

Base: match skin tone, matt
Blusher: soft natural shades
Eyes: Soft pinks, define with browns
Eyeline: Soft brown, smudged, take under lower lash
Mascara: Dark brown
Lips: Soft glossy pink

Design sheet for mature make-up by Julia Conway

* Do not over-highlight the frontal bone (brow bone) as this can accentuate a 'hooded' eye shape.

* When applying eye make-up you may need to lift the brow to remove creases from the eyelids to ensure an even application of shadow and eyeliner. Use multi-directional brush strokes to ensure all the tiny creases are filled with colour.

* Eyeliner is useful for defining the eyes, but make sure the effect is soft and smoky rather than hard and harsh.

* Define sparse eyelashes with dark brown or charcoal rather than black mascara, which can look too harsh. White or grey eyelashes often benefit from eyelash tinting.

Lips

* To avoid feathering, line the mouth with a lip pencil and apply foundation and powder over the outer lip area.

* Soft, slightly glossy colours for lips look best in natural tones.

* A strong red lipstick with white or grey hair pulled back from the face can look very classy, but it does not suit everyone and requires strong bone structure to carry it off.

Straight corrective make-up for male models

Foundation

A straight make-up on a male model should look completely natural on camera or on screen. The type of base that is used will depend on the condition of the model's skin and the amount of coverage required, but should always be applied sparingly. If the skin is in good condition all that may be required is a tinted moisturiser and a little concealer. If the condition of the skin dictates more coverage, it should only be applied to areas that really require it and be perfectly blended for an invisible finish. Do not forget the ears, or they will look very red on film or screen. Try applying bases with a natural sea sponge – this tends to give a lighter application. Mattifying pre-base products are useful to reduce surface shine.

Concealing

When carrying out straight corrective make-up application on men, you are not aiming to conceal 100 per cent of their imperfections. Rather, leaving 30 to 40 per cent of these flaws will create a more natural effect and retain a face's masculinity. It is the job of the make-up artist to be selective about which imperfections to conceal, but it is generally accepted that *completely* removing eye shadows and beard line will feminise the face. Therefore, it is usually more appropriate to *reduce* very dark shadows in these areas and concentrate on completely concealing unattractive skin blemishes, shaving cuts, etc., which will look unsightly on camera.

Using an orange-toned concealer prior to the application of foundation can reduce a heavy beard line on a man. However, concealing the beard shadow completely will feminise a man's face and should be avoided.

Powder

Powder should be applied as usual, but used particularly sparingly in the beard line. Never apply with a cotton pad or you will get fibres stuck to the skin's surface.

Eyebrows

To tidy brows they should be brushed through and any gaps should be filled with colour to match the natural brow. Sparse brows can also be strengthened in this manner. A clear mascara can be used to hold the brows in place.

Eyes

Male models with very blond lashes may benefit from a light coating of brown mascara.

Blusher

If a male model looks pale or washed out, the addition of a natural-coloured blush (bronzers work well) may help to brighten the complexion. It is important that the placement is correct to avoid feminising the features. The correct area of application is below the apple of the cheek, sitting just under the cheekbone towards the centre of the face.

Lips

A touch of clear lip balm helps to give the lips a healthy gleam.

Hairlines

Thinning hairlines can be corrected with various products.

Most professional male models and performers will be accustomed to wearing make-up. However, sometimes you may be required to apply make-up on members of the general public for television interviews, etc. In these cases tact and diplomacy may be required to encourage them to have products applied.

> **HANDS ON**
>
> Carry out a straight, corrective make-up on a male model. Aim to make him look healthy and attractive but completely natural.

Make-up applied on a male model

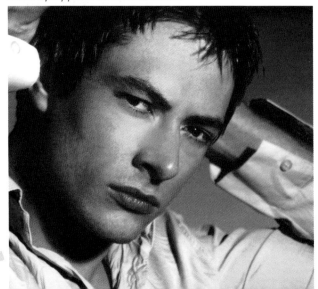

Make-up for children

If you are asked to apply make-up on children, it is important that the finished effect is kept very natural. Most children will not require much make-up – perhaps a little powder and cream blush if they are naturally pale. Remember that children's skin is generally more sensitive than adults', so try to ensure you use non-irritating, preferably hypo-allergenic products, and always follow stringent hygienic precautions.

Order of application for straight make-up procedures

1 Sterilise the equipment.
2 Sanitise the working area and set up a working station.
3 Wash your hands.
4 Protect the client's hair with a headband, net or sectioning clip as appropriate. Protect the client's clothes.
5 Carry out a cleansing routine if the client is wearing make-up. Tone and moisturise.
6 Analyse the client's skin type and note any areas that require correction, for example blemishes, face shape, features.
7 Discuss and agree the make-up plan with the client, stylist or photographer.
8 Apply foundation.
9 Conceal all blemishes and complete any corrective work necessary.
10 Apply crème or liquid blush at this stage of the make-up if appropriate.
11 Set the make-up with loose powder.
12 Apply highlighter and shader to contour the face if required. Crème contouring products are applied before the loose powder.
13 Apply blusher in the correct position according to the face shape and desired effect.
14 Brush through the eyebrows. Create the desired eyebrow shape using fine, feathery strokes with a pencil or shadow.

15 Apply the eye shadow.

16 Apply eyeliner if required. If using a pencil, ensure it is freshly sharpened.

17 Apply mascara.

18 Outline the lips with a freshly sharpened pencil to create the desired shape correcting any irregularities in shape, then fill with colour using a lip brush. Blot on a tissue, lightly powder and repeat the application. Alternatively, apply a lip sealer. Finish with a gloss if required.

19 Stand back from the client and check all areas of the make-up.

20 Make any necessary adjustments.

The above procedure is a guideline. When creating high fashion make-up, some stages may be omitted and extra stages added, for example the addition of glitter, iridescent liquid to the foundation, jewels, etc. **Additional media** can also be used to complement the overall design plan.

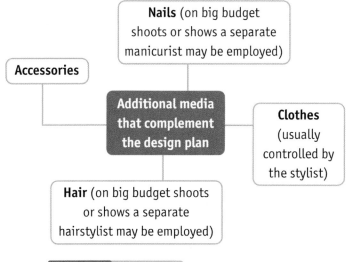

KEY NOTE

When working on location in hot and humid climates it is necessary to give careful consideration to the types of products you select. A general rule is that powder-based products will perform best under these conditions as crème make-up may melt and slide on the skin's surface. Never attempt to blot perspiration with powder – it will just 'cake' and ruin the make-up application. Always blot moisture with a tissue first.

REMEMBER

* Never use your fingers to decant products. Always gain the model's permission before using sanitised fingertips during make-up application.

* Keep your working area tidy and uncluttered at all times. Ensure waste products are immediately placed into the bin.

* Always use a powder puff or tissue when lightly resting your hand on the client's face.

* Always replace lids and close palettes immediately after use.

* Always use sanitised brushes and puffs.

* Dispose of sponges after use.

* Sharpen pencils before use to sanitise.

* Never blow on your brushes to remove excess powder. Instead, gently tap your brush on the edge of the workstation: any excess will drop from the brush.

Design principles when creating fashion and photographic images

So far in this chapter, we have looked at a how to apply make-up to create a number of different looks such as minimal, neutral, glamorous, etc. However, much of the work you will undertake as a creative make-up artist will rarely be this straightforward. Instead, you will be required to rely on your understanding of design principles to create new and exciting images. For every design you undertake you will be considering the basic elements of shape, texture and colour, and within these elements you must also consider the following design principles.

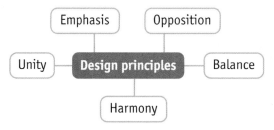

* **Emphasis** is the main focus of the design. Sometimes a design will have one area of emphasis, whilst on other designs there may be several areas of equal importance.

* **Harmony** describes visually pleasing elements of a design.
* **Unity** describes how the individual elements of a design work as a complete image.
* **Opposition** is based on contrasting visual elements with the design, for example light and shade, matt and iridescent, etc.
* **Balance** describes the visual emphasis and importance of two opposite parts of the design, for example the top and bottom half of the face and both sides of the face. This principle has been discussed in detail on page 00. All design should have a good sense of balance, however, this does not necessarily involve symmetry. Sometimes exciting imagery results from exploring asymmetrical balance.

HANDS ON

Developing and creating a design for a photographic shoot

This activity is intended to take you through the process of creating hair and make-up designs for photographic shoots. In addition to the information in this chapter, you will need to ensure you have read the section 'Contributing to the design process' in Chapter 6 (page 113). You will gain the most benefit from the exercise if you work as part of a team. Try to team up with a photographer, model and stylist to undertake the brief together. If you are at college, try approaching other departments to recruit fellow students. You can set your own budget for the project, but this must be done at the beginning of the activity and noted in the design plan.

Research the theme or concept

Carry out some research to ensure your design will meet the requirements of the brief. Begin by researching the magazine in question to establish their preferred style of imagery. You will find it to be very different from those found in magazines such as *Vogue* whose images tend to be more commercial. Then research images of birds of paradise and begin to gather thoughts on how this research may formulate into a make-up and hair design. If you are using additional media you may have to research where they can be obtained.

Develop a design plan

Next, create a design plan that contains the following information.

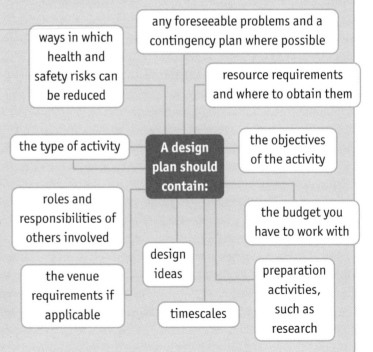

Identify the theme or concept of the photo shoot
⬇
Research the theme or concept
⬇
Develop a design plan
⬇
Create the design
⬇
Solve any problems that may occur
⬇
Evaluate the final design and make-up application

Stages of developing a design for a photographic shoot

A design plan should contain:
- ways in which health and safety risks can be reduced
- any foreseeable problems and a contingency plan where possible
- resource requirements and where to obtain them
- the type of activity
- the objectives of the activity
- roles and responsibilities of others involved
- the budget you have to work with
- the venue requirements if applicable
- design ideas
- timescales
- preparation activities, such as research

Identify the theme or concept for the photo shoot

You are working for a client who wants to create a set of avant-garde images for the magazine *Dazed and Confused*. The styling of the image is to be based on the theme 'Birds of Paradise'.

Create the design

Depending on the hair and make-up design you decide to create, you must consider the most suitable techniques to achieve the desired result and employ them effectively. You will also need to consider the choice of model carefully: their natural colouring and general appearance will naturally have an impact on the final result.

Problem Solving

Sometimes, problems occur even when careful planning has taken place. You may have to adapt your make-up design or product selection to the changing circumstance. If so, remain calm and professional and remember to keep others informed of your changes and concerns.

Evaluate the final design and make-up application

Once you have carried out this activity, you should evaluate your own performance and the finished image. You will also need to collect feedback from a number of people on the impact of the images. This is important if you are going to get maximum benefit from this exercise and improve your performance in the future. Feedback can be collected from the following sources:

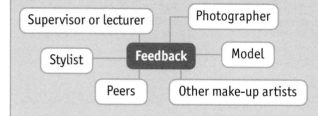

Try to assess and collect information about the following aspects of your work:
* your interpretation of the theme or concept
* the success of the finished result in comparison with your objectives
* the artistic quality of your work
* areas for improvement.

Most of the feedback you receive will be verbal, but it may be useful to make notes for future reference. Sometimes it is difficult to hear negative comments about your work, but as long as the feedback takes the form of constructive advice, this is an essential part of your professional development from which you will learn much.

You should also reflect on your design plan.
* Did you meet your objectives?
* Did the team carry out their roles and responsibilities effectively?
* Did you manage to stay within the set budget? Any overspending must be fully justified.
* Were you missing any resources on the shoot?
* Did any problems arise that you did not foresee?

Once the evaluation process is complete you should have identified clear opportunities for improvement in the future.

Knowledge Check

1 What type of foundation should be used on:

   a dry skin types?

   b oily skin types?

2 What is the function of foundation in make-up?

3 How are dark circles under the eyes hidden on:

   a dark skin tones?

   b light skin tones?

4 What are the drawbacks of using a shimmer base or powder?

5 What is 'ghosting' or 'flash back'?

6 Draw an illustration to show how you would contour

   a a round face shape

   b a square face shape

   c a long nose

   d a double chin.

7 When should crème blusher be applied in the make-up procedure?

8 Draw an illustration to show how you would contour

   a deep set eyes

   b close set eyes

   c small eyes.

9 Should dark, matt colours or light, glossy colours be used on small, thin lips?

10 What is the function of lip liner?

11 Why do we carry out a trial run for bridal make-up?

12 List the considerations when applying make-up to a mature model.

13 How could you conceal a heavy beard shadow on a male model?

14 List the main principles of design.

15 Why is it important to evaluate your work and whom could you ask for feedback?

Cosmetic camouflage

Cosmetic camouflage make-up refers to the art of concealing or disguising unwanted or undesirable 'marks' or disfigurements on the surface of the skin using specialised products. The aim is to create as natural a finish as possible. Clients with disfigurements can receive huge psychological benefit from using camouflage techniques. Types of conditions that may require treatment are: birthmarks, pigmentation disorders, scars, burns, varicose veins, tattoos and bruising. As a practitioner in cosmetic camouflage, you could find yourself working in hospitals or private clinics, in beauty salons, for the Red Cross, for St. John Ambulance or as a mobile freelance practitioner.

Aim and objectives

Aim of this chapter: to provide the underpinning knowledge and skills required to carry out a cosmetic camouflage procedure.

You should achieve the following **objectives:**

* Consult with the client and other involved people and organisations
* Discuss various conditions that may require camouflage application
* Plan the camouflage application
* Prepare the client and room for the camouflage application
* Select appropriate camouflage products, discussing types and availability

* Prepare the area to be camouflaged
* Apply camouflage products to restore skin colouration
* Instruct and advise the client in camouflage application and aftercare
* Discuss facial prosthetics and the work of maxillo-facial technicians
* Acquire knowledge of related anatomy and physiology.

To help you proceed through this chapter, re-read and familiarise yourself with sections from other chapters on the following:

* your responsibilities under health and safety legislation (Chapter 2, page 14)
* standards of hygiene and principles for avoiding cross-infection (Chapter 2, page 23)
* positioning of clients and correct posture when working (Chapter 2, page 26)
* the importance of keeping record cards (Chapter 2, page 30)
* the Data Protection Act (Chapter 2, page 31)
* disposing of waste (Chapter 2, page 16)
* contra-indications and contra-actions (Chapter 2, page 29)
* the importance of completing procedures in given time schedules (Chapter 3, page 00)
* communication and consultation techniques (Chapter 3, page 35)
* preparation of the client – maintaining client modesty and privacy (Chapter 3, page 39)
* colour theory (Chapter 5, page 70)

Client consultation

Clients will include men and women of all ages, and sometimes children. The one thing they will have in common is a desire to be helped to conceal a blemish or disfigurement. According to research, 30 to 40 per cent of adults and 75 per cent of children who have skin abnormalities will suffer from psychological problems. This often leads to a loss of self-esteem resulting in a withdrawal from social and working lifestyles. The use of camouflage techniques can be very successful in restoring a sense of confidence and acceptance within the community. The camouflage practitioner needs to be aware of the varying needs of individual clients and this is best achieved through a thorough consultation process.

Considerations when treating male clients

* They may be more inhibited than female clients.
* They may be more comfortable being treated in environments not traditionally associated with women, for example hospitals and clinics rather than beauty salons.
* They may feel uncomfortable if camouflage products are referred to as 'make-up'.
* They will require a totally natural finish.
* They may require more time to learn self-application techniques.

Considerations when treating female clients

* They may be less inhibited than male clients.
* They may be more concerned and embarrassed about their appearance than male clients.
* They may be more familiar with applying products to the skin and therefore more confident in self-application.

Considerations when treating children

* It is important to ensure they are not made to feel their disfigurement is unattractive or unacceptable or you may end up drawing their attention to the problem. After all, it will usually be the parents that have referred the child for treatment.
* They may be affected by peer pressure.
* Depending on the child's age, it will usually be the parent who is taught the application techniques.
* They will require a totally natural finish.

During the consultation

The following personal qualities are required of a camouflage practitioner.

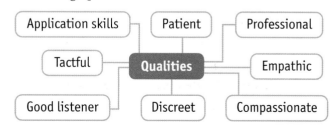

When you first meet your client it is important to allow plenty of time for the consultation. The client may feel embarrassed or anxious so it is important he or she does not feel rushed at any point. Creating a professional and relaxed environment is essential to allow the client to feel comfortable. It is also important to maintain the client's modesty and privacy at all times.

It may take some time to build a rapport with the client, but with time, patience and an empathic approach, most clients will be happy to discuss their problem. Never assume you know the reason for the client's referral. Always allow the client to tell you what that problem is or you may inadvertently cause further distress by pointing out a blemish that did not concern them rather than the actual cause for concern (which may initially be hidden beneath their clothes).

You should maintain a polite and friendly approach using effective non-verbal and verbal communication techniques, as discussed in Chapter 3 (page 35). You will need to discuss or consider the following points during the consultation process, using standard techniques of questioning, visual and manual examination and referring to existing client records and correspondence. It is important to show you are listening closely and to respond to the information in a sensitive manner.

1 Will you need to keep the client's source of referral informed of the treatment outcome? Clients may be referred to you from a number of sources:
   * hospital consultants (primarily dermatologists and plastic surgeons)
   * burns units
   * private clinics
   * GPs
   * the clients themselves
   * counsellors.

2 What are the client's camouflage needs? Remember, never assume but wait to be told.

3 Do you require medical permission before carrying out any treatment, for example when camouflaging moles? If in doubt it is best to obtain permission.

4 Are there any contra-indications present? Some conditions will require medical referral whilst others will restrict camouflage application.

5 Gather relevant medical information from the client that may affect treatment, for example find out if they are undergoing any medical treatment for the condition.

6 Gather information on current lifestyle, for example, how much time the client has to apply camouflage products in the morning. Does the client have an active lifestyle or particular hobbies, for example swimming, that will affect application techniques?

7 Does the client appear very nervous and anxious? How will you establish a rapport with the client that will make him or her feel more at ease?

8 Has the client had or used camouflage products before? This will help to establish what level of tuition will be required for self-application techniques?

9 Discuss and agree the treatment procedure and camouflage application plan. Will the client need to be shown self-application techniques or is the area to be treated inaccessible – in which case, will another person have to be shown?

10 Does the client have realistic expectations about the treatment? If not, then it is important to be honest and clearly explain the limits of the treatment.

11 What is the condition of the skin in the area to be treated? Some blemishes, such as scars and varicose veins, are sensitive to touch.

During the consultation it is important to make a written record of the information you have collected. This is best done on a client record or treatment card, which is then signed and dated by the client and yourself. This record card is kept in a paper or data-based filing system in line with the Data Protection Act 1998.

Record cards are important for camouflage procedures because:

* they act as a reference point for future appointments
* they contain important information about the client's background and history
* they act as a record of treatments you perform and their outcomes
* they act as a record of products used
* they act as proof that professional procedures have been followed in case of disputes and insurance claims – any correspondence should be attached to the card, for example medical letters.

have a record of all the information that has been collated, which has been signed and dated by both the client and the practitioner

At the end of the consultation the practitioner should:

be clear about the client's needs and requirements

be satisfied that it is safe to go ahead with the treatment

have realistic expectations of the treatment

feel his or her needs and concerns have been heard

At the end of the consultation the client should:

feel confident in the practitioner's ability to carry out the treatment

be assured that any information given during the consultation will be kept confidential

Treating clients with disfigurements

Initially, you may find treating scarred or disfigured clients difficult and you may feel out of your depth, embarrassed and worried about saying the wrong thing. You may also find it difficult to touch the affected area. However, if your clients sense your unease they will leave feeling resentful and awkward and will probably not return.

Many people make assumptions about people with disfigurements and this affects how they behave or think they ought to behave. For example, when treating a person with facial paralysis many people will assume they also have some sort of mental impairment and may shout or speak slowly to them.

The 'scared' syndrome

The charity Changing Faces suggests that on first meeting a client with a disfigurement a pattern of behaviour may emerge based on both parties feeling 'scared'.

A person with a disfigurement may	The camouflage practitioner may
S be **s**elf conscious	**S** **s**tare, be **s**ympathetic or **s**hocked
C feel **c**onspicuous	**C** be **c**urious
A feel **a**lone, **a**ngry, **a**nxious	**A** make **a**ssumptions
R feel **r**ejected	**R** **r**ecoil or feel **r**epelled
E feel **e**mbarrassed	**E** feel **e**mbarrassed
D feel **d**epressed or **d**ifferent	**D** feel **d**istressed

By extending the practitioner's communication skills, this pattern can be avoided and first meetings made more comfortable for both the client and practitioner. Important points to remember are:

* maintaining eye contact without staring
* not finishing the client's sentences if their speech is impaired
* not jumping to conclusions
* being supportive but not patronising
* ensuring your body language is welcoming.

Further information on providing good customer service for people who have facial disfigurements or unusual appearances can be obtained from the charity Changing Faces.

Liaising with other parties

As a camouflage practitioner you will often be required to liaise with a variety of other professional people and organisations when planning or carrying out treatments. It is important to be able to liaise with these parties in a professional and appropriate manner, and it is useful to keep copies of standard letters that can be used when contacting them.

Address
Date

Dear *(name of potential client)*

Thank you for your recent enquiry regarding the cosmetic camouflage service. The aim of the service is to temporarily restore the skin's appearance to normality with simple but effective camouflage techniques using specialised camouflage products. Treatable skin conditions include:

- minor skin blemishes and pigmentation disorders
- congenital disfigurements
- conditions resulting from trauma
- surgical procedures
- birthmarks
- tattoos.

A successful consultation will enable the client to carry out the treatment himself or herself after instruction and advice from a qualified practitioner. Prices for this service range from £** to £** and are confirmed on application.

I hope this information may prove useful and look forward to hearing from you again.

Yours sincerely

(Name of practitioner)

Example of a standard letter in response to an enquiry

Address
Date

Dear *(name of doctor)*

Re: *(name, date of birth and address of client)*

Following a consultation on *(date of appointment)* with the above patient for cosmetic camouflage treatment, I am writing to ask for permission to treat *(type of skin condition)* on the patient's *(area of body)*. The aim of the treatment is to temporarily restore the skin's appearance to normality with simple but effective camouflage techniques using specialised camouflage products.

I would be grateful if you could forward permission in writing for my records. If you require any further information, please do not hesitate to contact me.

Yours sincerely

(Name of practitioner)

Example of a standard letter asking permission to treat a client

HANDS ON

Researching useful sources

It will be useful to keep a reference file of organisations that can advise you and your clients.
To make a start, contact the following and ask them to send out some information:

* Changing Faces (produces excellent information about the psychology of facial disfigurement)
* Let's Face It (facial disfigurement)
* Raft (Restoration of Appearance and Function Trust)
* National Lichen Sclerosis Support Group
* Scar Information Service
* Cica-Care (treatment for scars)
* Vitiligo Society
* British Association of Skin Camouflage.

Conditions suitable for cosmetic camouflage

Skin conditions suitable for camouflage fall into three main categories: congenital, acquired and those resulting from trauma. Below is a list of some of the more common conditions and disorders Further details about these conditions can be found in Chapter 4, page 58):

* birthmarks
* chloasma
* vitiligo
* moles (with medical permission)
* port wine stain
* strawberry mark
* dilated capillaries (thread veins)
* varicose veins
* psoriasis
* non-infected acne vulgaris or acne rosacea
* pigmentation stains, for example from perfume or sun damage

* scars
* burns
* bruising
* tattoos
* post-operative trauma.

Term	Description	Example
Hypo-pigmentation	Loss of colour	Vitiligo, old scar tissue
Hyper-pigmentation	Increase in colour	Chloasma, port wine stain
Erythema	Reddening of the skin	Psoriasis, acne rosacea

Camouflage can be very effective in restoring the colouration of the affected area to that of the surrounding skin tone. Excellent results can be achieved when working on many of the above conditions if the skin in the affected area suffers from one of the three general visual colourations:

Camouflage application can prove less effective when in addition to the change in colour there is a change in texture. An example of this can be found when treating scars, where the skin is often indented or raised (as in keloid scars). In these cases, the condition can be much improved with camouflage application techniques, but the client should be informed of the treatment's limitations.

Depending on the area to be treated and requirements of the client, you may need to consider the following.

* If the condition appears on the face, you may need to leave additional time to teach straight make-up skills. You may also be required to apply minor prosthetics (false eyelashes for example) and the camouflage make-up will probably be applied by the client on a daily basis.

* Conditions appearing on body areas may be inaccessible to the client and therefore application techniques may need to be taught to a friend or relative.

* Waterproofing the make-up may be required if the client is active or sporty.

* The make-up may only be required for special occasions.

* Hairy areas may require the treatment to be modified.

* In any of these cases clients may require further additional consultations for winter or summer because of changes in the skin tone.

KEY NOTE

Camouflage products should never be applied on open skin lesions, unhealed scar tissue, infectious skin conditions or sore and tender areas.

Camouflage products

When covering up skin conditions and disfigurements it is essential that the correct products are used to produce optimum results. Ordinary foundations and concealers, even those that promote themselves as having excellent coverage qualities, will not be sufficiently opaque to cover up areas requiring camouflage and prevent the discolouration from 'bleeding back' through the application. Skin camouflage products are specially formulated to cover skin conditions and disfigurements; they are not the standard 'concealing' products that a number of high street cosmetic companies sell to conceal minor skin blemishes. Camouflage creams differ from ordinary cosmetics because they possess the following qualities.

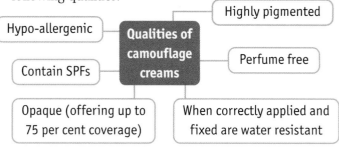

There are a number of ranges on the market, each available in a vast array of colours ensuring accurate skin matching is possible. Each brand has its own distinct texture, quality and consistency, and choice is down to personal preference. An increasing number of these are available on NHS or private prescriptions. Most of the brands listed below are available through mail order, chemists or specialised retail outlets.

Brand	Available on NHS prescription?	Notes
Covermark	Yes	Provides day-long cover SPF 15
Dermablend	Yes	SPF 15 Lasts 24 hours when applied correctly; easier to blend when a thin layer of moisturiser is applied first
Dermacolor	Yes (excluding fixing spray)	SPF 15 Lasts 24 hours when applied correctly; water-resistant when powdered
Keromask	Yes	Minimum of SPF Lasts for eight hours Not tested on animals
Veil	Yes	Sun protection from UVA and UVB Lasts 24 hours when applied correctly; tends to 'slide' on the skin in high temperatures and humidity, but is easy to blend on a drier skin type

Other brands include:

* Ben Nye
* Cinema Secrets
* Grimas Camouflage Make-up
* Jane Iredale Cosmetics
* Couvrance

* John Van G
* Matis
* Rita Roberts
* Screen Face
* Elizabeth Arden (Scar Cover)
* Clinique (Continuous Coverage Make-up).

> **KEY NOTE**
>
> Products should be stored in a cool, dry place when not in use.

> **REMEMBER**
>
> Ensure hygienic procedures are followed when decanting camouflage products. Always use sterile spatulas, never your fingers. Ensure you have a clean palette to work from when working on a client.

Most product ranges include a setting powder and recommend that it should be used along with the camouflage creams to ensure proper setting of the products. However, in my experience, any good quality powder normally does the job equally well. When choosing a powder look for the following features.

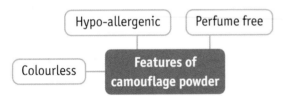

Some brands also manufacture **fixing sprays** that help to further set and waterproof the camouflage application. They are useful for returning a slight sheen to the skin, giving a totally natural finish.

Titanium dioxide and 'ghosting' or 'flash back'

Many products contain titanium dioxide and iron oxides. These are used in powders to reflect UV light and prevent photosensitive reactions. They are also used to give camouflage creams their opaqueness. These ingredients have two disadvantages.

When photographed (particularly when using flash light), these ingredients can cause 'whitening' and a pale, white bloom may be visible on the skin in the photographic image. This is known in the trade as 'flash back' or 'ghosting'. If you know your work may be photographed it is important to use products free of these ingredients.

When used on some skin tones (particularly black) these ingredients can give a greyness to the camouflaged area.

Durability of products

Most manufacturers state that their products, if set properly, will last on the skin between eight and 24 hours. However, certain factors will affect the durability of the application.

Factors affecting durability of camouflage application	Notes
Client's skin type	An oily skin type may cause crème-based products to 'slide'. Wiping the area with a skin toner prior to application may help.
Client's lifestyle (work and leisure activities)	Strenuous activities causing perspiration may cause the same problem as above. Although waterproofed applications should stay on through activities such as swimming, durability may be decreased.
Area of the body to be camouflaged	Some areas of the body are prone to rubbing and friction and this will reduce the lifespan of the application.
Care of application	Clients must be encouraged to follow aftercare advice. Any oil-based products will remove the application. When drying the area of application, the client should blot rather than rub.
Environmental conditions	Excessive heat and humidity may reduce the application's durability.

Removing camouflage products

As camouflage products are water-resistant once set properly, it will take more than water to remove them. The easiest method of removing them from the skin is to 'dissolve' them in an oil-based, non-irritating cleanser. Camouflage applications on the face should be removed daily; products on large areas of the body, which are time-consuming to apply, may be left on for a couple of days.

Planning and preparing for the camouflage application

Preparing the work area

It is important to ensure the area you are working in provides a comfortable and welcoming environment for your client.

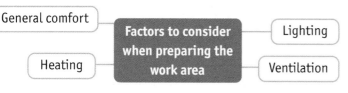

As with all make-up procedures, a good light source is essential for accurate skin tone matching. The type of light source should match the light in which the final camouflage application will be viewed – usually natural daylight. Other light sources give off colour casts that could adversely affect the skin matching process:

* tungsten (incandescent) lighting gives off a yellow colour cast
* fluorescent lighting gives off a green colour cast.

Preparing the client

It is important to ensure your client is comfortable and relaxed during the consultation and treatment.

Preparation of practitioner

It is important for the camouflage practitioner to be fully prepared for the treatment so that he or she comes across as professional and organised.

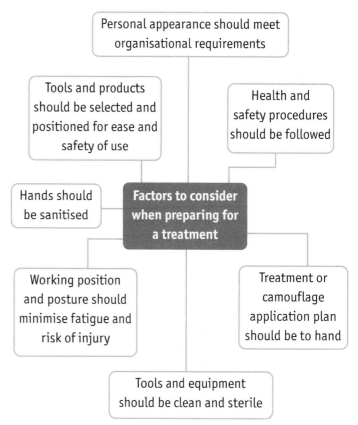

Neutralising colours

When attempting to neutralise predominant skin colours you will need to refer to the complementary colour rule.

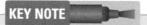
KEY NOTE

The technique of applying a layer of neutralising colour is only performed if skin matching alone will be insufficient to cover predominant colours.

The client should be facing the light source with no shadows over the area to be treated

The client should be positioned to avoid discomfort and injury

Factors to consider when preparing the client

The client's clothes and hair should be protected from products

The client should be checked for contra-indications

The client should undergo a full consultation on the first visit and a record card must be signed before treatment commences

Neutralising hyper-pigmentation

When covering skin areas that are hyper-pigmented you should begin by studying the colours that appear within the area. Once you have decided on the dominant colours you must then take steps to neutralise them prior to matching the area to the surrounding skin tone. It is important to look carefully at the colours you are trying to neutralise. Colours in the hyper-pigmented skin will not normally be in a true 'primary state'; they are more likely to be subtle mixes of secondary or tertiary colours. For example, a purpley-red will need to be covered by a mixture of yellow and green.

* To cancel out blue in the skin, apply a layer of muted orange camouflage cream.
* To cancel out purple in the skin, apply a layer of muted yellow camouflage cream.
* To cancel out green in the skin, apply a layer of rose (red, its true complementary, would be difficult to cover with the skin tone) camouflage cream.
* To cancel out yellow-orange in the skin, apply a pale lilac camouflage cream.
* To cancel dark brown areas on light skins, apply a layer of white camouflage cream mixed with a little of the matching skin tone crème mix.
* To cancel dark pigmented areas on black skins, apply a layer of muted orange camouflage cream.

For dark skin tones the orange can be mixed with a little of the matching skin tone crème mix to dull down the intensity of the orange.

Neutralising hypo-pigmentation

Apply a layer of muted yellow-orange (the darker the skin the more orange) prior to skin matching. When covering conditions where there is a complete loss of pigmentation, such as vitiligo, you can take the colour over the edges of the area – this will help to soften the demarcation line. Self-tanning products can also prove very effective on hypo-pigmented areas.

Neutralising erythema

To cancel out red in the skin, apply a layer of olive-green camouflage cream (a pure green would make the area look grey).

Once the neutralising layer has been applied, powder, blot with damp cotton pads and wait for ten minutes for the colour to settle. If the original colour is 'bleeding through', a further layer may be required, though this is not necessarily applied over the entire area. When you are happy that the skin colour has been successfully neutralised you can then skin match.

Skin colour matching

All skin tones originate from three basic colour mixes:

* yellow-brown (made up of a mixture of orange and green)
* red-brown (made up of violet and orange)
* olive-brown (made up of violet and green).

All skin tones are variations of these mixes.

* Sallow skin tones originate from the yellow-brown mix.
* Ruddy skin tones originate from the red-brown mix
* Olive skin tones originate from the blue-brown mix.

Begin by studying the skin tone – what colours can you see? Now look at your camouflage crème colour range and place a small amount of the colours that closely match the skin onto your palette (you may find it useful to hold your camouflage palette to the skin to help you decide). Working on a small area of the skin, near to but not on the treatment area, apply a little of the skin match colour. Blend the colour. If it matches the skin tone exactly and there are no visible demarcation lines, you can proceed to mix enough of the colour to cover the treatment area and then continue to camouflage the problem area. If the colour does not match the skin tone exactly, then make adjustments to the colour mix until the correct colour is achieved. This may require lightening or darkening the colour or changing the underlying tone, for example adding more yellow, pink, orange or olive.

Do not make the colour mix too complicated. Remember your client will have to buy each colour you use and eventually mix the colours himself or herself. Aim to achieve a correct skin match with a maximum of three colours.

Once the skin match has been applied, powder, blot with damp cotton pads and wait for ten minutes for the colour to settle. If the first layer has not fully camouflaged the area, a further layer may be required, though this is not necessarily applied over the entire area. Remember it is more effective to apply a few thin layers than one thick one. Indeed, applying several fine layers with a sea sponge results in a more realistic texture than trying to fully camouflage with a single blocked layer of colour. Remember to make a note of the colours and ratios of the mix. Once a successful skin match has been applied, you may then move onto the final stage of 'faking faults'.

The art of faking faults

Once a true colour match to the surrounding skin tone has been achieved, the practitioner or client needs to add normal variations in skin pigmentation to the camouflaged area to make the skin look real. This is called 'flesh impact'. Most skins have blemishes and areas of uneven pigmentation of some kind whether it be freckles or a beard shadow, dilated capillaries, moles, visible veins, etc. An area of skin missing these natural 'blemishes' will look distinctly strange and at odds with the surrounding skin tone. It is therefore necessary to fake these blemishes, a process known as 'faking faults'.

Faking faults can be achieved using a number of techniques. Fine stipple sponges or natural sea sponges are useful tools for applying texture and mottled colour. They are especially useful for re-creating the appearance of dilated capillaries. Freckles and moles can be painted on using a fine brush or the end of an orange stick. Veins can also be painted on.

Observe the surrounding skin tissue and try to recreate what you see. With careful observation and imagination, most 'faults' can be 'faked'. Be careful not to create the 'faults' in a uniform pattern – nature is rarely so ordered.

Covering a tattoo

As a camouflage practitioner, clients may come to you for advice on how to cover an unwanted tattoo. This may be for a special occasion, a wedding for example, or because the client no longer wishes the tattoo to be visible on a day-to-day basis.

As a media make-up artist you may be required to cover up a tattoo for a production. Permanent tattoos have become increasingly popular over the last decade, and more and more artistes and models, both male and female, are seen wearing them. However, a tattoo may not always be appropriate to the character or role they are portraying and it will therefore require covering for the duration of a production or photo shoot.

When covering a tattoo, using a skin tone match on its own over the design is usually insufficient to block out the strong colours found in most tattoos.

Many tattoos have intricate designs made up of a variety of colours that would be too time-consuming to cover in parts. Instead, go for the predominant colours and cover larger blocks of area, following the complementary rule. To cancel out black in a tattoo apply a layer of off-white camouflage cream.

Camouflaging scars

Scars are one of the more difficult conditions to camouflage for a variety of reasons.

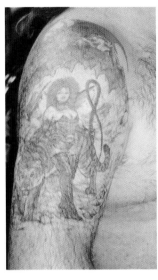

A tattoo

* Skin may be new and shiny making the products 'slide' and not fix to the surface. Applying a mattifying product over the skin prior to using camouflage products may help to reduce this problem.

* Skin tissue may be indented or raised making the area difficult to camouflage completely.

* Skin may possess a different texture to the surrounding area and appear puckered or loose.

* Skin may be sensitive to touch.

* Skin may change as the scar heals, making regular appointments necessary.

Although pigmentation in a scar can usually be treated successfully, camouflaging an indented or raised scar has limited success. The technique that can be used is based on the theory of light and shade: shading an area will make it recede, whilst highlighting an area will bring it forward.

To camouflage an indented scar apply a shade of camouflage crème one to two shades lighter than the skin tone to the inside edge of the scar (this area will look naturally darker than the surrounding skin).

To camouflage a raised scar apply a shade of camouflage crème slightly darker than the skin tone to the raised edge of the scar (this area will look naturally lighter than the surrounding skin).

The client and practitioner will have to decide whether the result of using the above technique is worth the extra time involved when applied on a daily basis.

Teaching clients to apply camouflage products

Almost all of your clients will require tuition in self-application of the camouflage products as most will want to apply them every day. It is important to remember this when carrying out the camouflage application. Several steps should be taken to ensure the clients leave confident in the knowledge they can perform the procedure themselves.

* Give the client a mirror so he or she can watch what you are doing throughout the procedure.

* Explain what you are doing at each stage of the procedure.

* Keep the application as simple as possible, using as few colours as possible.

* Give the client a list of the colours used and a sample of the skin match mix, so the client can compare this with his or her own attempt at home.

* Ensure you provide the client with comprehensive homecare advice, including information on where to obtain the products. You may wish to consider creating a standard advice sheet containing useful tips for self-application and homecare to give to your clients at the end of the consultation.

* Always check the client's understanding of the process and ability to apply camouflage products before he or she leaves.

STEP-BY-STEP   Applying camouflage

Equipment required

* Cleanser
* Cotton buds
* Brushes, sponges, stipple sponges or natural sea sponges
* Toner
* Velour powder puffs
* Moisturiser
* Tissues
* Mirror (hand held)
* A selection of camouflage products
* Water spray

* Record card or referral letter
* Spatulas
* Clips for hair
* Small containers for samples
* Damp cotton wool pads
* Gown or towel to protect clothes
* Client advice sheet

You may also need extra items to meet an individual's needs, for example false lashes.

1 Cleanse and wipe the area with cotton wool soaked in toner to remove surface oil. Apply a thin layer of moisturiser if required.

2 Study the area to be treated. Note the predominant colours. If neutralisation is required, block out using a thin layer of the complementary-coloured camouflage cream. If neutralisation is not required go to Step 4.

3 Set with powder using a velour powder puff and wait a few minutes before brushing off any excess powder. Blot with damp cotton wool pads and leave for ten minutes to see if any original skin colour 'bleeds through'. If this is the case, add another thin layer and set as above.

4 Whilst you are waiting for the neutralising layers to set, begin to mix up a colour that matches the surrounding skin tone. Try to keep the mix as simple as possible for future reference.

5 Apply, using a brush or sponge, a thin layer of skin tone matching camouflage cream. Blend to avoid any hard edges.

6 Set with powder and wait a few minutes before brushing off any excess powder. Apply further layers as required, making sure you set and wait a few minutes between each layer.

7 Carefully note any blemishes and pigmentation changes in the surrounding skin tone and 'fake some faults'. Set with powder and wait a few minutes before brushing off any excess powder.

8 Spray the area lightly with water and blot dry with a tissue. This eliminates the 'powdery' look to the skin and helps to maintain 'flesh impact'.

9 An optional final stage is to apply a fixing spray.

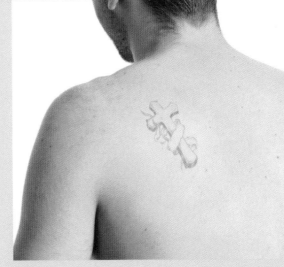

Before

Ensure the work area is kept in a clean and tidy condition through the procedure and that wastage of products is kept to a minimum. Remember to make a record of the specific colour and products used, describing how you mixed and applied the products. If the client suffers a contra-action, act promptly following the usual recommendations (refer to Chapter 2, page 30).

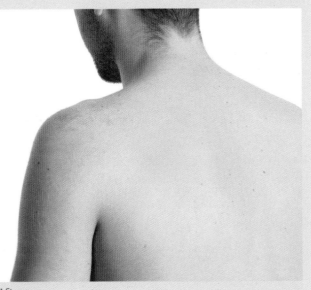

After

KEY NOTE

Camouflage application using airbrushing techniques and products has become very popular recently. Airbrush products are ideal for camouflage because they are water resistant, have longevity and are smudge proof. Sealers can be sprayed over the colour products to waterproof the area. As airbrush products are matt, cosmetic grade oils are available to restore a natural sheen to the skin. Further information about airbrushing can be found in Chapter 16 (page 374).

Aftercare advice

You should inform the client of the following aftercare points.

* The do's and don'ts to avoid premature removal of the products:
  * Do not use any oil-based products on the camouflaged area.
  * Do not use any soaps or shower gels on the camouflaged area.
  * The camouflage make-up is water-resistant (waterproof in some cases), but will need to be gently patted dry with a towel. Rubbing may dislodge the make-up.
* How to remove the products:
  * Gently massage the area with a cleansing cream (preferably oil-based).
  * Wipe off with damp cotton wool.
  * Tone the area with a light astringent.
  * Apply a skin moisturiser if required.
* Recommended frequency of re-application (daily on facial areas, up to a couple of days on body areas).
* Sources of further information.

It is good practice to write to clients confirming outcomes of the consultation.

Address
Date

Dear *(name of client)*

Following our successful camouflage consultation on *(date of appointment)*, I can now recommend the following products for home use:

(list of camouflage products and quantity required)
(ratio of colour mixes).

Apply the products as explained during the consultation and described on the advice sheet attached. If you have any problems do not hesitate to contact me on the above telephone number.

I have forwarded my recommendations to your GP as the above products are all prescribable.

Yours sincerely

(Name of practitioner)

Example of a standard letter to a client following an appointment

You will often be required to write to other contacts such as doctors following camouflage application.

Below is an example of a standard letter.

Address
Date

Dear *(name of doctor)*

Re: *(name, date of birth and address of client)*

Following a successful consultation on *(date of appointment)*, with the above patient for cosmetic camouflage treatment, I am now in a position to recommend the following products for home use, which are available on prescription.

(list of camouflage products and quantity required).

If you require any further information, please do not hesitate to contact me.

Yours sincerely

(Name of practitioner)

Example of a standard letter following an appointment with a referral

Clients with prostheses

As a camouflage practitioner, you may come across clients who wear prostheses. A prosthesis is an artificial appliance, usually made of silicone rubber, that replaces the human form. Examples are:

* artificial limbs
* artificial breasts
* wigs
* dental prostheses
* artificial eyes, noses, ears, etc.

Facial prostheses are made and fitted by a maxillo-facial technician. These technicians are trained in both medicine and dentistry and are highly skilled in creating realistic-looking prostheses for the face. If a client removes a prosthesis during the consultation it is important not to look embarrassed or shocked.

Additional cosmetic techniques

As a camouflage practitioner, there are a number of additional minor cosmetic techniques that you could offer your client:

* manicures to distract from disfigurements on the hand
* false lash application for clients who have sparse or missing lashes
* make-up techniques to correct lip lines, apply eyebrows, etc.

Knowledge Check

1 List three sources of client referral for cosmetic camouflage treatment.

2 List four personal qualities required of a cosmetic camouflage practitioner.

3 List three requirements of camouflage products.

4 List two brand names available on NHS prescription.

5 How would you neutralise blue in the skin?

6 How would you neutralise a purpley-red colour in the skin?

7 List three difficulties in camouflaging scars.

8 Describe how you would set camouflage crèmes.

9 List four skin conditions you may be asked to camouflage.

10 What disadvantages does titanium dioxide have?

11 Describe how you would advise a client to remove a camouflage application.

12 Why is it important to keep a record card?

13 How would you ensure you avoided cross-infection between clients?

14 What would you do if a client suffered a contra-action?

Further information regarding skin camouflage and possible career routes in this specialist area can be obtained from:

British Association of Skin Camouflage
P O Box 202
C/o Resources for Business
South Park Road
Macclesfield
Cheshire
SK11 6FP

Changing Faces is a national charity that supports and represents people with facial disfigurements. For information and advice, contact:

Changing Faces
Tel: 0845 4500 275
Email: info@changingfaces.co.uk
Website: www.changingfaces.co.uk

Techniques for creating special effects

The question the make-up artist should be asking is 'Do I really need to use special effects for this make-up?' Invariably the simplest option is often the most preferable in terms of cost, time and comfort of the model. However, having said this, special effect make-up does have an important role to play. It can:

* assist the portrayal of particular characters
* be visually exciting to an increasingly demanding audience
* create realistic dramatic effects
* create unrealistic dramatic effects.

Aim and objectives

Aim of this chapter: to provide the underpinning knowledge and skills to design and create a variety of special effects with make-up, safely and effectively.

You should achieve the following **objectives:**

* List and explain the use of products and equipment used in common make-up special effects
* Use the products and equipment safely, effectively and in a cost-efficient manner
* Prepare the performer for a safe and comfortable make-up application
* Block out eyebrows
* Change features using putty or wax

* Apply ready-made prosthetics and blend with the surrounding area
* Make, fit and apply colour to bald caps
* Dress, apply and maintain facial hairpieces
* 'Lay on' loose hair
* Create a variety of casualty effects using direct-applied make-up
* Remove products and effects safely.

Equipment and products

In addition to the equipment described in the previous chapter required for basic and fashion make-up application, there are many more products to explore in the art of special effects. Many companies specialise in manufacturing products for the make-up artist. These products come and go, are updated and improved, are renamed and re-launched, and are often sold under various pseudonyms. This can often lead to confusion for the training or newly qualified artist.

Generally speaking, most of the products available will fall into one of the following categories.

Product	Properties and uses	Examples of products currently available
Prosthetics	Can be made from latex, rubber, gelatine or foam latex. Applied to the skin using adhesives in order to change the appearance. Effects can be subtle or dramatic.	Ready-made prosthetics are widely available in all shapes and sizes. For a truly professional fit or for more unusual pieces, prosthetics can be made to measure.
Lace facial	Human or yak hair is knotted onto lace that can then be adhered to the skin using adhesives. Various shapes and styles are available in a variety of colours.	Ready-made pieces are widely available in all shapes, colours and sizes. For a truly professional fit or for more unusual pieces, pieces can be made to measure.
Crepe hair	Sold in braided form to give it a curl. Can also be straightened using a steam iron. Applied directly to the skin to 'lay on' hair. Can also be sewn into bald caps.	Widely available in varying lengths and colours.
Skin adhesives	Glue suitable for use on the skin. Available in varying strengths. Mainly used to fix lace pieces, loose hair and prosthetics in place. Water-based adhesives are available for sensitive skins, but these tend not to have the strength of others. Spirit gum (also known as Mastix), prosthetic adhesive (often latex based) and medical adhesives (silicone based) are stronger in this order, offering superb adhesion with the skin.	A vast array of products is available from each of the major manufacturers. Examples include Pros-Aide (prosthetic adhesive) and Telesis (silicone adhesive). Choice is down to personal preference and specified use.
Adhesive removers	Designed to remove or thin adhesives. Ensures skin and appliances are effectively cleaned of adhesive. Always use the right remover for the adhesive used.	Examples include MME (Mild Mastix Remover), Pro-clean, Ben Nye Bond-Off, Mavidon
Grease paint / crème make-up	To provide colour on the skin or over a prosthesis. Natural or fantasy colours available. Water-in-oil consistency. Applied directly, does not require water. Available in either 'stick' or 'compact' packaging. Some manufacturers sell 'palettes' or 'colour wheels' containing colours for specific use, e.g. bruise wheels, beard cover, old age, beard stubble.	Kryolan Supracolour, Grimas Crème Make-up, Ben Nye Crème FX Wheels.

Product	Properties and uses	Examples of products currently available
Cake make-up	To provide a coloured base on the skin. Natural or fantasy colours available. Also available in metallic, iridescent or UV. High powder content. Applied with a damp sponge. Usually found in 'compact' packaging.	Otherwise sold as Pancake – widely produced by all manufacturers.
Water paints	To provide colour on the skin or over a prosthesis. Natural or fantasy colours available. Also available in metallic, iridescent or UV. Mix with water and apply with a sponge or brush. 'Compact' colours require water to be added, but are also sold in pre-mixed bottles that can be applied directly.	Kryolan Aquacolour, Fardel Liquid Colours.
Prosthetic make-up	Special make-up to add colour to latex and foam pieces. Usually very 'oily' in texture but provide excellent coverage. Not suitable for use directly on the skin. Natural or fantasy colours available. Available in 'kit form'.	RCMA Appliance Foundations, Kryolan Rubber Mask Grease Paint, PAX (Cinema Secrets). Works on both prosthetic pieces and skin. It is less oily and heavy than traditional prosthetic make-ups and easier to use.
Silicone paints	Exciting, new make-up product used to colour and paint prosthetics and the skin. Gives an incredible 'flesh-like' translucent appearance. Covers tattoos, colours foam latex, gelatine, plastic and silicone appliances. Can also be used to add colour to hair.	Reel Creations, Temptu Pro and Premiere Products (Skin Illustrator) manufacture a number of palettes.
Moulding wax and putty	Used for build-ups and moulding features, e.g. noses, warts, swellings, etc. Usually sold as putty or wax and often in varying consistencies, e.g. soft or firm. Also available in clear or coloured form.	A variety of waxes and putties are available. Choice is dependent on preference of texture and budget.
Eyebrow plastic	A very firm wax used to block out the eyebrows. If unavailable it is possible to use a thin slither of a firmly textured moulding wax.	Widely available.
Sealer	Used to 'seal' moulding putty or wax prior to the application of make-up. Can also be used on its own to cover sparse eyebrows.	Widely available.
Liquid latex	The most useful and widely used product in the art of special effects with a number of uses, e.g. to mould noses and bald caps, for build-ups (many casualty effects can be created from latex). Thickened latex can be used to hide joins between a prosthesis and the skin. 'Old Age Stipple' is diluted latex, often coloured, which can be used around the eyes to create an ageing effect. Latex can trigger severe allergic reactions in some people.	Widely available.
Bald caps	Used to cover hair giving the appearance of a bald head. Can be made from latex, rubber or plastic.	Widely available.

Product	Properties and uses	Examples of products currently available
	Using plastic has the advantage of being able to 'melt' the edges using acetone, providing an ultra-fine join with the skin. Hair can be added to the bald cap if required – useful for giving the appearance of alopecia.	
Bald cap plastics	A liquid plastic used by make-up artists to make bald caps.	Available in thick or thin formulas. DBA Cap Plastic and Glatzan L are a couple of examples.
Collodian	A clear liquid which, when painted onto the skin, contracts creating the illusion of 'contracted' scar tissue. Can cause skin reactions.	Widely available.
Scar material	Used to create the illusion of raised or incised scar tissue, depending on the product and its application.	Tuplast via Kryolan. RCMA also have scar material.
Tear stick	Used by actors to bring tears to the eyes. A menthyl stick applied directly around the eyes (only a small amount is usually required).	Widely available.
Fake blood	A vast array of non-toxic blood products are on the market. Some are more staining on the skin and clothes than others. Running blood is usually available in light and dark. Congealed blood is also available along with 'wound filler' to fill open wounds. A special product for use in the eyes is 'Eye Blood'. 'Fix Blood' creates dried blood on the skin. Blood can come premixed or in powder form.	Widely available. Think about the effect you want to create and choose the most suitable product from the vast array on the market.
Tooth enamel	Use to discolour the teeth. Never to be used on capped teeth. Available in a variety of colours, the most popular being black to give the illusion of missing teeth, and 'nicotine' to create stained teeth. Also available in gold and silver.	Widely available.
Glycerine and gelatine	Once mixed and heated these can be used in the simulation of scars, burns, lumps, blisters, etc. Glycerine on its own mixed with water is useful for creating sweat on the skin. Gelatine can also be used to mould a prosthesis.	Sold separately but often available in convenient mixtures ready for heating – Gelglyk is an example of this.

There are hundreds of products available on the market today, and their quality is constantly improving. Each make-up artist will have a different list of 'favourite products' from the next. Experience at handling different brands and products will eventually result in your own list of 'favourites'.

Try not to stay with one particular brand – you will often find that your favourite moulding wax will be a different brand to your favourite water-based make-up – and listen to your colleagues, who will be able to recommend products they have used. Always keep up-to-date with new products on the market and try them out – don't just take the advertisers at their word.

Your budget will obviously have a say in what products you choose to keep in your kit or purchase for a job. You generally get what you pay for, but remember that the best is not necessarily the most expensive. It is also important to use the products economically.

Always turn up to jobs with products that have earned your trust. Trying out a new product during production is asking for trouble and may prove to be an expensive mistake.

REMEMBER

There are serious health and safety implications when using many of the products listed above. Refer back to Chapter 2 (page 18) for a reminder about COSHH regulations and remember to follow manufacturers' instructions for use and storage.

It is always a good idea to give product allergy checks to any model you intend to treat with special effect materials. This should be done well ahead of when you actually intend to use the materials so alternatives can be found if tests are found to be positive. Remember it is always better to be safe than sorry. People can suffer extreme allergic reactions to products such as latex. Finally, always record the details of any tests you carry out. Can you remember why? If not refer back to Chapter 2 (page 30).

HANDS ON

Researching suppliers

- Research outlets that supply make-up products for special effects.
- Ask them to send you an up-to-date price list and order form.
- You can then create a 'resource' file, which will be useful when sourcing products and equipment for jobs and re-stocking your kit.

Preparing the model and maintaining a safe working environment

The following considerations should be taken into account when preparing a model for special effect make-up.

- ✱ The materials chosen must be safe for use on the skin and appropriate to the performer's skin type, the area of skin, the role, the effect to be achieved and the cost requirements.

- ✱ The model may be required to sit in the make-up chair for lengthy periods of time so thought should be given to the position of the model to minimise personal discomfort.

- ✱ The model's hair and clothing must be protected sufficiently.

- ✱ A good relationship should be maintained at all times to ensure the performer's continuing co-operation.

- ✱ Communication is essential and the model should be kept informed of the make-up application process at each stage.

- ✱ Materials must be used as directed, all the manufacturer's guidelines must be observed and contact with the inside of the eye should be avoided.

- ✱ Hygiene precautions should be followed to avoid cross-contamination.

- ✱ The skin should be prepared for application according to the type of contact material to be used and the skin type of the model. This will usually begin with a cleanse, tone and light application of moisturiser that is blotted or powdered to ensure there is no residue on the skin's surface. If harsh products are being used or the skin type is sensitive, a thin layer of barrier cream is advisable. This layer should then be powdered.

- ✱ Do not forget to carry out skin tests to establish allergies and sensitivity to products.

KEY NOTE

Should any disruption in the make-up process take place, for example an unexpected skin reaction or disintegration of the make-up during shooting, it is important to make the make-up supervisor or production manager aware of the circumstances as soon as possible.

Always keep accurate records of methods and processes used to allow future replication and ensure continuity in a production.

We will now look at how we can put these products to good use.

Blocking out eyebrows

This is a useful technique used by make-up artists when the natural eyebrow needs to be hidden or re-defined in a different position. Sometimes just part of the brow requires blocking; at other times the entire length needs taking out. This technique is often used in 1920s period make-up, ballet and dance, or when you wish to make the face look less human.

STEP-BY-STEP | **Blocking out eyebrows using wax and sealer**

Equipment required

* Eyebrow brush
* Wax or eyebrow plastic
* Vaseline
* Spatula or modelling tool
* Sealer
* Powder
* Camouflage cream in the appropriate colour
* Make-up as appropriate

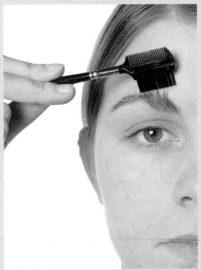

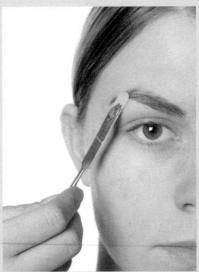

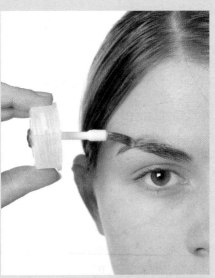

1 Cleanse and tone the area to remove any surface oil, dirt and make-up. Comb the eyebrows up and outwards in order to flatten the natural brow as much as possible. This is particularly important with thick or heavy brows.

2 Place a small amount of wax or eyebrow plastic onto a palette. Use a spatula to manipulate the wax until it has softened slightly. Using the edge of the spatula or modelling tool apply the wax over the eyebrow, keeping the wax as flat and thin as possible – this will prevent cracking later on. Use a little vaseline or lubricating jelly on a finger-tip to smooth the applied wax. Try to avoid getting too much wax on the surrounding skin but make sure you trap the hairs at the outside edge.

3 Brush sealer across the wax and when completely dry, apply make-up.

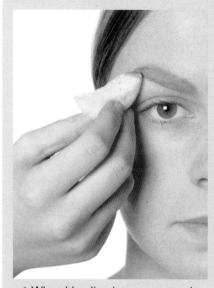

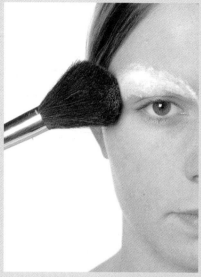

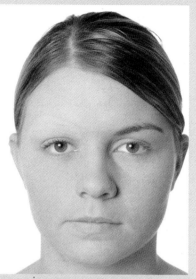

4 When blending into any natural skin tone, first apply a pink base. This 'kills' (hides) any darkness caused by the underlying hair. Camouflage make-up has the best coverage. Make sure you keep the pink to areas of darkness only. It may not be necessary at all on blonde hair.

5 Apply a light dusting of powder.

6 Apply a layer of make-up to match the surrounding skin tone. Remember to powder between additional layers of cream-based make-up.

If you are creating a fantasy effect, you can simply apply the chosen make-up medium over the blocked out area.
The wax and sealer can be removed with surgical spirit.

KEY NOTE

If redrawing eyebrows in a different position, paint them in rather than using a pencil. A pencil will dislodge the soft wax underneath and spoil the effect. Paint will simply glide over the made-up surface and create a smooth finish. Remember you are creating an illusion – the eyebrows you paint on will detract from the blocked out area.

HANDS ON

Following the step-by-step demonstration, block out the natural eyebrows on a model. Take a photograph of your work as a record.

Evaluation

Study your work carefully and make a list of the aspects of the blocked out eyebrow you are pleased with and the aspects you think could be improved. Then state how you will make these improvements next time. To help you, the table on the next page lists common problems and ways of avoiding them in the future.

Common problems	Troubleshooting
Applied the wax too thickly to the natural brow	Use the edge of a spatula or a modelling tool to apply the wax. Press quite firmly but check you are not causing any discomfort to the model.
Took the application of wax too far over the edge of the natural brow.	Be more careful in your application. Use the natural brow as your guideline.
Make-up difficult to apply over covered eyebrow – wax and sealer started to dislodge during application .	Make sure the sealer is thoroughly dry before applying make-up. Use a stippling action when applying make-up with a sponge to this area. Do not drag the area. Alternatively use a brush with a light touch
Make-up has not covered brow sufficiently	Have you used the pink base to hide any darkness prior to applying a skin tone match? Make sure you powder between every layer of crème make-up applied.

KEY NOTE

If the eyebrows are sparse or fine then 'soaping' the eyebrows alone may be sufficient to block them out. If this is the case, soak a bar of soap in hot water and use your spatula to apply the soap. The soap dries and hardens quite quickly. Sealer may be applied afterwards.

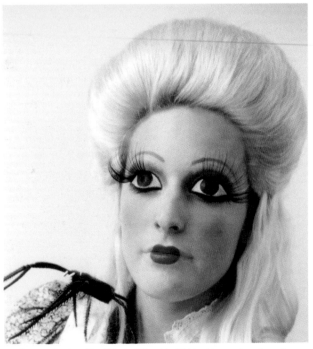

Make-up design for 'Little Miss Muffet' – the natural eyebrow has been blocked out and re-drawn in a new position

Changing the features with wax or putty

This is a useful technique used by make-up artists when the natural features need to be changed. The most common use of this technique is to make minor changes to the shape of the nose. Because of the weight of putty and wax, any major changes to facial features would be better attempted with the application of pre-formed prosthetic pieces.

Working with wax or putty is the first step to character building and opens up the world of prosthetics. It is important to become familiar with the moulding medium – there are many brands of wax and putty to choose from and textures vary from firm to soft. Choice of moulding material will once again be down to personal preference, budget and suitability to the task at hand.

STEP-BY-STEP | Changing the shape of the nose using wax or putty

Equipment required

* Research material
* Cleanser, toner and moisturiser
* Spirit gum or medical adhesive
* Wax or putty
* Vaseline or other lubricating jelly
* Spatula or modelling tool
* Sealer
* Powder
* Camouflage cream in the appropriate colour
* Make-up as appropriate

Research the shape of the nose you want to create (this may include sketches). Have your design or reference material to hand.

1 Apply a barrier cream and powder thoroughly. Apply spirit gum or medical adhesive. Cotton wool fibres placed in this can help adhesion. Allow the spirit gum to become tacky before proceeding. (Some make-up artists use a slither of wax over the area to adhere to instead.)

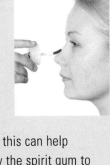

2 Build up the shape with wax or putty. A small amount of Vaseline or lubricating jelly rubbed into your fingers will stop the wax adhering to your fingers. It will also help you to blend the wax, therefore giving you more control. If the wax is particularly hard prior to application, warm a small amount in your hands. Use both your fingers and modelling tool to shape. Blend the edges finely – there should be no obvious demarcation line. Check the nose shape from all angles.

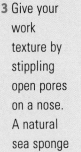

3 Give your work texture by stippling open pores on a nose. A natural sea sponge is useful for this.

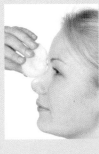

4 A sealer (Pros-aide works well) may then be applied prior to make-up application. Take the application slightly onto the skin surface.

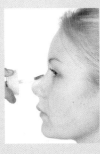

5 Powder well, pressing into the edges.

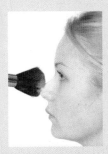

6 Apply colour to the putty or wax using your chosen medium. The putty or wax can be covered with any medium – foundation, watercolour, cream make-up, camouflage, etc. The new nose shape is now complete.

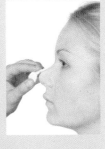

To remove the wax or putty it should be lifted gently from the skin. Any residue can be removed with surgical spirit.

HANDS ON

Following the step-by-step demonstration, change the natural shape of your model's nose. Take a photograph of your work as a record.

Evaluation

Make a list of the successful and unsuccessful aspects of your work. Think about how you could improve the finished result. Below is a troubleshooting table listing common problems and their causes.

Common problems	Troubleshooting
The nose moves and lifts off the face during facial expression.	The wax or putty was taken too high over the bridge of the nose. Facial expressions such as frowning, etc. will cause movement in this area and will dislodge the moulding material.
The wax or putty is not staying on the nose at all.	Did you apply adhesive first and wait for it to become tacky before applying the moulding material? Try applying a slither of wax over the adhesive and building the nose in stages.
	Is the final shape of the nose too large? Remember that the weight of the putty or wax makes it inappropriate for very large nose shapes.
Make-up is difficult to apply over the wax or putty.	Make sure the sealer is thoroughly dry before applying make-up. Use a stippling action when applying make-up with a sponge to this area. Do not drag the area. Alternatively, use a brush with a light touch. Try not to let the wax or putty spread beyond the area you are attempting to

change the shape of. You can use a little surgical spirit to clean up any residue wax or putty from the surrounding area.

Make-up has not covered the wax or putty sufficiently.	Have you used the pink base to hide any darkness prior to applying a matching skin tone?
	Make sure you powder between every layer of make-up you apply if you are using cream-based make-up.
The wax or putty is difficult to work with.	If you are working in a warm environment, a firmer textured wax or putty is the preferable moulding material. A softer textured option would become very sticky and difficult to work with. If the wax or putty is cold and very hard, warm it in your hand before you start to work with it and use Vaseline to help smooth whilst working.

KEY NOTE

To save time the make-up artist could mould the desired nose shape onto a plaster life cast of the artiste (see Chapter 16 for further details) prior to the call time. The nose area of the life-cast would be covered with a tissue and the moulding material applied and sculpted on top. To remove from the cast, the tissue is peeled off the cast and then off the base of the nose. The sculpted piece is then transferred onto the artiste's actual nose, adhered in the usual way and blended away at the edges before being coloured.

Colouring wax, putty or prosthetics

If you are blending into a natural skin tone, it is best to stipple colour onto the prosthetic piece. A sea sponge or 'stipple sponge' is useful for achieving this. Stippling the colour on results in 'breaking up' the colour. If several colours are layered in this way the prosthetic will take on a very natural appearance, mimicking natural skin which is also a mixture of tones rather than a single flat colour. Remember to powder between layers of cream-based make-up.

Before attempting to match the prosthetic to the surrounding skin colour, first apply a pink (rose) base. Camouflage has the best coverage of the

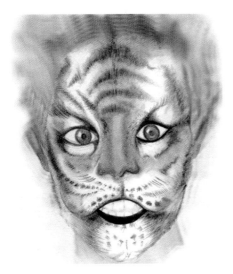

Worksheet for make-up applying a ready-made prosthetic piece by Julia Conway

cream-based make-ups (Dermacolor D32 or Veil 'Rose' are both excellent camouflage colours for this purpose.) This colour 'kills' (hides) any darkness caused by the prosthetic piece and simulates the colour of a blood supply, missing from a prosthetic piece but apparent in skin, giving the area a more organic appearance.

If you are creating a fantasy effect, you can simply apply the chosen make-up medium over the area. Many types can be used and your choice will depend on the desired result. Water-based paints, cream-based make-up, camouflage make-up, prosthetic make-up, silicone paints and airbrushed paints are all suitable for covering sealed wax or putty.

On prosthetics many types can be used and your choice will depend on the desired result. Water-based paints, cream-based make-up, camouflage

make-up and prosthetic make-up are all suitable for covering prostheses. On prosthetics Many make-up artists prefer to thin these make-ups with 99 per cent alcohol and apply them in washes. Silicone paints, tattoo inks and airbrush paints are all very popular in industry, as they are translucent by nature and can be applied over the prosthesis creating realistic skin effects.

In television and film, most appliances are tinted a base flesh colour then painted. Pieces can be pre-painted prior to application, which means the model has to spend less time in the make-up chair. In this case, the pieces should be fixed using an appropriate make-up sealer to improve durability and resist damage.

The application of ready-made prosthetics

Your make-ups can be made more life-like and three-dimensional by first applying a prosthetic piece. There are many ready-made pieces to choose from such as noses, eyepieces, animal faces and ears. These may be formed from various products, the most common being foam latex, gelatine, foaming gelatine or silicone.

When you have designed your make-up on your worksheet you must then choose a suitable prosthetic piece. For example, to begin with you may choose an upper lip piece to recreate an animal, or you may choose a witch with a nose and chin.

The next step is to set out all the materials needed, together with your design sheet, and you are ready to begin.

KEY NOTE

* Opaque lets no light through.
* Translucent lets some light through.
* Transparent lets all light through.
* Human skin is semi-translucent, falling somewhere
* between opaque and translucent.

STEP-BY-STEP | **Changing the model's features using ready-made prosthetics**

Equipment required

* Research material or worksheet
* Cleanser, toner and non-oily moisturiser
* Tissue or cotton wool to pad out prosthetic piece if required
* White pencil
* Adhesive (spirit gum, Pros-Aide (not on gelatine) or surgical adhesive)
* Make-up for coverage as appropriate

* Damp lint-free cloth or powder puff
* Prosthetic piece
* Appropriate product for blending edges (see below)
* Sealer
* Powder
* Prosthetic edging brush or small spatula

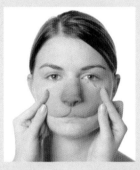

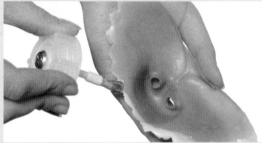

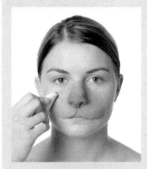

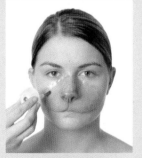

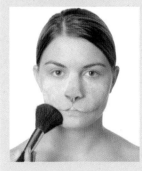

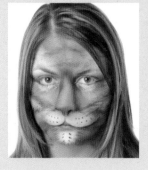

1. Cleanse, tone, apply barrier cream and powder thoroughly. Pad out large latex prosthetic pieces with tissue or cotton wool (avoid cotton wool around the nose as it will tickle your model) so they stay firm.
   Decide where you will stick the piece by holding it in different positions. Mark on a guideline in white pencil.

2. Apply adhesive to a single point on the prosthetic that will act as an anchor point. Do not glue the edges yet but secure the bulk of the piece in place. If applying a nose piece, make sure you line up the nostrils first and stretch the piece up to avoid pleating. Check the position of the prosthetic piece from all angles.

3. Apply adhesive under the edges of the piece (only to the scalloped edges on latex pieces), let it go tacky and then press the piece into place. A damp piece of lint-free cloth, sponge or powder puff is ideal to press any edges that require adhesive into place. Alternatively, roll the end of a brush over the edge. Press firmly until the piece adheres to the skin. It will take a few seconds to adhere, so be patient. Any edges that persistently work loose can be stuck down by applying more adhesive to the area. Pre-made pieces do tend to be a little crude around the edges, which are often scalloped, so they are quite hard to disguise.

4. Disguise prominent edges by blending as described below. For this demonstration a latex piece has been used.
   Seal the piece with Pros-Aide, apply over the prosthetic and immediate surrounding skin. Allow to dry.

5. Powder generously, pressing into the edges.

6. Apply colour to the prosthetic piece with your chosen medium.
   Complete the design.

Type of appliance	Blending edges	Adhesion
Gelatine prosthetic piece	Blend with witch hazel. Apply to the edges with a brush and work as required.	May be glued with a number of adhesives – Pros-Aide, Telesis, even spirit gum if needs be.
Latex prosthetic piece	Use a prosthetic filler and fill upwards from the skin onto the piece. Examples of prosthetic fillers are: Pros-Aide cream adhesive Liquid latex thickened with Cabosil (an agent used with paints, resins and make-up to form a smooth paste. A face mask should be worn when using Cabosil).	Pros-Aide and other prosthetic adhesives work best.
Silicone	When applied correctly, edges can be made undetectable without the use of make-up or ridge fillers.	Pressure-sensitive silicone adhesives, e.g. Telesis, or water-based acrylic adhesives.

HANDS ON

Following the step-by-step demonstration, change the natural shape of your model's features using prosthetics. Take a photograph of your work as a record.

Evaluation

Make a list of the successful and unsuccessful aspects of your work. Think about how you could improve the finished result. On the next page is a troubleshooting table listing common problems that occur when applying prosthetic pieces and their causes.

Common problems	Troubleshooting
The prosthetic piece moves and lifts off the face during facial expression.	The piece was not adhered to the skin sufficiently. Check the skin is cleansed and oil free before the piece is applied. Any oily residue on the skin will act as a barrier and prevent proper adhesion. Ensure the adhesive goes tacky before attempting to secure the piece to the skin. Was the adhesive sufficiently strong? Water-based products, although good for sensitive skins, do not have the strength of other products.
The edges are wrinkled and do not lie flat.	Take your time when securing the piece. Work your way around the piece, pressing the edge into place and ensuring it is flat before moving to the next section. Ready-made pieces are not ideal as they come in a size to fit all and are not specifically made for your model. The 'fit' may be causing problems and wrinkling can occur if the piece is too large.
The edges are not blending with the surrounding skin.	Some ready-made prosthetic pieces have crude edges that are very difficult to blend. Check you are using the correct blending medium. As a last resort use a clever make-up design to help distract the eye from the edges.
Make-up is not covering the prosthetic piece.	Ensure you have sealed the piece. Try using a stippling rather than dragging action if using a sponge. A number of thin layers is always better that one thick application.

* Prosthetic pieces need constant attention. They will lift from the skin when there is constant facial movement.
* Do not cut the edges of the prosthetic piece. The edges are tapered to allow for easier blending into the surrounding skin. Cutting them will leave you with a hard edge that will be difficult to blend.
* It is always better, when you have the experience or contacts and the budget, to cast the model's face and make the prosthetic to fit the model perfectly. This will always look more natural.
* Always consider the comfort of the model. After all, the model is the one who will be wearing the prosthesis, often for many hours at a time. If you are covering the nose, always ensure an adequate airway. Most ready-made prosthetics leave the nostril area uncovered, but do check with your model that he or she can breathe through the nose comfortably.
* A special brush is available from some suppliers that is designed to apply adhesive under the edges of prosthetics. It is angled at 90° to enable easy application. Always clean your brushes immediately after using adhesive.
* Pros-Aide when white is not very sticky. Wait until it goes clear (and very sticky) before attempting adhesion.
* You can overlap prosthetics if required.

REMEMBER

Many of the products used to apply prosthetics could be dangerous if used in a reckless manner. Check the manufacturer's guidelines and demonstration, and take note of COSHH warnings before using any products. Be extra careful when working around the eyes. Remember to carry out and document allergy tests before starting any procedures on a model.

Removing the prosthetic piece

Apply a suitable remover for the adhesive used. By their very nature, adhesives are water- and sweat-resistant and a specialised remover will be required. Use a cotton bud soaked in the remover and gently ease under the edge of the piece. Wait for the remover to do its job, and then gently roll the cotton bud to release the piece from the skin. Slowly and gently work your way around the edge of the piece. Do not pull the prosthetic away as this may damage or tear the skin. Extra care should be taken on areas around the eyes and where hair is present. Once the piece is removed, gently clean the area of any residue adhesive and soothe the skin with a gentle lotion.

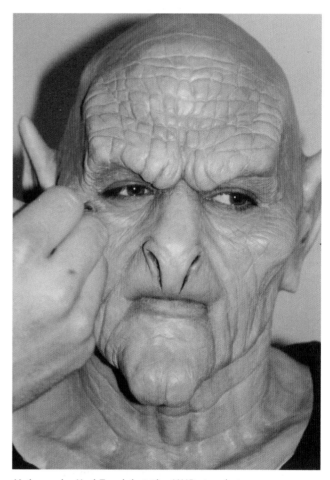

Make-up by Karl Zundel at the MUD stand at the European Make-up Artist trade show

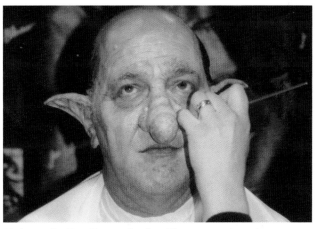

Make-up by Zoe Hay at the Joe Blasco stand at the European Make-up Artist trade show

Adding hair to prosthetics

Hair can be added to prosthetic appliances using a hair punching tool (available from special effects suppliers). This is a time-consuming process but has very realistic effects in the hands of an expert. The technique works well on materials such as latex, foam latex, plastic, gelatine and silicone. The point of the tool is very sharp so great care is required during use.

* Hair is placed across the prosthetic surface where you wish it to be inserted.

* The tool is put across a strand of hair and the hair is pushed into the surface of the prosthesis. It is important to push the tool in the direction that you want the hair to appear to be growing out.

* The tool is withdrawn and the hair should stay in the prosthesis.

* The hair can be glued in place if required, but this is often not required or practical.

With imagination, practise, talent (and big budgets) the possibilities with prosthetics are limitless.

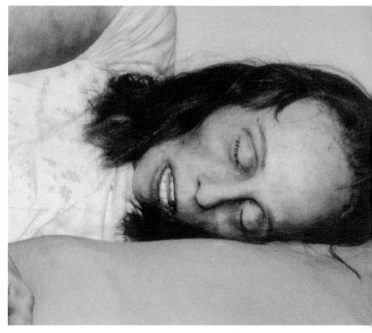

Big budget example of hair punching from the film '28 Days Later'

Bald caps

Bald caps are a very versatile medium to work with. They form the basis of many creative fantasy make-ups. In addition, hair can be added to create the effect of alopecia, which is useful in ageing make-ups.

Almost any colour medium can be applied to the cap to give it colour and texture for example ordinary make-up foundations (well powdered), camouflage make-up (excellent coverage), watercolour, grease-paint, silicone paint, airbrush paints, etc.

STEP-BY-STEP | Measuring and making a bald cap

Equipment required

- ✳ Gel or wax
- ✳ Cling film
- ✳ Wide sellotape
- ✳ Scissors
- ✳ White pencil
- ✳ Black marker pen
- ✳ Head block made of either red plastic (economical) or porcelain (expensive but provides an ultra smooth surface)
- ✳ Vaseline
- ✳ Wax
- ✳ Coarse nail file

- ✳ Powder
- ✳ Liquid cap plastic or glatzan
- ✳ Cap plastic application brush
- ✳ T-Pin (optional)
- ✳ Tissues

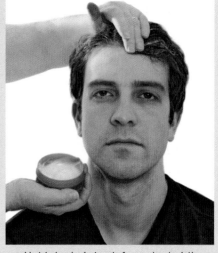

1 Hold the hair back from the hairline with gel or wax.

5 Cut slits across the middle of the ear shape and lift off the model's head.

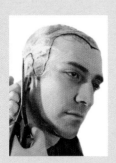

6 Cut around the drawn-on hairline (do not cut out the ear shape).

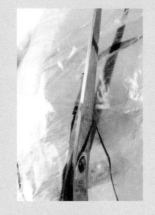

7 Place on a head block. Draw around the cap with a white pencil, leaving a 2 cm excess. Keep it long at the back (this is so when it is stuck down, it is not stuck to the nape hair). You may need to tape the slits across the ear shapes back together to get the accurate hairline. Remove the template from the block.

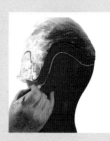

10 Wait for the cap plastic to dry completely and then powder generously ('slapping' the block all over with a loaded powder puff will work well and leave the right amount of powder on the head).

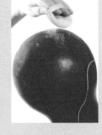

11 Apply the second layer in the same manner, this time working across the pattern from side to side (this increases the strength of the bald cap and reduces the risk of missing bits of the block between strokes). Wait for it to dry completely and then powder generously.

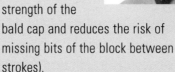

12 Apply the third layer, as the first, this time starting approximately 3 cm inside the front hairline. (This ensures a thin edge on the bald cap for a more realistic application). Wait to dry completely and then powder generously.

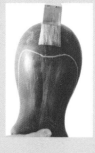

2 Place cling film around the artiste's head, wrapping it over the ears. Make sure the edge of the cling film is well over the hairline.

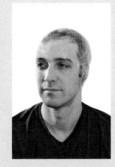

3 Cut lengths of thick sellotape. Place the tape right on the edge of the cling film, tightening the cling film to the shape of the

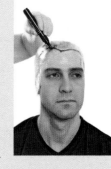

head. Overlap the lengths of tape, working over the entire head and tightening as you go. When you finish, the cap should feel quite stiff.

4 Mark on the hairline in a black marker, going around the base of the ear, but also draw the ear shape in (this makes it easier

to line up on the head block). Keep the hairline long at the back.

8 If using a red head block, file down any ridges or raised areas. If any unevenness remains, apply wax over it, blending the edges well (otherwise your bald cap will be marked by the raised areas). Apply a thin layer of Vaseline over the marked pattern on the block. This acts as a release agent. Blot excess Vaseline with a tissue and powder well.

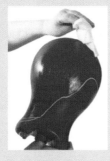

9 Take the cap plastic and pour some into a glass bowl. Apply a thin even coat with a 'bald cap application brush' (if unavailable, a good paintbrush will suffice) from the centre of the front hairline to the nape, going in one direction. Repeat all over the head working within the white pencil line and going from the centre to the sides of the front hairline. **Work quickly and try not to overlap your strokes.** Try to avoid overloading your brush. Try to avoid overloading your brush. Do not let any brush hairs get stuck in the cap plastic as it will ruin the final result.

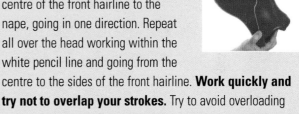

13 Apply the fourth layer as the second layer, starting about 3–4 cm inside the white pencil. Wait for it to dry and then powder generously. Continue for five to eight layers, depending on the thickness of the layers and how thin you want the final bald cap to be. Don't forget to powder between the layers. The last layer should cover the crown of the head only for added strength. Try to leave overnight to dry completely. Clean your brush immediately in acetone.

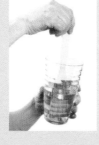

14 To remove the cap from the block, powder well, then start to peel back the edges (a T-Pin can be useful for initially lifting the edge from the block), powdering underneath as the cap is lifted from the block.

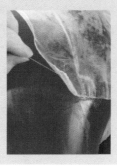

15 When removed, powder well both inside (matt) and outside (shiny). Pack out with tissues and store.

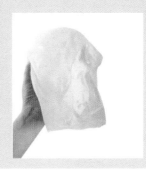

Common problems	Troubleshooting
The cap template is too big or too small for head block.	The head blocks are supplied in different sizes. Measure the circumference of your model's head and use a head block that has a similar circumference.
The completed cap is too short at the back.	It is important to leave extra length at the nape of the neck. It is often advisable to extend the cap plastic application to the base of the head block.
The completed cap is imprinted with ridges and other raised areas.	Do not forget to file the red head and apply wax over any remaining raised areas before applying the liquid plastic. Alternatively, use a porcelain head block.
The completed cap is rough and uneven in thickness.	This could be for a number of reasons. The brush is overloaded with cap plastic causing a thick application and air bubbles. Individual strokes were overlapped as the cap plastic was applied. Strokes were applied too slowly, allowing the cap plastic to begin to dry mid-stroke. This causes a rough, bobbly texture.
The completed cap has holes.	Some parts of the head block were missed during the application of liquid plastic. Ensure you alternate layer direction, i.e. front hairline to nape, then in the next layer side to side.
The cap tears on removal.	Handling of the cap was too rough during removal from the block. The cap should be eased off slowly and carefully. The cap may have been too thin. Next time apply a few more layers.

HANDS ON

Following the step-by-step demonstration, make a customised bald cap for your model. Take a photograph of your work as a record.

Evaluation

Make a list of the successful and unsuccessful aspects of your work. Think about how you could improve the finished result. Opposite is a troubleshooting table listing common problems.

KEY NOTE

Some make-up artists like to use a matt cap plastic for the first layer of application on the head block. This leaves the bald cap with a matt surface which make-up often adheres to better.

The liquid plastic can be coloured before application. Various forms of pigments, for example pancake scrapings, prosthetic paints or specialised pigment powders, can be added to the liquid and mixed thoroughly. The completed result will be a coloured bald cap. The strength of colour will depend on the amount of pigment used. To maintain a semi-translucent appearance, some make-up artists will paint a layer of aqua-colour make-up on a porcelain head block before applying the first layer of matt liquid plastic. When the cap is peeled off it is coloured.

Just like a wig, a bald cap can be repaired. So that it can be reused, a bald cap will sometimes need to have a new edge added around the hairline. This can be achieved by fitting the cap onto a Vaselined and powdered head block. Liquid plastic is then painted onto the front hairline overlapping the existing cap and extending onto the block as required. A couple of layers should suffice.

REMEMBER

* Liquid plastic gives off very strong fumes and therefore should only be used in well-ventilated areas.
* Precautions should be taken to ensure that plastic in its liquid state does not come into contact with the skin as it may cause irritation.

Bald caps are generally thicker for theatre (some can be almost like a swimming cap), and thinner for television or close-up work. They are generally made of plastic, but can also be made from rubber latex. New products are constantly being introduced onto the market and these should be tried and tested by the up-to-date make-up artist. Although ready-made bald caps can be bought from make-up suppliers (at varying cost), they are easy and economical to make. Making your own will also ensure a perfect fit on your model.

Adding hair to a bald cap

Hair can be added to the bald cap to give an appearance of alopecia or other fantasy effects. Human hair, yak hair and crepe hair can all be used for this purpose and can be added in the following ways.

* By inserting the hair into the cap itself. This will give a very realistic effect close-up but can be time consuming. The knotting hook is very sharp and should be used with great care.

1 Take a knotting hook and holder (available from wig suppliers).

2 Take some hair – the amount will depend on the effect you want to create. A finer, more realistic appearance will result from using just a few strands of hair each time.

3 Pick up the hair with the knotting hook and push it through the bald cap.

4 Grasp the hair protruding through the underside of the cap and pull it through until there is enough to stick down with adhesive. Once the cap has been fitted this will not show.

5 Trim the hair to the desired length and style.

* Alternatively, hair can be 'laid' onto the bald cap and glued in place. This is a much cruder way of applying hair to a bald cap but can work well for large theatres, where the result will not be viewed close up.

STEP-BY-STEP | **Fitting a plastic bald cap on a model**

Equipment required

* Plastic bald cap
* Water spray
* Hair gel
* Hairbrush
* Scissors
* Skin adhesive
* Lint-free cloth or damp powder puff
* Acetone
* Tissues or towel
* Cotton buds
* Make-up of your choice

1 Start with a cleansed, toned and lightly moisturised face. Dampen down and gel back the hair from the hairline. With short hair this is very easily done. Long hair should be kept as flat as possible to the head by sectioning the hair down the centre, from the forehead to the nape of the neck, and then swirling the hair around the head in opposite directions. More gel should be applied to help secure or flatten the hair. Hairgrips should never be used under bald caps as they can work loose and pierce through the cap. Ask the artiste to hold the cap at the front with his or her finger while you stretch and manoeuvre the cap into position. The cap should be smooth with no wrinkles.

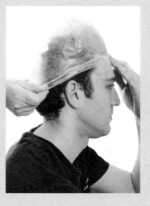

2 Cut around the ear hole just inside the edge of the ear so that the cap tucks behind the ear. Take time getting this right.

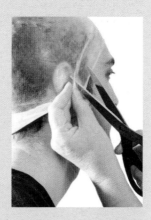

3 The cap is glued down using skin adhesive. Apply to the centre of the forehead first, using the skin adhesive sparingly, then pull the cap down around the ears and secure in the same manner. Use a lint-free cloth or damp powder puff in cap into position. Before gluing the back, ensure the model's head is level to prevent wrinkles.

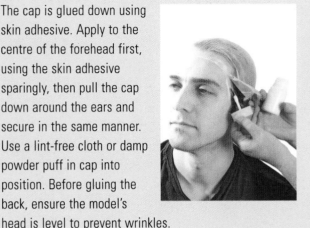

4 Blend the edges of the bald cap with acetone on a cotton bud. Ask the artist to hold a tissue or towel over the face to protect him or her from the risk of dripping acetone. Try to avoid touching the skin directly with the acetone, but keep the application on the edge of the bald cap itself.

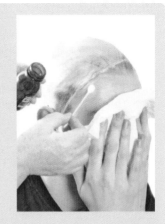

5 The bald cap is now ready to have make-up applied. If you are blending into a natural skin tone, apply a pink (rose) base before matching to the skin tone. This 'kills' (hides) any darkness caused by the underlying hair. Powder generously and dust off excess.

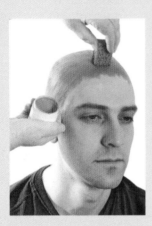

6 Apply a colour matching the skin tone. Powder between the layers of cream-based make-up. The final layer of application should be taken over the cap and face to provide perfect colour matching. For a fantasy effect, you can simply apply the chosen make-up medium over the bald cap and face.

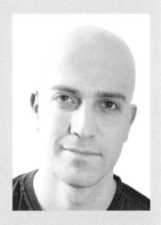

HANDS ON

Following the step-by-step demonstration, fit a plastic bald cap on your model. Take a photograph of your work as a record.

Evaluation

Make a list of the successful and unsuccessful aspects of your work. Think about how you could improve the finished result. Opposite is a troubleshooting table listing common problems.

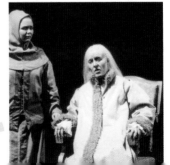

Old age stage make-up for a performer in her twenties is enhanced by the use of a bald cap with hair inserted to give the impression of alopecia

Common problems	Troubleshooting
The bald cap is too big or too small for the model.	The red head blocks are supplied in different sizes. Measure the circumference of your model's head and use a head block that has a similar circumference. Alternatively, make a template of your model's hairline.
The cap looks wrinkled on the head.	Ensure the cap is stretched over the model's head so it fits snugly and the model's head is level before attaching the cap with adhesive.
There is a gap around the ear.	Make sure the ears are lined up before attempting to cut and glue the cap. Make sure you cut just

inside the edge of the marked ear hole. The ear can then be eased through the hole and the edge of the bald cap can be hidden behind the ear itself.

The edge of the bald cap will not disappear.	If the bald cap is made of plastic the cap edge may have been made too thick. The edges of rubber latex bald caps will not blend with acetone, but can be disguised by stippling liquid latex over the edge.

KEY NOTE

Although using acetone is currently the most successful way to blend the edges of a plastic bald cap, there is concern in some areas of the industry about the safety of using such a potent product on the skin. Check the policy of the particular studio you are working for before using acetone on a performer. The risk of irritation can be minimised by ensuring the acetone is applied to the edge of the bald cap and not to the skin itself. All COSHH regulations should be followed.

Removing the bald cap

(Please refer to 'Removing the prosthetic piece', page 220.)

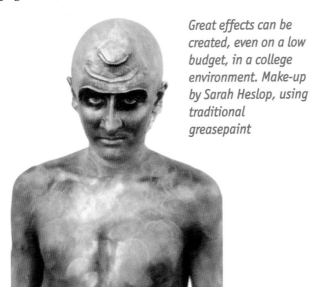

Great effects can be created, even on a low budget, in a college environment. Make-up by Sarah Heslop, using traditional greasepaint

Directly applied casualty make-up effects

Without the use of pre-made prosthetic pieces, directly applied casualty make-up is a frequently used special effect for the make-up artist working in television, film and theatre. There are many different ways to achieve similar effects and all make-up artists will have their own techniques and favourite products to help them achieve the appropriate effects, which may vary from dramatic alterations to minor 'on set' changes. In this section, we will look at the most commonly used effects from minor injuries to more severe effects such as full thickness burns. Remember, you are trying to create an illusion. There is nothing to be gained from overcomplicating a make-up effect if it won't be seen. Use what is appropriate, safe and time effective and do not experiment with new products or techniques on set.

Researching reference material

As with all aspects of your work as a make-up artist, it is important to research all the effects you are trying to create. Medical journals (though not for the squeamish) are an excellent source of reference material. You cannot hope to create realistic effects without fully appreciating what the real thing looks like.

HANDS ON

Researching casualty effects

Start to collect images of real injuries, wounds and skin diseases. In addition, start to collect information about the work of other make-up artists. Trade magazines are a useful resource for this information. Keep all the information you have collected in a reference file.

Understanding the injury when designing the make-up

In order to create realistic effects it is important to understand the injury. There are several questions you should be asking yourself when designing the make-up.

* What caused the injury?
* How old is the injury and how would it heal?
* Is the injured person dead or alive?
* Is the performer male or female? You do not need much casualty make-up on a woman to create a dramatic effect.
* Where is the injury on the body? Wounds should always be in the right place – this goes a long way towards convincing the audience it is realistic.

Production requirements

It is important to liaise with the production team to ensure the effects you are creating are appropriate. Points to consider are budgets, time constraints, film certification, television watersheds, target audience, etc. You do not want to create a dramatic effect that will land the production in trouble with the censors. It is very easy to 'over-do' casualty effects, but restraint should be shown, particularly for realistic productions such as medical dramas.

Products and materials for directly applied casualty make-up

The products most commonly used in direct application are briefly discussed in the table at the beginning of this chapter.

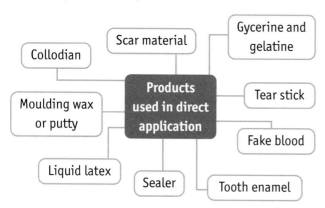

It would be useful to look at a couple of the products and their uses in closer detail.

Uses of gelatine and glycerine

Gelatine and glycerine are harmless to the skin and can therefore be directly applied to create a number of casualty effects ranging from skin diseases and blistering to third degree burns. It can be pre-coloured before application (with food colouring or special pigments, or even fake running blood) or make-up can be applied on top. The main advantage of gelatine and glycerine applications is their semi-translucent quality and it is important to bear this in mind when choosing make-up to colour the application. Gelatine and glycerine mixtures can be bought pre-mixed (Gel-Glyc, Gelfix or Gelskin) and are simply heated up and applied. However, it is easy and economical to make your own mixture.

Gelatine-glycerine recipe for direct application on the skin

Use equal quantities of gelatine powder and glycerine (approximately 1 tablespoon of each should be sufficient for a small application). You will also need water, colour pigments (if required) and a small saucepan and hob.

1 Protect the model's clothing.
2 Cleanse the area to be covered in order to remove any residue oil and make-up.
3 Mix equal quantities of glycerine and water and heat them in a small saucepan on a hob (or mix them in a smaller bowl and place in a larger bowl of boiling water to melt if a stove is not available).
4 Sprinkle gelatine powder onto the hot water and glycerine and mix together. Continue to heat gently until the mixture clarifies (goes clear).
5 You may add more water at this stage to obtain the desired consistency – the mixture should run gently off a spatula.
6 Add the colouring pigment if required and mix well.

The mixture is now ready to be applied to the skin. It can be applied using a spatula, brush or pipette. It can be spread on the skin and sculpted into shape only when it is warm. After setting on the skin, the gelatine mixture can be worked with a heated stainless steel modelling tool to create the shape required.

On its own, glycerine can be used to create tears; mixed with water it can be applied with a spray bottle to simulate sweat on the skin.

KEY NOTE

* This mixture can also be used in a mould for more exact shapes such as eye pouches and scars. It is used cold and fixed with adhesive.
* On the plus side, gelatine is semi-translucent, is fast and easy to produce, adheres easily to the skin, takes most make-up applications and its edges are easily blended. On the negative side, gelatine does not move that well, can melt if used in a very warm atmosphere, for example under stage lights, dries out when exposed to heat, is heavy in large applications and smells awful, although essential oils can be added to the mixture to help cover up the smell.
* Heavy applications can be fixed to the skin more securely by first applying a thin coat of spirit gum and attaching cotton wool fibres onto the layer of glue before applying the gelatine mixture. The cotton fibres act as an anchor and prevent the gelatine from lifting from the skin. If the area of application has heavy body hair, then spirit gum alone should be used as the hair will act as an anchor.

REMEMBER

The mixture can be very hot and burn the skin on application if precautions are not taken. It is very important that you test the temperature of the mixture on yourself before applying it to your model. The mixture should gently run off the spatula during application, feel warm but not burn and set quickly on the skin. Test the temperature on the inside of your wrist using a small amount of mixture. *Be careful* – if the mixture is very runny, allow it to cool before applying.

Blood products

There are many considerations for the make-up artist when choosing blood products.

* What age is the injury – is the blood wet or dry?
* Is the wound deep or superficial – is venous or arterial blood colour required?
* Does the blood suddenly appear or does it flow slowly?
* Often the make-up artist will require several products to create a realistic effect.

Some knowledge of the blood system is valuable to the make-up artist. Re-read the section on the blood system in Chapter 4 (page 63) before attempting to design any casualty make-up using blood products.

Running blood

Usually water-washable and stain-free on the skin.

* Some types are washable from fabrics – check instructions before use.
* Available in drying and non-drying formulas with varying flow rates.
* Most spread easily.
* Safe to use on the skin and around the mucous membranes (again, check instructions about use in the mouth).
* If blood is accidentally splashed into the eye, it should be rinsed immediately with an eye bath, although any irritation is usually minor.
* Available in light and dark colours.

Crusty blood

* Usually latex-based.
* Used when scabby, dried blood effects are required.
* Dries very quickly.
* Safe on the skin but should be avoided around the mucous membranes and eyes.
* Removed using Pro-clean.

Fix blood

* Used when a waterproof and long-lasting casualty effect is required.
* With a plastic-like material as a base, fix blood is more irritating than other blood products and should not be used around the eyes or mucous membranes.
* Removed using Pro-clean.
* Available in light and dark.

Woundfiller

* A congealed, slow drying product used to fill open wounds.
* Available in light and dark.

Fresh scratch

* A fast drying, stiff paste useful for creating scab effects.
* Once dried it is smear- and rub-proof.
* Removed with an oil-based cleanser.
* Can stain so check before use.

Blood capsules

* Creates an effect of bleeding from the mouth.
* Gelatine capsules are filled with blood for internal use and sometimes a saliva-stimulating ingredient.
* The capsules should be chewed just before the effect is required.

Blood sachets and blood bladders

* Fine plastic film bags filled with blood, which break easily under pressure or with explosive squibs.
* Designed for external use only.

Eye blood

* Blood approved for use in the eye.
* Effect lasts for between 10 and 20 minutes.
* Has a short shelf life.

Blood powder

* A powder that is almost invisible on any light skin tone or foundation base.
* Activated into a blood product when water or transparent jelly is added.

Creating different effects using casualty make-up

Numerous effects can be created using casualty make-up. The following section aims to take you through the process of creating a variety of effects. Remember there are often several ways of creating the same effect and each make-up artist will have his or her preferred techniques and products. Use the following as a guide. When you have gained some experience and confidence in using the materials, try experimenting and come up with your own solutions to creating realistic effects.

Bruises and black eyes

It is very straightforward to create bruises on the skin. Unless a major swelling is involved, make-up colour alone can create very realistic effects. The important factor is to make sure the colours are correct. A new bruise will be a very different colour a week later due to the healing process. It is important you understand the stages of these colour changes, particularly for requirements of continuity in television and film. As a bruise heals it changes colour as follows:

* various shades of red, turn to
* reddish-blue or dark purple, turns to
* brown, turns to
* yellowish green, turns to
* yellow.

When creating a bruise, it is important to consider what caused the bruise as this could affect the shape and severity. You will often be required to create bruising around the site of more severe injuries, for example a deep wound. If you study a bruise, you will notice that it is irregularly formed with a depth of colour that fades at the outside edges. Semi-translucent make-up colour lends itself to creating realistic-looking bruises. Make-up can be applied with sponges, brushes or clean fingertips and should be well blended. Minor swelling can be introduced by applying a touch of Vaseline over the area.

Suggested make-up routine for a black eye on a light skin tone

1 Paint crimson-red in the deep corner of the eye socket.

2 Paint red-crimson under the eye pouch.

3 Paint deep purple under the lower eye-socket and on the inner corner of the eyebrow, and suggest a circle to create an under-eye pouch.

4 Fade out the crimson into a more subtle reddish colour.

5 Use a greenish tinge under the outside corner of the eyebrow and eye.

6 Use a yellowish tinge out from the green.

7 If the eye looks too colourful or the colours look disjointed, take a stipple sponge and blend. If

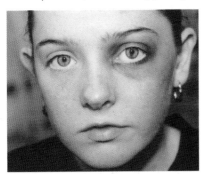

you want the bruise to look swollen, apply some Vaseline over the make-up to create the shiny, stretched surface of a new bruise.

A black eye created with greasepaint

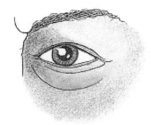

Make-up for a black eye and a bruise

For dark skin tones, omit the green and yellow stages and concentrate on using blacks, blues and purples to create the desired effect.

Shock and illness

This is an effect that you will often have to use in conjunction with other casualty effects. A person suffering a severe burn or wound will normally display symptoms of shock. Severe blood loss will also lead to changes in skin colour. There are various ways of creating a look of shock or illness. Here is one example.

1 Apply a pale foundation sparingly and take it over the lips. You will need to blend down to the costume line.

2 If the natural skin tone contains a lot of red or pink, you could stipple green over these areas to strip the colour.

3 Leave the areas under the eyes free of foundation – this will add to the 'ill' effect by leaving the natural shadows.

4 Further shadows can be added if required using a little grey or brown make-up under the outside corner of the eyes, in the lower socket circle and around the nostrils.

5 Add a little red greasepaint close to the top and bottom lashes and also to the nostrils.

6 If you are trying to create the effects of long-term illness, hollow out the temples and under the cheekbones.

7 If the model is supposed to be feverish, add some redness high on the cheekbones using a fine stipple sponge.

8 For serious illness add a little blue to the shading colour (4) and in addition, apply to the lips.

9 Powder if required.

10 Perspiration can also be added if required.

Shock, created as described above

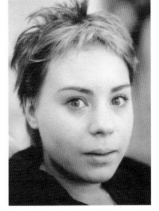

Tears and perspiration

A spray bottle filled with half water and half glycerine can be used to denote perspiration. A dropper with pure glycerine can be used to create tears from the corners of the eyes. Vaseline can also be used to create shine and is useful for holding the 'perspiration' in place, particularly on the forehead and upper lip.

A tear stick irritates the eye causing it to water when held close to the eye area. Adding a little red make-up around the eyes will increase the effect.

Broken noses

The illusion of a broken nose can be created through the use of light and shade (see below).

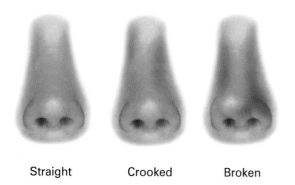

| Straight | Crooked | Broken |

Creating a broken nose using light and shade

If the nose is freshly broken you will need to add swelling, using wax or putty, and redness to the skin tone.

Discoloured and missing teeth

Special coloured tooth enamel can be applied to teeth to create the impression of missing or discoloured teeth. Although the effect works well from a distance, close-up it tends to look rather crude. The effect also needs constant maintenance. Black is used to create missing teeth; yellowy-brown is used for discoloration, for example if the person is a heavy smoker. Gold and silver are also available. The enamel should always be used sparingly. Under no circumstances should tooth enamel be applied to capped or false teeth as it will cause permanent staining.

1 Check the model does not have capped or false teeth in the area you are working.

2 Ask the model to dry the tooth with a cotton bud.

3 Paint enamel onto the tooth close to the gums.

4 Ask the model to rub the tooth gently with the fingertip. Leave it to dry.

5 To remove the enamel, put a small amount of surgical spirit on a cotton bud. Rub this over the tooth.

Grazes

Method 1

1 Spread latex on to the chosen area.

2 Take an orange stick and roughen the surface by rubbing it backwards and forwards over the substance.

3 Leave it to dry.

4 Take a brush and apply red make-up into the grooves.

5 Apply spots of running blood over the rough area. This gives a fresher finish.

6 Remove with Pro-clean.

Method 2

1 Apply deep and bright red make-up blending at the edges.

2 Using a brush paint on a 'Fresh Scratch'.

3 Apply spots of blood on the area.

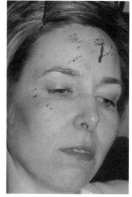

A simple graze

4 Texture can be added, for example make-up imitating dirt and gravel, etc.

5 Remove with surgical spirit.

Scratches

1 Draw a line of scar material on the skin. Do not make the scratches too uniform or they will not look realistic.

2 Working quickly, take a modelling tool and lightly cut down the middle of the line through the scar material.

3 Take some Pros-Aide and lightly stipple over the opened scar material to seal it.

4 Once dry, apply skin-toned make-up over the scratches. If using cream-based make-up, fix with powder, fixing spray or a liquid make-up sealer.

5 Once dry, colour the scratches with red make-up and then a much darker red in the centre to show depth. Add some spots of blood to the scratches, but do not over do it

6 Remove with Pro-clean.

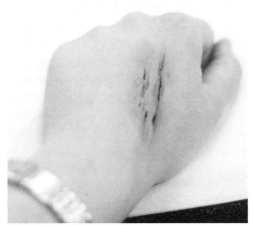

A simple scratch

Minor cuts and wounds using a gelatine mixture

1 Sketch out the shape of the injury for reference.

2 Create a background colour with make-up.

3 Apply an uncoloured Gel-Glyc or Gelmix mixture over the background colour.

4 Apply some mixture which is coloured red.

5 Blend the edges with witch hazel.

6 Apply Pros-aide over the application and slightly onto the surrounding skin.

7 Allow to dry and dust generously with powder, pressing into the edges.

8 Apply make-up over the application.

9 Add some blood products according to the type and age of the wound, for example wound filler, running blood.

10 Remove by lifting gently from the skin and cleaning with Pro-clean.

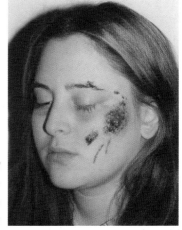

A minor wound created using a coloured gelatine and glycerine mixture

Deep wounds

Putty, Derma Wax or Morticians Wax can be used for building up an area, which can then be cut into a deep cut or wound.

1 Apply some red and dark red make-up onto the area of the wound.

2 Smooth wax onto the area, building up the area to create a 'swelling'. Follow the natural contour of the area, for example arm, neck. Blend the edges using some Vaseline or lubricating jelly.

3 Cut a wound into the wax with a palette knife or modelling tool.

4 Gently pull back areas of the wax as necessary to create the desired effect.

5 Apply Pros-aide to seal, taking it slightly onto the surrounding skin, and allow to dry completely.

6 Powder generously, pressing into the edges.

7 Stipple pink or rose-coloured make-up over the wax.

8 Set with powder, fixing spray or liquid sealer as appropriate.

9 Stipple make-up on top of the wax to match the surrounding skin tone.

10 Seal again.

11 Choose a red-tinged make-up and stipple it around the wound to create a bruised 'fresh wound' effect.

12 The wax wound is then coloured dark red and filled with 'wound filler'.

13 Running blood is added at the end using a pipette.

14 Remove by lifting gently from the skin and cleanse with Pro-clean.

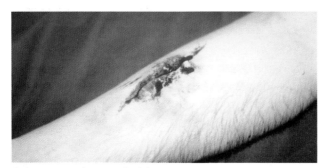

A deep wound created with wax

Stitched wounds

1 Redden the area slightly with make-up.

2 Use double threaded black cotton or thick thread. Make knots at regular intervals along the thread and cut the thread halfway between the knots. The sections you are left with should look like those illustrated below.

3 Using a fine brush draw a line of scar plastic or latex.

4 Working quickly (before the line of plastic or latex dries), press the stitches into the line. The knots should be stuck down at approximately 1 cm intervals.

5 Randomly apply more red make-up around the outside of the stitch line.

6 Draw on stitches across the wound on either side of the cotton knots with black cake eyeliner and a fine brush.

7 Put a small drop of congealed blood around the base of the knots.

8 Cut any long ends of cotton until they are all the same length – they should look neat.

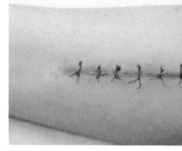

A stitched wound created as described

9 Remove by lifting the stitches from the skin and cleanse with Pro-clean.

Bullet wounds

1 Dab adhesive (Pros-Aide or spirit gum) onto the area.

2 Mould some wax or putty into a small ball and stick it onto the glued area.

3 Take a cork (or similar shaped instrument) and press it into the putty to create a 'well'.

4 With some Vaseline or lubricating jelly, smooth the putty surface and blend out the edges.

5 Seal with a thin layer of Pros-Aide, taking it onto the surrounding area slightly.

6 Powder generously, pressing into the edges.

7 Use red make-up to redden the area and dark red in the centre of the well to add depth.

8 Fill the well with a small amount of wound filler and fix blood.

9 Add a small amount of running blood to the wound.

10 Remove by lifting gently from the skin and cleansing with Pro-clean.

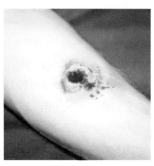

A bullet wound created as described

Scars

Scars are formed as part of the normal skin's healing process. They are made up of a mixture of fibrous tissue and blood vessels. Generally, new scars are red and raised, but over a period of time they become flatter and pale. This healing process can take anything from a year to eighteen months. However, scars can take on many different forms. They can be indented (atrophic), protruding (hypertrophic) or keloid (common in black skins). Pigmentation can also be altered.

Hypo-pigmentation is the loss of colour compared with the surrounding skin.

Hyper-pigmentation is an excess of colour compared with the surrounding skin.

As with many of the other casualty effects, make-up artists will use a variety of techniques to create scars. Below are a couple of suggestions.

New hypertrophic scar

1 Choose the position of the scar. Using scarlet or crimson lake make-up colour, draw a line blending the edges.

2 Apply latex or scar plastic along the line. Whilst it is still wet, shape it with a modelling tool.

3 Paint more crimson lake around the edges of the material in a random fashion. Blend a little scarlet red as well so it looks sore. Leave it shiny.

4 If the scar is from a stitched wound, you may wish to add deeper red points at regular intervals along the scar material.

5 Remove with Pro-clean.

Old hypotrophic scars

1 Using make-up, paint a line in a colour lighter than the skin tone. Blend the edges.

2 Paint Collodion onto the line and leave it to dry. Collodion will make the skin 'pucker up' creating a hypotrophic effect.

3 Apply a light grey or brown colour around the edges of the Collodion and a slightly deeper

shade randomly down the centre of the scar to accentuate the depth.

4 Powder well all over; this will help add to the 'aged' effect.

5 Remove with Pro-clean.

KEY NOTE

Collodion can also be used around the edges of scar plastic, tuplast or latex to create contracted skin on older hypertrophic scars.

REMEMBER

Collodion is a harsh product that can cause irritation on the most robust skins. Before proceeding with the full application, it is wise to carry out a small patch test on a discreet area. On the face, Collodion can leave temporary erythema after removal and should therefore be used with extreme caution. If in doubt, try applying latex to stretched skin for a similar effect.

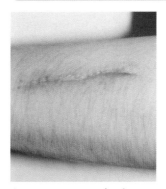

A new scar created using scar material

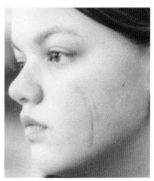

An old (hypotrophic scar) created using Collodion

Burns

The severity of burns is classified as follows.

* A **superficial** burn affects the top layer of skin only (epidermis). The skin looks red and is mildly painful. The top layer of skin may peel a day or so after the burn but the underlying skin is healthy. It does not scar. Sunburn is a good example.

* A **partial thickness** burn causes deeper damage. The skin forms blisters and is very raw, red and painful. However, some of the deeper layer of

skin (the dermis) is unharmed. This usually means the skin can heal well without scarring unless the area of the burn is large.

* A **full thickness** burn damages all layers of the skin. The skin is white and waxy or charred black. There may be little or no pain as the nerve endings are also destroyed.

* Electrical burns can cause damage inside the body even if there is little damage to the skin.

It is important to have images of all these types of burns in your reference file so that when you are planning your make-up you can create an effect that is as realistic as possible. Again, you will need to understand the cause and severity of the burn before you start to plan the application.

Suggested procedure for superficial burns (sunburn) using latex

1 Redden the area with make-up.

2 Sponge on three to four layers of latex, making sure each layer is dry before applying the next.

3 Pinch the latex and move it in a circular pattern until it blisters.

4 Paint under the latex with more make-up.

5 Remove with Pro-clean.

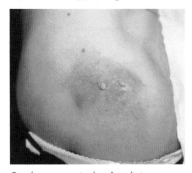

Sunburn created using latex

Suggested procedure for partial thickness burns using gelatine

* Redden the skin.

* Make a fairly runny gelatine and glycerine mixture. (You can add more water to help create a runnier mixture, which is good for creating a 'water blister' effect.)

* Splatter the mixture from about 10 cm above the area – let the mixture run off a spoon or spatula and fall onto the skin. The lesions you create should not be too raised.

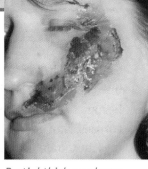

* Redden the area around the blisters. Do not make them look too uniform, otherwise they will look false.

* To make a blood blister, take a hairpin and push runny or congealed blood under the gelatine mixture.

Partial thickness burns created with a gelatine and glycerine mixture

* Remove by gently lifting the gelatine from the skin and cleanse with Pro-clean.

Full thickness burns can also be created using make-up, a gelatine mixture, blood and black hairspray to simulate charring.

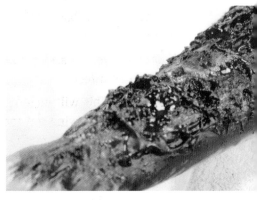

Full thickness burns created with a gelatine and glycerine mixture

HANDS ON

Skin diseases and disorders

Using research as a starting point for your work Chapter 4 'Anatomy and Physiology' will provide a starting point), recreate several skin diseases and disorders using the techniques you have practised in class. The photographs below provide some suggestions.

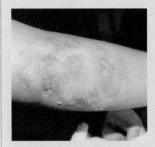

Psoriasis created using latex

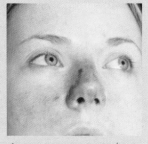

Acne rosacea created using greasepaint and a stipple sponge

Death and corpses

Creating the illusion a dead person requires changing the skin tones. The flesh of a light-skinned person becomes grey, purple and yellow. Studying images of corpses, though unpleasant for most of us, is the only way to really appreciate the changes we need to make. As usual, planning the make-up is very important. You will need to consider factors such as:

* What caused the death?

* Are there any wounds or marks on the body?

* How old is the corpse?

Although creating a realistic-looking corpse takes much planning and experimentation, a corpse-like effect can be achieved using the following procedure.

1 Apply a 'death flesh' base. Take any natural colour out of the lips.

2 Stipple on grey, yellow and purple tones to create a mottled affect.

3 Define the face. This will include deepening the eye sockets and hollowing out the temples and cheekbones. If visible, the neck and clavicles will also need definition.

4 The hands will need defining, and the roots of the nail-beds will need to become deeply discoloured.

5 Powder the skin to create a matt, dull appearance.

6 Although hair continues to grow for some time after death, you may wish to lightly powder the hair to take the shine and lustre down.

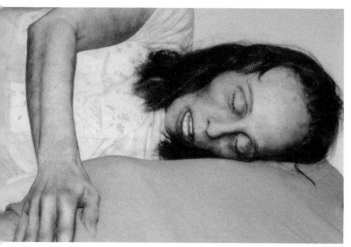

An example of a corpse created for the film '28 Days Later'

> **HANDS ON**
>
> Research the effects required when transforming a dark-skinned performer into a corpse.

You may also wish to try out the following casualty effects and add them to your portfolio:

* glass wound

* compound bone fracture

* split lip.

> **KEY NOTE**
>
> * Materials and techniques should be chosen to achieve the desired effect.
> * The effect must meet the requirements of the on-screen image.
> * The effect must be achieved within the allocated time and budget.
> * The degree of the effect must be suitable given the watershed (television) or certificate (film) and production requirements.
> * The final effect must look realistic and natural on screen or camera.
> * It should be possible to repeat the final effect accurately at a later date if required. Records of work should be maintained for this reason. All aspects of continuity should be considered and recorded.
> * Don't use good brushes with latex – it will ruin them.
> * For distance shots and extras just use lots of blood.
> * When working on a sensitive area (generally speaking the face and neck of any woman), use latex rather than scar plastic – but if you can get the correct effect, it is best to use wax or gelatine.
> * Do not put materials such as blood, latex, etc. down the sink, as they will block it. Dispose of them appropriately, following COSHH guidelines.

Facial hair application, removal and maintenance

Facial hair is associated with fashion and should always suit the period of the production. You should research the period, but also make sure that you do not make everyone look exactly the same. Facial hairpieces are available as beards, moustaches and sideburns, and are either bought off the shelf or made to order. For leading men in televisions and film, hair (usually yak) is knotted onto the finest lace. A number of copies of the facial hairpiece would be made as fine lace is delicate and the pieces would probably not last long. Extras can get away with heavier lace. Theatre lace, which is much coarser, is only suitable for large auditoriums where there are no close-ups.

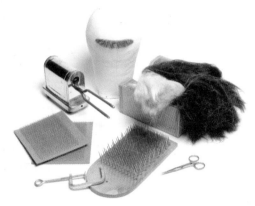

A selection of equipment required for applying facial hair. From top centre clockwise: a malleable block; hair; hairdressing scissors; a hackle and clamp; drawing mats; heated tongs

Ordering a customised lace facial piece

When the budget of a production allows, it is preferable to order customised facial hairpieces, particularly for leading performers. This will result in the correct hair and lace colour and a better fit on the performer's face. It will also create a more comfortable, natural and realistic effect. As a make-up artist ordering facial hair pieces from a wigmaker you will need to know how to take measurements from the performer to ensure a perfect fit. You cannot afford to get it wrong as a customised beard costs between £300 and £400.

Making a pattern for a lace beard

1 Place a piece of cling film over the bottom half of the performer's face.

2 Cut lengths of thick sellotape.

3 Ask the performer to open his mouth – this will help with comfort when wearing the piece and allow room for flexibility.

4 Place tape under the chin, then over the chin up to the mouth, sideburns and under jaw, tightening the cling film to the shape of the face as you go and overlapping the lengths of tape. When you have finished, the cap should feel quite stiff. If you want the beard to go down the neck, apply tape here also.

5 Check the performer will not shave any natural sideburns off if the proposed beard meets them.

6 Mark on the required hairline in a black indelible marker.

7 Cut away any excess cling film.

8 Send the pattern to the wigmaker with details of hair colour and choice of lace.

A moustache pattern can be achieved in a similar manner.

Simple beard measurements can also be taken:

* from sideburn to sideburn under the chin

* from the lip to the end of the beard line under the chin

* from back jaw bone to back jaw bone going round the front.

A beard is always made up of four to five colours and is always lighter around the edges. Study the performer's natural hair colour and ask what colour his facial hair is naturally. Consult the wigmaker with regard to colour matches. Tail yak hair is mainly used to knot facial hairpieces; belly yak is sometimes used for very young men or for edges as it is softer.

Finally, you will need to choose the lace. This will need to be as close a colour match to the skin tone as possible. It is sometimes useful to send a sample of the performer's base colour to the wigmaker to match. The weight of the lace will depend on how close-up the facial hairpiece will be viewed.

STEP-BY-STEP | Dressing and applying a moustache

Equipment required

* Plastic skin or Pros-Aide
* Base
* Lace facial piece
* Matt adhesive

* Lint-free cloth
* Tail comb
* Hairdressing scissors

* Heated tongs
* Tissues
* Plastic spray or hairspray

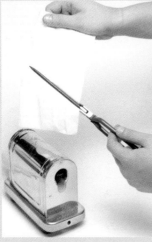 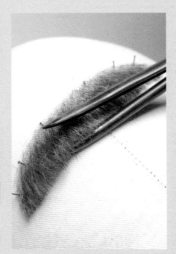 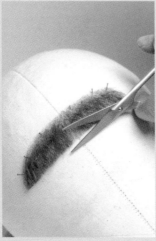 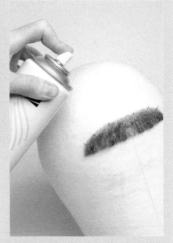

1 Facial hair can be dressed using small heated tongs. The temperature of the tongs should be tested on a tissue first to avoid burning the hair.

2 Create some 'lift' at the roots of the moustache with the tongs.

3 Facial hair sometimes needs to be trimmed with hairdressing scissors. This can be done before or after application on the performer.

4 Spray the moustache with plastic spray (or hairspray) to set in damp weather and prevent 'droop'.

5 Before applying the moustache gown the model. Make sure the skin is clean and free of grease. Men should be clean-shaven, although models should be advised not to shave *directly* 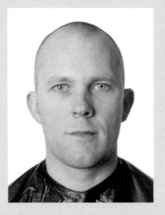 *before* applying facial hair as the adhesive will sting the area. If the model has shaving cuts, 'plastic skin' can be painted over the area to act as a barrier, and Pros-Aide adhesive should be used in preference to spirit gum or medical adhesives.

6 Apply a base if required (this is sometimes required to hide a natural beard line). Do not apply to the area where the lace will be stuck but blend away. Position the piece on the actor's face to check for size, etc. before applying adhesive. When you are happy, apply one of the following matt adhesives with a brush.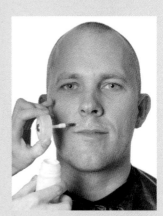
Matt spirit gum: apply a thin layer to the skin, tap with your finger to take away the shine and to make it tacky. Apply lace piece.
Pros-Aide (allows some movement as it is flexible): apply to the skin and allow to go clear before positioning lace piece.
Telesis 5 Matt Lace Adhesive: apply to the skin, wait a few moments and then apply the lace piece. Can be applied to lace as well for extra adhesion.

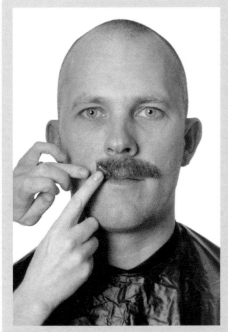 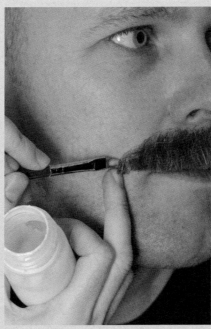 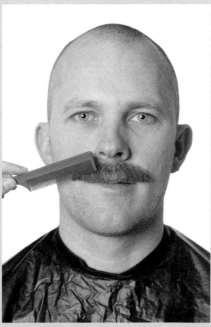

7 Place the piece into position. Make sure the lace is stuck firmly to the skin all over. Press down the edges with a tail-comb or lint-free cloth, for example silk or muslin.

8 Apply more adhesive to the edges as required, taking care you do not stick hairs, but ensuring the edges are all stuck down. Allow to dry, then test by pulling at the piece gently.

9 Trim as required and tidy the moustache using a tail comb.

KEY NOTE

A hard lace edge can be softened by overlaying with loose hair (see the section on 'Laying on a beard', on the next page.

Sideburns

For side burns in film or television, lift the natural hair and place the piece so the natural hair falls over it. If necessary, cut or shave a small section of the natural hair away where the piece will actually be stuck down (you do not need to do this for stage). Comb down the actor's own hair to hide the join. Make sure the two sides match each other. There should be no visible join between the sideburns and the natural hair.

Full beards

To apply a full beard, use the same method as applying sideburns, but the mouth should be open during application to allow for greater flexibility and movement. Opera singers are better off with beards made in several pieces as this allows for greater flexibility and movement of the face.

Removing facial pieces

1 Using appropriate adhesive remover, take a brush to stipple the edge of the lace to loosen it.

2 Work slowly around the edge until the piece can be gently peeled off, whilst holding the skin taut.

3 Wipe over the area with a tissue. Remove any sticky areas with a little more remover.

4 Tone the skin to remove any last traces of remover.

5 Clean the lace with acetone or adhesive remover on a stiff brush, working from the edge of the lace inwards (this prevents fraying). Heavily soiled pieces can be soaked first.

6 Pin the moustache to a malleable block (a soft canvas block shaped like a chin) and re-dress.

STEP-BY-STEP | Applying stubble

If stubble is required, it is obviously much easier for the performer to grow it. But sometimes it is necessary to apply the effect of stubble on a performer, for example when transforming a female to a male or when the shooting schedule affects continuity. For large theatre, applying a blue or grey greasepaint with a stipple sponge may be adequate, but for television, film and close-up work a more realistic technique is required. It is important to study some images of real stubble growth to ensure your work takes on a realistic appearance.

Equipment required

* Stipple wax
* Finely cut human or yak hair in a variety of colours
* Knotting lace (approximately 10 cm square)
* A large brush

1 Apply stipple wax to the area.
2 Finely cut the hair to resemble stubble, about 2-3 mm long. It is best to use human or yak hair in different colours for a natural effect.
3 Place knotting lace, cut to approximately 10 cm square, over the area. Start in an area that will allow you to work logically.
4 Brush on hair over the lace with a large brush.
5 Lift the lace gently from the skin.
6 Move onto the next area until complete.
7 Make sure the actor is told not to touch his face or attempt a kissing scene.
8 Stubble can be removed using a heavy-duty cleansing cream. Follow this by toning to remove any last traces of cleanser.

KEY NOTE

Dark-haired performers may benefit from a light stippled application of blue or grey greasepaint to create the effect of a five o' clock shadow prior to the application of stubble paste.

Laying on a human or yak hair beard

STEP-BY-STEP | Preparing the hair

Equipment required

* Selection of hair (using different colours makes the hair 'alive')
* Heated tongs (small barrel)
* Tissues
* Hackle (to mix hair) – see REMEMBER box on the next page
* Drawing mat

1 Choose a selection of hair in different colours to suit the model. Check your reference file and question the model to assist you.

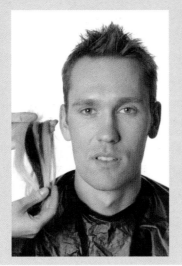

2 Tong the hair to create waves (facial hair is not naturally straight). Test the temperature of the tongs on tissue to avoid scorching the hair. Pinch the tongs together along the length of the hair, working on small areas at a time. Work each area several times. This coarsens the hair for ease of use and a natural looking finish.

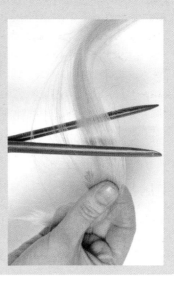

3 Secure the hackle to a worktop and ensure it is fitted with a safety cover when not in use. Line the hackle with a sheet of tracing paper by pushing it over and down the points (take care when doing this). This keeps the hackle clean and makes it easier to remove hair from the hackle after use.

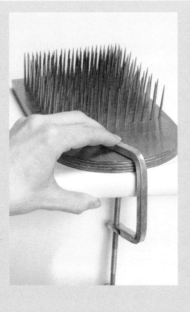

4 Take equal portions of each of the hair colours. For example, with a blonde beard start with browns, then take reds and finally blonde for the top. Keep the hair close at hand and make sure each colour is kept separate.

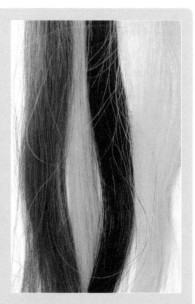

5 Place a sample of the first hair colour in the hackle, grab hold of the end and drag it out through the points of the hackle. Keeping hold of the end of the hair, 'flick' the hair back into the hackle, twisting as you go. Then take a sample of another hair colour and add this to the hair in the hackle. Repeat this action several times, adding more hair as you proceed a little at a time. The hair colour should be mixed but not too thoroughly, so each colour has a positive effect rather than a muddy one.

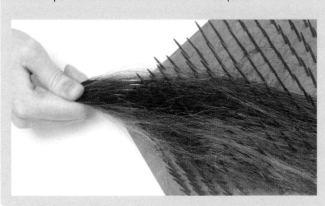

6 When you are satisfied with the colour mix, remove the hair from the hackle and transfer it to a drawing mat to secure it.

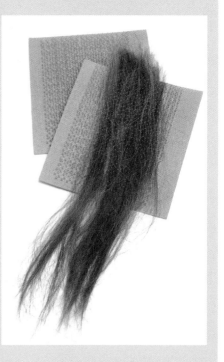

STEP-BY-STEP | Laying on a beard

Equipment required

* Adhesive (spirit gum or Pros-Aide both work well)
* Acetone
* Vaseline
* Cotton wool

* Hairdressing scissors
* Hair (colours mixed)
* Facial hair tongs
* Tissues

It is important to work from both sides to:

* protect your back from postural damage
* see your work in the mirror clearly (you cannot see if you are leaning over)
* avoid the intrusive body language of leaning over someone.

1 Take some hair. Soak a pad of cotton wool with acetone. Spread Vaseline over another. Keep these to one side. Hold the scissors in the thumb and third finger. The lower blade remains straight; it is the upper blades that do the moving. Ensure the model is comfortable. Push natural sideburns up with a comb and anchor the hair behind the ear with the comb (this is to avoid a gap between the natural hair and false hair).

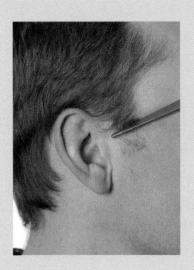

2 Brush adhesive onto the skin in the final desired shape. At first, when you are working slowly, you may find it easier to apply a section at a time to prevent it from drying.

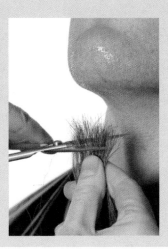

3 Spread the hair between the thumb and fingers. Cut the ends at the angle you are directing it onto the skin.

4 Starting at the bottom and following the diagrams below, push the hair onto the adhesive with the edge of the scissors.

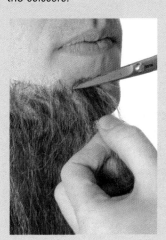

5 Cut the hair to the desired length. Repeat working upwards, cutting the hair shorter as you go up. You may apply more adhesive if required. Use the acetone and Vaseline-soaked cotton wool to clean the scissors of adhesive as you go. This enables you to work cleanly and neatly.

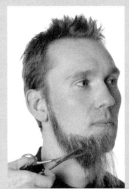

6 Remove any stray hairs. Press into place with a lint-free cloth or damp powder puff. Remove the comb from the natural sideburns and take the natural hair down over the laid-on hair. Comb through gently to remove any loose hairs. If required, apply more hair to gaps, etc.

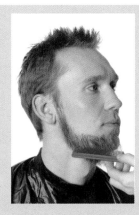

Hair can be removed by easing it off and wiping over the skin with appropriate remover. Tone and moisturise well afterwards.

KEY NOTE

You can angle hair to change the direction of hair growth so it looks natural.

If you have to dress the hair, use a comb as a barrier between the tongs and the skin and **proceed with caution**. Alternatively, spray the hair with plastic spray or hairspray and shape with the fingers.

A natural hairline is lighter in colour at the edges and less dense. Bear this in mind when creating a 'laid on' beard.

Laying hair directly onto the skin may sometimes be the preferred way of creating the effect of facial hair.

✳ You may need to create facial hair on a performer unexpectedly with no time to order or make a lace piece.

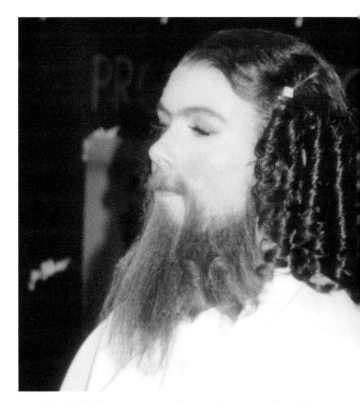

'Bearded lady' by Zoe Hay at the Joe Blasco stand at the European Make-up Artist trade show

* It creates an ultra-realistic effect and is suitable for occasions when even the finest lace would create a problem.

It is vital to study beard growths so you can lay hair in the direction of natural growth. Start collecting photographs of beards from newspapers, magazines, etc. and store them in your resource file for future reference.

It is also important to prepare the hair first – work with a variety of colours for a more natural finish.

Working with crepe hair

You can also lay on a beard using crepe hair. Crepe hair is more economical to work with but does not give such a realistic effect as human or yak hair for close-ups. It is therefore suitable for theatre. Although crepe hair is laid on in the same manner as shown one the previous pages, the hair is prepared in a different manner.

Crepe hair is supplied in lengths and is braided around string. Begin by selecting the appropriate colours for your performer, then cut the strings of the braid and gently unbraid the hair. Because the hair has been tightly braided it will be curly in texture and will therefore need to be straightened. To straighten the lengths of hair, take a steam iron and gently press whilst holding the hair taut. It is important to leave a kink in the hair as facial hair is not naturally straight.

Do not cut the hair but gently pull it from the ends. The hair should break away in approximately 12 cm lengths. Gather the hair together and comb through it gently to remove any tangles and short hairs.

To mix the hair colour, take several sections of different-coloured straightened hair and hold them together. Gently pull the hair apart with the other hand and then bring the two sections back together again. Repeat this action several times until the colours are mixed. The hair is now ready to lay on.

Knowledge Check

1 What points should you take into consideration when positioning a model for special effect make-up application?

2 Why is it important to communicate effectively with the performer during application?

3 When preparing the skin appropriately for special effect application, what should you take into consideration?

4 Why is it important to use products economically?

5 How can you ensure the make-up is sustained under different shooting conditions?

6 Why is it essential that the completed special effects meet the design plan and production requirements?

7 What procedure should be followed if there is any disruption in the make-up process?

8 Describe how to remove prosthetics causing minimal discomfort to the performer.

9 List the health and safety aspects that are particularly relevant to special effect make-up.

10 Describe the types of discomfort that could be experienced by the performer when applying and fixing a prosthetic and how to alleviate the problem.

11 List three types of adhesive and their appropriate removers.

12 Describe the use of sealers and block release agents.

13 List three different materials used for making prosthetics.

Body art

Body art, where the entire body becomes the artist's canvas, can be one of the most expressive and creative forms of make-up artistry. This chapter begins by looking at the historical and cultural influences of this art form and then proceeds through the most commonly used techniques such as creating tattoos, statue effects, painting on clothes and camouflaging the body within the immediate environment. Once these basic techniques have been mastered the make-up artist can move on to other projects involving experimentation and visual illusion, limited only by the imagination.

Aim and objectives

The aim of this chapter is to provide you with an understanding of the basic techniques required to undertake body art briefs.

In achieving this aim you will complete the following **objectives**. You will be able to:

* evaluate the historical and cultural influences of body art
* discuss developments within contemporary body art
* undertake body art giving due consideration to the care of your model
* discuss various techniques and products used in body art
* create a temporary tattoo using a method suitable for the requirements of the design brief
* create a 'bronze bust' effect on a model
* paint clothes on a model's body, successfully rendering folds in fabric
* camouflage a body with a background.

Historical and cultural influences

From the beginning of our history, humans have been piercing, tattooing and painting their bodies as part of a conscious effort to express themselves and the significance of their bodies. Across the continents and centuries, body art has attained diverse cultural significance. Messages of an individual's social status within a community, political or religious interest, stages of personal development or significant events have been expressed visually on the skin, bringing together and identifying cultural groups spanning time and continents.

Traditionally, colour has always played an important part in the decoration process. Primitive humans used natural pigments such as ochre and manganese to create a varied palette. Colour was thought by some cultures to have magical properties. When applied to the body it was thought to offer the wearer protection, luck, fertility and even divinity. Because of this, decorating the body often became a major part of rituals and ceremonies for many tribes across the world.

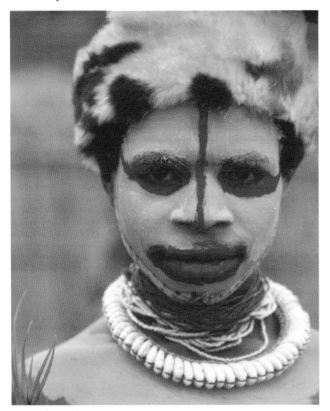

Tribal body decoration

Another form of skin decoration – scarification – may seem barbaric to modern Western culture, but it needs to be taken in the context of its own social and cultural background. In West Africa, scarring is a form of tribal initiation and a sign of bravery. Done with razor blades, the painful process starts at puberty and continues into adulthood. Each tribe has distinctive designs.

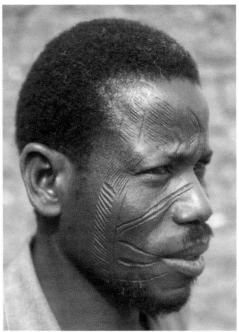

Example of scarification

Markings indicate the wearer's village and clan and include black magic symbols to keep away evil spirits. The markings can also show the social prestige of the wearer.

Permanent tattoos are another form of body decoration which remains popular today. Historically, tattoos were used across many cultures for many of the reasons described above. However, one particular culture to embrace the art of tattooing is that of the Japanese.

From the sixth century, tattooing in Japan was used as a form of punishment to distinguish criminals from the rest of society and 'mark' the despised lower classes. However, as the power of the common people in Japan grew in the eighteenth and nineteenth centuries, horimono, or traditional Japanese tattoos, began to flourish as an art form. Based on images from watercolour

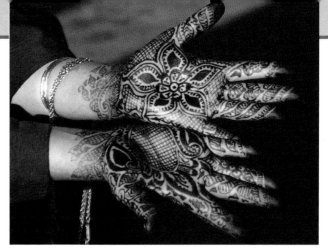

Example of traditional mendhi

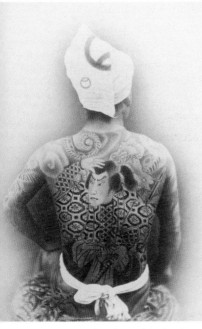

Example of zenshin-bori

paintings, woodcuts and popular picture books of the time, the ultimate reward for the long endurance of pain would be an elaborate tattoo. Many tattoos were full body, called zenshin-bori, and included the face.

Another traditional technique of body decoration that has become popular in Western culture in recent years is that of henna painting. Henna has been discovered as a form of decoration on Egyptian mummies, suggesting that the use of henna in this way dates back to around 1200BC.

The prophet Mohammed dyed his hair and beard with henna, popularising the art in Saudi Arabia around the year 632AD. As a result, Muslim women also began to stain their hands and feet. Traditionally, henna is used to decorate the hands and feet for ceremonies and celebrations in Eastern households. Henna application has no class boundaries; the majority of women have henna applied at least twice a year.

Henna powder is made from crushed leaves of the henna plant, Lawsonia inermis. The plant grows in hot, dry climates in countries such as the Sudan, Egypt, India, and North African and Middle Eastern countries.

Henna is traditionally applied to the hands and feet but designs vary from region to region. Most Indian and Pakistan designs are composed of intricate, repetitive patterns created by line work and teardrops, whereas in North Africa the patterning tends to be very geometrical in style with attention being paid to solid border work.

KEY NOTE

If you would like to research or learn more about the history of body art, there are a number of books on the subject. A particularly useful reference is *Decorated Skin: A World Survey of Body Art* by Karl Groning, published by Thames & Hudson (1997).

Contemporary body art

Throughout the twentieth century, communities from every region in the world have settled in the West influencing styles of body decoration.

Henna art became popular in the late 1990s when celebrities such as Madonna began to wear 'mendhi' designs. The fashionable enthusiastically embraced eastern traditions, but most Western women chose to paint their henna decorations on areas of the body that Asian women would never contemplate painting. In the West, the belly button proved to be a popular place for a henna design, whilst the back offered an expansive canvas for larger and more intricate designs. These are both areas of the body that are definitely out of bounds for traditional henna designs. In terms of the designs themselves, Celtic designs and Chinese letters have become popular with both men and women, along with traditional tattoo designs such as flowers and animals.

Permanent tattoos remain the mark of people who want to either express their individuality or make a statement about their identity. Tattoos have always come in and out of fashion, but in the Western world were originally associated with soldiers and sailors. Since then, and until quite recently, tattoos were associated with unruly groups such as the 'Hells Angels'. In the world of the motion picture the anti-hero often wears a tattoo; it seems to represent the slightly dangerous, unsavoury character. In the 1970s and early 1980s rebellious rock groups were seen wearing them. The era of 'punk' and 'skinheads' brought tattoos to the street where they were worn by unconventional men as well as women to complement their body piercings and shocking hairstyles. However, in the late 1990s there was a re-emergence of the permanent tattoo, this time as a mainstream fashion item. Now it had less of an 'unsavoury' reputation, teenagers and their parents were seen visiting tattoo parlours together for a small design – flowers or hearts for the ladies, Celtic designs for the men.

The traditional association of body decoration with rituals and ceremonies has largely been lost (perhaps with the exception of theatre make-up, carnivals and face painting at sporting events). More frequently it has been turned into an expression of individuality and creativity – an art form – and has been heavily influenced by developing technologies such as airbrushing.

Techniques of body art

Being able to apply make-up to the body in a creative way is a skill that is most useful to the make-up artist. There has been an increase in the popularity of this art form over recent years, particularly in the commercial environment, with a number of companies employing make-up artists for their promotional campaigns.

Body art is really only limited by your imagination. However, this chapter looks at some ideas that have been explored by make-up artists so far. First it is important to establish some ground rules for body art.

Care of the model

Your canvas is not a piece of paper – your client will have needs and requirements.

* Consider your model's modesty. A gown or wrap is a useful item to have around for breaks in the session. Try to ensure areas of the body you are not working on are covered up – large towels are useful for this.

* As your model will probably be undressed for at least some of the session, ensure the temperature of the room is comfortable. If you are using water-soluble paints, mix them with warm rather that cold water – your model will really appreciate this.

* When working on areas such as the breasts on a woman or the inner thigh and lower stomach of a man, be aware that your model may feel self-conscious or embarrassed. You can make the model feel more at ease by ensuring you work quickly and confidently. Maintaining an air of professionalism is very important.

* Full body painting sessions can sometimes take many hours. Make sure you give your model lots of short breaks and try to vary the model's posture throughout the session. Be aware that some positions may be more comfortable than others. Ensure the model is fed and watered!

* Effective communication with the model at all times is very important.

> **KEY NOTE**
>
> If the body you are working on is hairy, you may have to ask the model to remove the hair before you begin painting.

Products and techniques

Almost any traditional make-up medium can be used – water-paints, grease-paint and cake-make-up are all suitable. More specialised products such as camouflage make-up, silicone paints and airbrush make-up can also be used. Your choice will often depend on personal preference, the suitability of product properties and the requirements of the project brief.

In addition to painting, try experimenting with other materials to create unusual designs and wonderful textures – working with natural clays such as Fuller's Earth can create wonderful tribal or statue effects; gold and silver leaf will create beautiful polished effects; loose powder colours can add shimmer, depth of colour and texture. Your imagination is really the only limitation. Try visiting a haberdashery store for inspiration – feathers, material, zips, buttons and flowers can all be applied to the skin with suitable skin adhesives.

Project and client briefs

It is important to consider the nature of the project brief before launching into a design.

* Is the make-up being completed for still photography, video or film?
* Will the model be static or moving around?
* Will the shoot be on location or in the studio?
* What light source is there?
* How long will the make-up have to last?
* Will the make-up need to be waterproofed?
* What is the budget?
* How long do you have to complete the make-up?

Where practical it is very important to plan a job in as much detail as possible. It goes without saying that the larger the task, the more preparation is required. Yes, a client will want you to be creative and produce a wonderful make-up, but just as importantly they will require the job to be done efficiently, within budget and on schedule.

Creating temporary tattoos

Despite becoming more acceptable as a fashion item the tattoo can still give off mixed messages, and this is largely due to the design of the tattoo. Think about the different designs of tattoos you

have seen in everyday life, motion pictures or magazines. What impression of the wearer did they give you?

HANDS ON

Researching tattoos

Research and collect tattoo designs that you associate with the following:

* convicts
* soldiers
* female bikers
* mainstream fashion
* contemporary pop-stars.

There are various ways of creating tattoos for television, film or photography from simple ready-made transfers to intricate hand-painted designs and even rubber stamps. When creating a tattoo, a few key points must be taken into consideration.

* Will the tattoo need to be recreated on more than one occasion? If so, you must take photos of the tattoo to ensure that you recreate it in the same position. Would a transfer or stamp be time saving and ensure continuity when working with a design that will have to be reproduced time and time again?
* Are there any time restrictions? A hand-painted design may take much more time to create and time is always money.
* Should the tattoo look old or new? Old tattoos are more faded and frequently have a blue or green outline.
* What type of character is the tattoo for (biker, thug, pop-star or everyday person)?

When all of these points have been considered you will be able to decide the best method to use when designing your tattoo.

Applying a temporary tattoo

1 Choose your design and sketch it onto paper. When both you and the client are happy with the design it can be drawn freehand onto the

area of the skin, or if the design is quite complicated, *carbon paper* can be used. When using carbon paper make sure you place the carbon firmly where the tattoo is required. A small amount of oil can be placed onto the skin first; this will enhance the impression left by the carbon paper. Alternatively, *stencils* can be used. These can be bought or made yourself. Temporary tattoos can also be bought in *transfer form*, but the designs are sometimes limited. Semi-permanent tattoo kits are also available, lasting three to five days. *Air-brushing* tattoos using stencils is a more recent method of application (see Chapter 16 'Advanced techniques for the make-up artist', page 368).

2 You can then fill in the design with colour. A blue or black ballpoint, non-toxic felt tip pens, grease paint, water paints (mixed with fixing spray or liquid), eyeliners, special tattoo pens or ink can all be used for this purpose.

3 Powder the area well once the design is dry; this seals the design and gives a more natural looking result.

4 Fixing spray can also be used for a longer lasting finish.

Tattoos required over a lengthy period of time

For motion pictures or television productions tattoos will sometimes be required every day for a substantial period of time. In these cases it is advisable to have a customised rubber stamp of the design made up for ease of application.

The rubber stamp is inked and applied to the artiste's skin.

Colour the tattoo with your chosen medium – felt tip pens (non-toxic) or tattoo inks are particularly useful as they are longer lasting.

Powder when dry to give a slightly 'worn' feel to the tattoo.

Colouring a tattoo

Look carefully at the colours of a real tattoo. Many tattoos (particularly as they age) are made up of predominately blues and greens. It is important to study the real thing if you are going to create a convincing fake! See also how the colours have a translucent feel to them allowing the colour of the skin tone to radiate through. Choose your materials carefully, making sure they are appropriate for your requirements.

Water-based paints work well for one-day fashion shoots, where designs need to look realistic but can be removed quickly. Mixing the paints with fixing spray or liquid rather than water will prevent smudging. Tattoo ink colours are translucent, which means the texture of the skin shows through, giving them a very realistic appearance. The ink is smudge proof and normally lasts two to three days on the skin. Eyeliner pens are easy to use for simple designs and are smudge proof. However, they have a limited colour range. Grease-based make-up can be messy to use and needs much powdering and fixing. However, camouflage make-up such as Derma-Color, Veil or Dermablend are long lasting, water- and smudge-resistant when set with fixing powder, and can be useful for creating tattoos and any other type of body art. Non-toxic felt-tip pens are also excellent for creating tattoos as they give a translucent finish and are easy to use, cheap to buy and long lasting. However, they are sometimes difficult to remove, so get permission from the artiste before using them.

STEP-BY-STEP Applying a temporary tattoo

Equipment required

* Surgical spirit or alcohol skin wipe
* Tattoo design
* Carbon copy paper
* Ink pen
* Wet cotton bud
* Colour medium of your choice
* Translucent powder (not containing titanium dioxide or iron oxides)
* Fixing spray (optional)

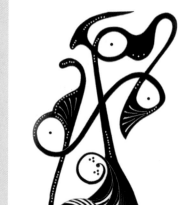

Masculine tattoo design by Julia Conway

Feminine tattoo design by Julia Conway

1 Ensure your model is comfortable (particularly when painting more obscure areas of the body) and you have a safe working position. Clean the skin with surgical spirit or an alcohol skin wipe. This removes any grease from the skin and will help make the tattoo last longer.

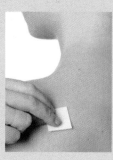

2 Choose your design. Using an ink pen, draw or trace your chosen design on carbon paper with a piece of blank paper underneath so the pattern goes through.

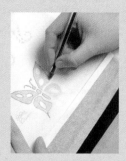

3 Lay the carbon paper against the skin and dab the back with a wet cotton bud (not soaking or the ink will run). This transfers a clear outline onto the skin.

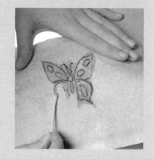

4 Fill in with colour using your chosen medium.

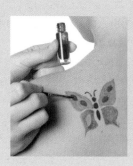

5 Powder the tattoo when dry to set and take away the 'new look' of the colour.

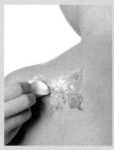

6 The tattoo will last longer if you use a fixing spray.

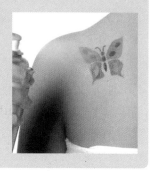

Aftercare

Remember to give your model some aftercare advice to ensure the tattoo lasts.

* Avoid getting soap or shampoo on the skin.
* Avoid getting oil-based products on the skin.
* Do not rub the skin.

If you wish to remove the tattoo, you can wipe the design off with either make-up remover or surgical spirit depending on the medium used to colour the design.

Alternative methods of applying temporary tattoos

Using a stencil

Find a design and copy it onto a sheet of acetate with a waterproof felt-tip pen. Cut the pattern out carefully using a sharp scalpel knife. Attach the stencil to the skin, taking care the whole stencil is stuck down. Use your chosen medium to fill it in with colour.

Using a transfer

Choose a design. Lay the transfer against the skin, making sure the entire surface is in contact with the skin. Dab the back with a wet cotton pad soaked in surgical spirit (or follow the manufacturer's instructions). Carefully peel off the transfer backing.

Freehand

It is useful to make sketches of the design on paper beforehand. An outline of the entire design should be marked on the skin before any colour is filled in. This makes mistakes easier to rectify. Work from the furthest part towards yourself, so you do not smudge your work as you go.

Airbrushing

This method uses stencils, a compressor and specially formulated cosmetic paints. Colour is applied through an airbrush under pressure. The practice of airbrushing is discussed further in Chapter 16 'Advanced techniques for the make-up artist' (page 368).

HANDS ON

Apply a tattoo on a model. Take a photograph of your work as a record. Use an example from above or design your own.

Evaluation

How did you get on? Learning to evaluate our own work is an essential part of the learning process. Study your work carefully and make a list of three aspects of the tattoo you are pleased with and three aspects you think could be improved. Be honest when evaluating your work.

Once you have reached your own conclusions ask the opinion of someone else – perhaps a fellow student, tutor or friend. The person you choose should be someone you can trust to be honest with you. Listen to the comments and take them on board.

Think about how you could make improvements and overcome problems you may have encountered. Did you smudge your work? Remember to work from the furthest point towards your working position.

Remember your canvas is not a piece of paper that you can turn and move easily around. Make some notes – these will be useful for the future to ensure you do not make the same mistakes again. Try this activity again in a week or so, and remember practice makes perfect.

KEY NOTE

Professional tattoo transfers are available that are easy to apply and great for continuity. Check your resource file for suppliers.

Creating a statue effect

There are many ways of creating statue effects in body art. The technique you choose will often depend on the type of statue you want to create. Real statues can be formed from a variety of materials, for example bronze or marble. Statues are often a good starting point for full body painting as the process is fairly straightforward and can be achieved in a relatively short period of time.

STEP-BY-STEP Creating a bronze bust effect on a model

Equipment required

* Gown for the model
* Towels or paper roll to protect surrounding surfaces
* Products to style the model's hair
* A couple of large sea sponges
* Gold watercolour body paint
* Bronze watercolour body paint
* Large powder puff

* Gold loose powder
* Small sea sponge
* Dark brown watercolour body paint (small to medium)
* Small paintbrush
* Black watercolour body paint (small)
* Props – in this case ivy coloured with gold or bronze hair spray

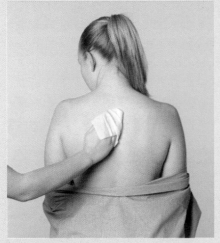

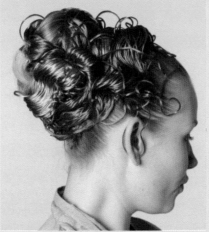

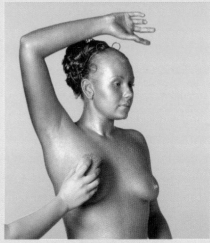

1 Prepare your work area and protect surrounding surfaces such as furniture and floors. Ensure the model's skin is clean and free from any oily reside such as body lotions. Make the model comfortable. This make-up works best if the model is topless.

2 Prepare the model's hair – braiding, twists or waves work well. Study pictures of real statues and try to recreate the effect of the hair having been sculpted.

3 Apply the gold body paint to the skin and hair using a large sea sponge. Work quickly and cleanly. Try to ensure an even coverage. Work down to the hips at the front and back.

4 Take the bronze body paint and stipple over the gold. The application should be heavy in some areas (giving dense coverage) and lighter in others (allowing more of the gold to show through), particularly where you want to accentuate 'planes' of the body, for example the top of the cheekbones, on the collarbones, etc. The effect should be a pleasing graduation of gold and bronze tones over the entire body. Allow to dry.

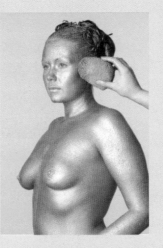

5 Take the dark-brown body paint on a small sea sponge and stipple on areas of shadow. Remember, you are trying to create a 'sculpted' effect and accentuate the body's surface planes.

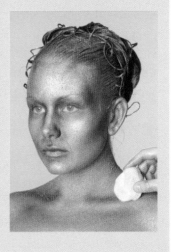

Excellent areas for this are under the cheekbones, above and under the collarbones, around the nostrils, in the eye sockets, around the nipples, between the fingers, between braids or twists in the hair, etc. Do not make the colour look too 'blocked' but keep the stippled effect, allowing some of the gold or bronze to show through.

6 With the large powder puff pick up some gold loose powder. 'Buff' areas of the skin that are predominately gold with a gentle rubbing action. The paint should take on a highly polished, highlighted effect.

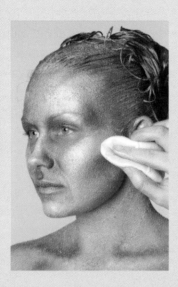

7 Take the black body paint and sparingly stipple in small areas to accentuate the areas of shadow and add more texture. Add some broken lines with a small paintbrush to emulate the texture created by the sculptor's tool. Good places for these lines are from the corner of the mouth, from the nipple, from the corner of the eye and through the hair onto the face.

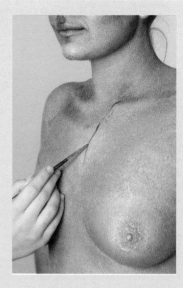

8 Complete the make-up by adding props as appropriate. In this case ivy has been coloured with gold and bronze hair spray and used as a prop. Ensure you spray in a well-ventilated area.

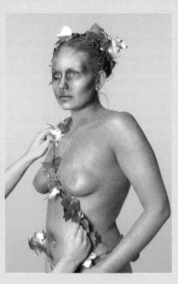

9 For an authentic finish, spend some time considering the pose of your model. Ask the model to close his or her eyes for the photograph or the effect will be ruined.

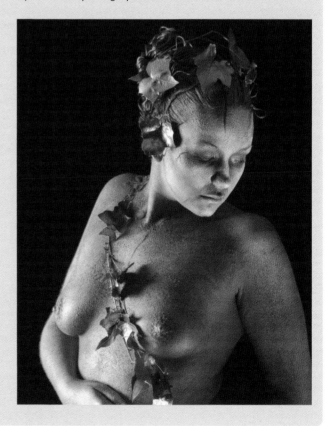

Painting clothes on the body

Before beginning to attempt to paint clothes onto the body, it is important to have an understanding of how fabric can be rendered. You will need to practise this on paper before attempting it on a live model.

Fabric has no form of its own; instead it takes on the form of whatever lies beneath it. The easiest way to approach the task is first to break down the folds and tonal areas into a line drawing, then you can move on to add tones, colour and detail. You should find that this way of working is successful, even for very complex clothes or patterned fabrics.

Once you feel confident about drawing fabric on paper, you can move onto a live canvas.

If you are not a confident artist in the traditional sense, it is often easier to start with a simple item of clothing such as a t-shirt or bikini top and sarong. Begin with some actual clothes and ask your model to wear them whilst you take a Polaroid or digital photo. This will act as an excellent reference throughout the painting process. Study the image, looking at where the folds lie and noting areas of light and shade. Recreating these realistically will give your painting a three-dimensional effect. Now choose your medium, prepare the work area, ensure your model is comfortable and begin to paint. Make sure you take a photograph of your finished work for your portfolio.

HANDS ON

Drawing fabric

* Start with a plain piece of cloth, such as a large handkerchief. Pin it to a wall in front of you and arrange the fabric in folds to create interesting but simple shapes. You may find it useful to adjust the lighting in the room so the cloth is lit from an angle.

* Draw a contour sketch, loosely outlining the main tonal areas and folds as in the example. Use thin, light lines to define the areas of light and shade. Use stronger lines to represent the folds of the cloth.
* Block in the tones.
When you have mastered the technique try again using a larger, patterned piece of material.

Sketches by Julia Conway

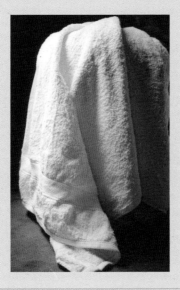
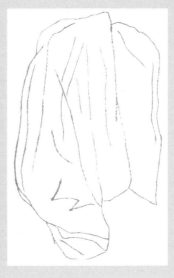
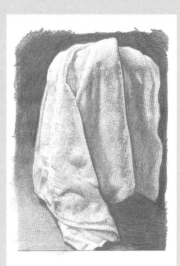

Camouflaging the body with a background

Another popular theme for body artists is camouflaging the body into a chosen background. In order to do this successfully you must use your skills of observation. The following points should be considered.

* Colour – an accurate recreation of the background colour is vital.

* Texture – is the background smooth or rough, shiny or matt, etc.? The choice of products will be important for this.

* Pattern – a highly patterned background may be time consuming and difficult to recreate.

* Will you focus on a section of the body or include the whole person?

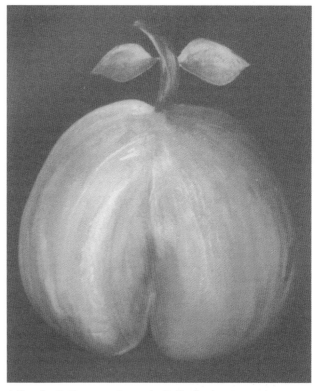

A Peachy Bottom: make-up by Julia Conway

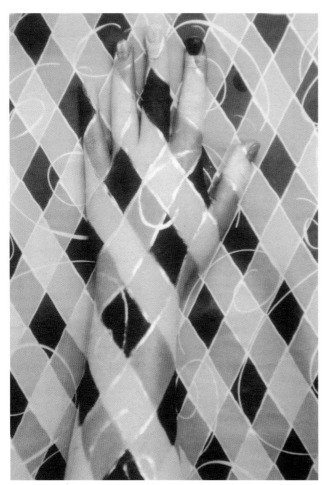

Student's work showing a hand camouflaged into a patterned background.

Interview with body artist Carolyn Cowan

Why did you choose a career in make-up and body art?

I had a friend who was a decorative paint finisher and became inspired by her. I left home at the age of eighteen and began travelling with an Italian punk band – the lead singer was very beautiful with amazing bone structure and I began to apply crazy make-ups and paint to her face. She let me do what I wanted to her, which gave me a chance to experiment with ideas.

How did you initially get your portfolio together?

I got together with a girlfriend who was a photographer and started to photograph the make-ups I was creating. I eventually ended up with a small portfolio of her work, completely self-directed and non-commissioned.

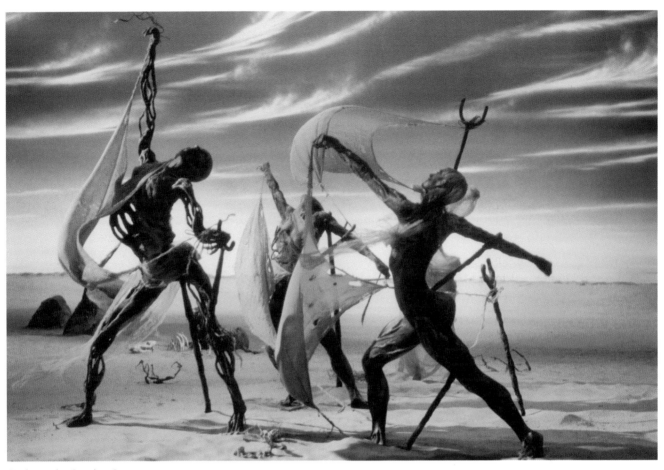

Body art by Carolyn Cowan

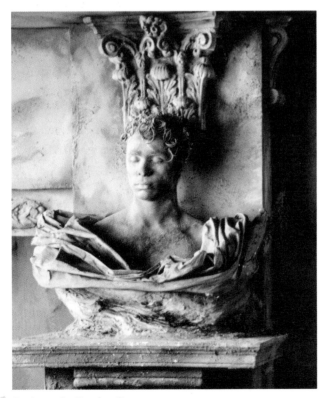

What was your first big break?

I sold my belongings to buy a plane ticket to Milan and arrived with little money, not knowing a soul and with nowhere to stay. The next day I took my portfolio of work to Italian *Vogue* (I always believed in starting at the top). I was booked immediately and worked every day for the next five months, working with some of the best photographers and models in the world.

On returning to England from Italy, I was signed up by 'Sessions' (the top agency in London at this time) and continued to work with photographers such as Bailey, Testino, Saunders and Nicholson.

At this time, music videos were becoming popular and I was commissioned to work on the Duran Duran video *Rio* and Elton John's *I'm Still Standing*. Following this I went on to create make-ups for big advertising campaigns such as Guiness

Body art by Carolyn Cowan

(the ones based on the Salvador Dali paintings) and Natrel. You have successfully carried out some very complicated jobs in you career. What has been the greatest challenge professionally?

A large proportion of jobs require problem solving, but the Natrel campaign, where models were required to look like extensions of trees, was the most complicated, purely because of the scale, time and continuity involved in the shoot. The make-up was 360° full body painting and the morale of the models had to be maintained (they couldn't sit down for hours at a time). The shoot had to be based entirely around the make-up. The make-up needed to be maintained for up to 10 hours between six make-up artists, in a heated tent. Meetings with the director and art director were vital to ensure there were no misunderstandings.

What has been a highlight of your career so far?

Working with Queen and Freddie Mercury on the *I Want to Break Free* video – they were so charming, friendly and enthusiastic.

Have you ever had a job go wrong?

For a video, the client wanted two models, one male and one female, painted (full body) as the 'King and Queen of Hearts'. I spent time creating a pure white base with 2-3 inch red hearts all over the base. During this time the models were flirting with each other. When I finished, I left the room and while they were alone, they decided to have sex. The make-up was a complete mess when I returned – I packed my bag and left!

Occasionally celebrity clients can be difficult, particularly if they have woken up in a bad mood. This can sometimes make life a little difficult. One male actor (who shall remain nameless) gave me one hour to impress him before he would let me do what I was commissioned to do. So, I applied a giant Chinese dragon tattoo to his body and painted

it with oranges and gold. Luckily he liked it, so he let me continue with the job I was being paid for.

Your portfolio demonstrates an ability to create beautiful make-ups from a remarkable variety of products and materials. Do you have anything in your kit that is indispensable?

Yes – my brushes. I have an amazing collection each with a specific task for applying paint and make-up. They are made up of make-up brushes and traditional art brushes.

Where does your inspiration come from?

Nothing is new, everything comes from other things. I often find inspiration in books and works of art. My travels around Africa have inspired my series of 'tribal' body art images.

Children are also a great inspiration as they are usually very in touch with their imagination. Give them a set of body paints and a mirror and see what they create.

Is there anything you haven't done that you want to do?

I am lucky enough to be in a position where I can pick and choose what I want to do – I will only take on jobs that challenge or excite me. I mainly act as a consultant now and run body painting master classes.

A large proportion of my body art is non-commissioned work. Over the years I have developed a passion and flair for photography and many of my favourite images are designed, painted and photographed by myself.

There are currently a couple of ideas that I want to explore, inspired by paintings by the artists Giuseppe Arcimboldo and Salvador Dalì. I also want to explore the use of plants and flowers as materials in body art.

Do you have any advice for those starting out as body artists?

1 Find a good photographer to record your work – your make-up is only as good as the two-dimensional image you are left with. Never forget about the importance of light, both in creating your make-up and recording it.

2 'Look people in the eye'. You cannot hide from your insecurities and you need to instil confidence about your work in those around you. You will only achieve this through your own security and confidence. A model will be more co-operative if they have confidence in you.

3 Use your mirror as it will help you see your mistakes that will be blaringly obvious on the final 2-D image.

4 Keep your tools clean – it is unacceptable to work with dirty equipment.

Follow the links from www.heinemann.co.uk/ hotlinks to Carolyn Cowan's website, where more images of her work and details about her masterclasses can be found.

Knowledge Check

1 List three aspects of client care particularly relevant when carrying out body art.

2 List five considerations when preparing for a project or client brief.

3 Discuss the advantages of using a rubber stamp for applying temporary tattoos.

4 Discuss the importance of props when completing a design.

5 Why is it important to consider the script and the character a performer is portraying when applying a tattoo design?

Hairstyling for the make-up artist

More and more jobs require the make-up artist to work on both hair and make-up so hairstyling skills are important in order to secure regular work. Generally, the make-up artist will not be required cut, colour or perm a client's hair (though there are exceptions to this, particularly when working on postiche). It is more likely that the make-up artist will be required to set, style and dress the hair; these are the techniques discussed in this chapter.

Aim and objectives

Aim of this chapter: to provide you with the knowledge of different hairstyling techniques so that you may create a range of hairstyles in your role as a make-up artist. Before you begin working through this chapter, you must ensure you are familiar with the information found in Chapter 2 'Health and safety' and Chapter 3 'Establishing positive relationships'.

You should achieve the following **objectives:**

* Evaluate a client's hair type and texture
* List the common contra-indications to hairstyling procedures
* Describe the critical influencing factors when styling the hai
* Choose appropriate tools and equipment
* Describe the functions of various hairstyling products
* Perform a shampooing and conditioning treatment
* Wet set the hair using appropriate techniques to meet a design plan or client requirements
* Perform a blow-dry on hair of various lengths
* Carry out various sectioning and winding techniques.

* Pin curl the hair
* Finger wave the hair
* Dress the hair according to a design plan or client requirements
* Style the hair using various types of heated equipment
* Evaluate the health and safety risks and precautions when using heated equipment
* Dress long hair using a number of techniques
* Apply temporary colour to the hair
* Break down a hairstyle so that it may be recreated accurately
* Produce a range of hairstyles for your portfolio

Before beginning the practical activities in this chapter you may wish to consider obtaining a hairdressing practice head block and clamp, available from hair and beauty suppliers. These blocks, made from human hair, are available in various hair lengths and are useful for practising the different techniques described in this chapter.

Remember to check your posture when working on the hair. If your client is seated in a make-up chair, remove the headrest and lower the seat to its lowest setting. Your client should be at a height that allows you to work comfortably without placing any strain on your back or upper body.

Hair types and textures

The basic structure of the hair and hair growth is discussed in Chapter 4. The section below looks at the characteristics of different hair types and textures.

Hair may be described as healthy, meaning it is in good condition, or unhealthy, meaning it has undergone damage to some degree. The cuticle scales of healthy hair lie flat, reflecting the light and giving the hair shine. On unhealthy hair the cuticle is roughened or raised, causing light rays to scatter and giving the hair a dull appearance. The condition of the cuticle is referred to as the hair's porosity.

Curly hair, even when it is in good condition, will not appear as shiny as straighter textures because the surface is uneven, causing the light rays to scatter.

Healthy hair is a reflection of good health, a good diet and the correct use of hair care products. One or more of the following can cause damage to hair:

* chemical damage (caused by the overuse of chemicals such as colouring, perming or relaxing)

* physical damage (caused by heated styling techniques, or rough handling)

* environmental conditions (UV damage)

* ill health (including certain medications).

If a client you are working on has damaged hair, it is important to try to establish the cause and offer advice on how to avoid further damage in the future. Damaged hair will also be more fragile and will therefore require careful handling by the make-up artist.

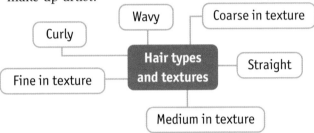

Hair texture refers to the thickness of individual hairs. Coarse-textured hair has a wider diameter than fine-textured hair. The texture of hair may vary on different areas of an individual's head, with finer hair often found around the front hairline.

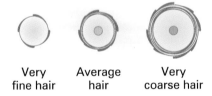

Hair texture

Do not get hair texture confused with **hair density**, which refers to the number of hairs on an individual's head. The average number is about 100,000 to 150,000, with blondes usually having the most and redheads the least. Hair may also be curly, wavy or straight.

These characteristics will help to determine the hairstyling techniques and styles suitable for your client. However, you can also alter the texture of the hair using styling products and particular techniques.

Elasticity of hair

The cortex makes up the bulk of the hair and gives the hair its strength and elasticity. This is the part of the hair where the changes take place that allow the hair to be permanently and temporarily styled. The cortex is structured from bundles of parallel fibres that are made up of smaller fibres. Minute chains of molecules (polypeptide chains) hold the cortex together. These chains are made up of amino acids and are held together by two types of cross linkages or bonds: hydrogen bonds, which are broken by water, and disulphate bonds, which are unaffected by water.

Hair that is soaked in water can be stretched to up to one and a half times its normal length. The unstretched hair is referred to as alpha-keratin (or a-keratin) and the stretched hair is referred to as beta-keratin (or b-keratin). The change from a to b-keratin is referred to as the alpha-beta transformation. Care must be taken not to overstretch the hair, which would cause breakage. The more water content the hair receives, the greater the stretch on the hair; the dryer to hair, the less the hair will stretch.

Testing the hair's elasticity

Prior to setting or styling the hair it is useful to assess the degree of damage to the internal structure. Take a couple of strands of wet hair between your thumb and fingers. Pull the hair gently. The hair should stretch slightly but then return to its original length. If the hair does not return to its original length or if it snaps, this means the hair is in poor condition and will be prone to overstretching and / or breaking during the setting or styling process.

Contra-indications specific to the scalp and hair

As with any make-up procedure where the client's skin should be checked for contra-indications (refer to Chapter 2, page 29), the make-up artist undertaking hairstyling procedures should check the client's scalp and hair for conditions that may prevent or restrict setting or dressing techniques from being applied. Some of the more common conditions are described in the table below.

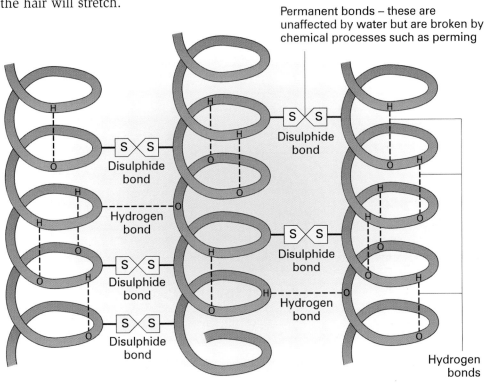

Permanent bonds – these are unaffected by water but are broken by chemical processes such as perming

Disulphide bond

Disulphide bond

Hydrogen bond

Disulphide bond

Disulphide bond

Disulphide bond

Disulphide bond

Hydrogen bond

Hydrogen bonds

Polypeptide chain   Polypeptide chain   Polypeptide chain   *Polypeptide chains and bonds*

261

Condition	Description	Referral required?
Head lice	A parasitic infestation. The females lay eggs (nits) which take the appearance of small white or grey specks. These stick to the hair close to the scalp and cause itchiness. Cross-contamination may occur via direct or indirect contact (infected brushes etc).	Refer to a pharmacist for treatment. All hairstyling procedures should be avoided.
Alopecia areata	Bald patches, thought to be caused by stress or shock. However, some cases seem to have no obvious explanation as to the cause.	Refer to a trichologist.
Diffuse alopecia	Gradual hair loss affecting females that is caused by hormonal changes, e.g. following pregnancy, during the menopause, when taking the contraceptive pill. May also be caused by certain medications.	Refer to a GP or trichologist.
Fragilitis crinium	Split ends caused by harsh physical or chemical treatment, or long intervals between haircuts.	Refer to a hairdresser for regular cutting and conditioning.
Dandruff	Dry, flaky scalp, sometimes accompanied by itching, caused by overproduction and shedding of epidermal cells.	Severe cases should be treated by a trichologist.
Seborrhoeic dermatitis	Yellowish, greasy scales that flake from the scalp and stick to the hair shaft causing itchiness and inflamation. Caused by overproduction of sebum, accompanied by dandruff.	Refer to a trichologist
Sebaceous cyst	A lump under the surface of the skin caused by a blockage of the sebaceous gland. They range in size from 1 to 4 cms. Hair follicles become 'strangled' on larger cysts, preventing hair growth.	Refer to a GP for removal if they become infected or unsightly.
Trichorrhexis nodusa	Hair becomes swollen and roughened, causing splitting along the hair shaft. Caused by harsh physical or chemical treatment.	Refer to a trichologist in severe cases. Apply reconditioning treatments.

In addition to the above conditions, you should also ensure you are familiar with the following contra-indications which are discussed in Chapter 2 (page 29):

* scabies
* ringworm
* impetigo
* folliculitis
* psoriasis
* eczema and dermatitis.

Critical influencing factors

When deciding on appropriate hairstyles and styling techniques for your client there are a number of considerations you should take into account.

Production or brief requirements

The hairstyle must meet the design plan and any continuity requirements. A very complicated hairstyle may look fantastic, but may not be easy to recreate at a later date (see Chapter 6, page 104, for further information on continuity). Hairstyles can generally be classed as classic, period (historical), fashion and avant-garde, and will often require some research.

Hair characteristics and condition

It is important to look at the hair during the initial consultation and check its porosity, density, texture, amount of curl and elasticity, as these characteristics will affect the choice of hairstyle and hairstyling techniques. For example, a head of fine, sparse hair will require different handling from a coarse, dense hair type. Fine-textured hair is often hard to curl, so may need smaller rollers or a smaller blow-drying brush to obtain a satisfactory curl. Coarse hair may need larger rollers or a larger brush to hold the extra bulk of the hair. Naturally curly or permed hair requires larger rollers or blow-dry brushes to smooth out the existing curl. Straight hair requires smaller rollers or brushes. Over-porous or damaged hair tends to loose some of its elasticity and may not wet set so well as it takes longer to dry. It does respond well to heated styling techniques, but extra care should be taken so as not to cause further damage. It may also be helpful to note any previous and existing chemical treatments as these will affect the hair characteristics.

Length of hair

The longer the hair, the older it is and the more damage it is likely to have sustained in its lifetime. Check the entire length of hair for damage when assessing the hair during the initial consultation.

Hair may be one length or layered, meaning it has different lengths around the head. The length of hair will have to be considered when deciding on appropriate styles, dressing techniques and tools.

Very short hair may be too short to curl, and longer hair may tend to drop after styling because of the extra weight. Any length of hair can be blow-dried, but each length will require very different styling techniques to achieve satisfactory results.

Scalp condition

The scalp should be discreetly checked for contra-indications during the initial consultation. Any problems should be dealt with in the usual way (see Chapter 2, page 29). The condition of the scalp – which may be normal, dry, oily or affected by dandruff – will affect the type of products used rather than the actual hairstyling techniques. Care should be taken if any irritation or sensitivity is present.

Growth patterns

Hair growth patterns are caused by the distribution and angle of the hair follicles and may affect the type of style you can successfully create on your client. Where possible, it is always advisable to work with the natural growth patterns as the hair will be easier to control and maintain. If you comb the hair in different directions and lift it to assess the natural hair distribution, strong patterns such as partings, double crowns and cowlicks will be clearly visible.

* A **double crown** will affect the way the hair lies on this area. Setting with a couple of rollers will create some movement and encourage the hair to lie better. Partings can also be altered to disguise the double crown pattern.

* A **cowlick** affects the fringe area with the hair tending to grow more strongly to one side. Working with this natural movement when styling the hair will make the hair easier to work with and maintain.

* A **widow's peak** also affects the front hairline and will make a difference to the appearance of the finished style. Work with rather than against the widow's peak when styling the hair.

* **Nape whorls** should be considered when dressing long hair. Check which way the hair is growing and try to adjust your style accordingly.

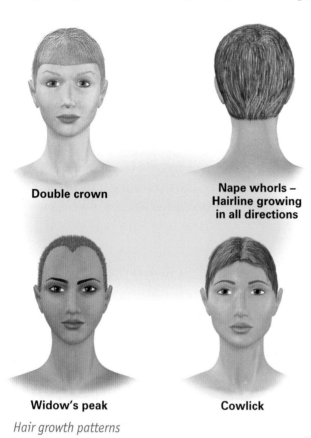

Double crown

Nape whorls – Hairline growing in all directions

Widow's peak

Cowlick

Hair growth patterns

Face shapes

Basic face shapes are discussed in Chapter 8 (page 154). As with make-up application techniques, face shapes in hairstyling are very important. Choosing to style the hair in particular ways can help to bring balance to a client's face and draw attention to or away from facial features.

* The oval face: This already has balance, so the hair can be styled in any way. Drawing the hair back and away from the face will emphasise its shape. Consider using styling techniques to draw attention to specific features, for example a fringe will highlight the eye area.

* The round face: The hairstyle should add height and width at the top of the head, but be kept close at the sides. Avoid straight fringes.

* The heart-shaped face: The hairstyle should remain close to the head at the forehead, and should add width to the jaw line. A true heart-shaped face will also have a widow's peak.

* The pear-shaped face: The hairstyle should create the illusion of width at the forehead whilst making the jaw line appear narrower.

* The oblong face: The hairstyle needs to add width but not height. A fringe will help to reduce the length of the face. You should aim for fullness and softness at the sides.

* The square face: This face shape needs soft, rounded lines that taper at the jaw line to hide the angular structure. Try to add a little height but no width to the hairstyle.

Oval face shape

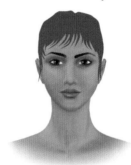

Will suit any hairstyle

Round face shape

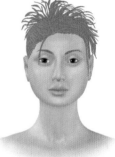

Lots of height, half fringe and soft tendrils to hide roundness at jaw line

Square face shape

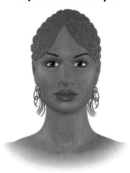

Corners need to be 'cut off' when dressing the hair i.e. fringe and soft tendrils to soften the squareness

Oblong face shape

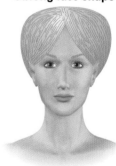

Width required to balance out the length no extra height, as this will elongate the face

Hairstyles for head and face shapes – female

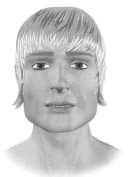

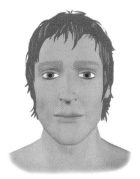

| Square face | Oblong face |

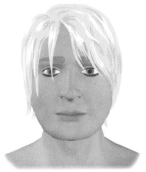

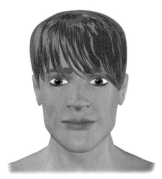

| Round face | Oval face |

Hairstyles for head and face shapes – male

Facial features

* A prominent nose can be disguised by avoiding hairstyles that are drawn back from the face or have centre partings. A long fringe can also help to disguise a large nose.
* Large ears can be kept covered by hair.
* A fringe can disguise a high or receding forehead.
* Low foreheads and hairlines should have the hair swept away from the face.
* Short necks should have the hair dressed off the neck.

Tools and equipment

Using the correct tools is vital when styling and dressing hair if you are to achieve satisfactory results.

Tool	Description
Blow-drying brush	Used to achieve a smooth finish. They come in a variety of sizes with varying amounts and types of bristles. A popular brand of brush is 'Denman'.
Vent brush	Have open spaces at the back to allow airflow during blow-drying. Use to create broken-up styles for a soft, casual effect.
Circular brushes	Used to create curls, flicks, waves and volume. Available in a variety of styles; the smaller the brush the tighter the curl. Hair length and type will also affect the choice of brush.
Paddle brushes and finishing brushes	Used to create a smooth finish and to brush out sets. Smaller brushes can also be used to sculpt hair, backcomb, etc.
Combs	Tail comb: Used for setting and sectioning the hair; the tail is useful for tucking the ends of the hair cleanly round the roller and creating partings. Dressing-out comb: Used for combing, backcombing, dressing out and teasing the hair. Rake comb: Used to disentangle the hair after shampooing. Have wide-spaced teeth to avoid overstretching and breaking the hair. Pin tail comb: Use for setting and sectioning the hair.
Afro comb	Used to disentangle curly hair.
Sectioning clips	Used to hold sections of hair out of the way whilst styling or dressing the hair.
Rollers for wet setting	Available in various sizes for different degrees of curls. Can be smooth or spiky.
Velcro rollers for dry setting	Produce soft curls with body and bounce. Can only be used on dry hair.

Pins	Geisha pins, straight pins, wavy pins, fine pins. Used to secure hair when dressing. The size of the pin will determine how much hair it can hold. Available in a range of colours.
Hairgrip	Used to secure long hair when dressing. Available in a range of colours and sizes.
Double-pronged clip	Made of metal or plastic, used to secure the hair when pin curling.
Hair bands	Used to hold the hair in ponytails or secure braids, etc. Ensure bands are non-snag so the hair is not damaged.

KEY NOTE

The choice often facing the hair stylist is whether to buy natural or artificial bristle brushes. Natural bristles are softer and are said to promote shine to the hair. However, they are fairly expensive to buy and take longer to get used to working with. Artificial bristle brushes (usually nylon) are less expensive and grip the hair well but are thought to be firm and inflexible. Brushes with a combination of both types of bristle are a good compromise. A good brush will grab the hair and allow the hair to move through the bristles easily.

REMEMBER

Electrical equipment should be cleaned regularly with surgical spirit. Never use water, as there will be a risk of electrocution. All electrical equipment must comply with the Electricity at Work Regulations 1989.

Heated styling equipment

Equipment	Description
Tongs	Used to create curls. The type of curl will depend on how the hair is wound onto the barrel and the size of the barrel. The smaller the barrel, the tighter the curl.
Spiral tongs	Used to create spiral curls.

Straightening and flat irons	Temporarily straighten the hair. Available with ceramic or metal plates. Ceramic is less damaging to the hair.
Crimping and waving irons	Give the hair texture depending on the shape of the plates.
Heated rollers	Give, curl, volume and root lift. Available in various sizes for different effects. Fixed in place with pins or butterfly clamps.
Hot brush	Gives curl volume and lift. Available in different sizes.
Flexi-shapers	Give a variety of effects depending on application. Good for creating spirals to soft curls.
Hairdryer	Choose a drier with a range of heat and power settings. Usually fitted with a nozzle to give direction to the airflow when styling.
Diffuser	Attachment for a hairdryer, used to blow-dry curly hair by using a 'scrunching' technique. Helps to avoid frizziness whilst creating volume and lift.

Products for styling and dressing hair

A wide range of products is available to assist you when styling and dressing hair. Although different brands will refer to their products using a variety of names, the majority of styling products will have one or more of the following functions.

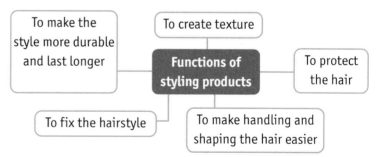

For all the above types of product it is important to follow the manufacturer's instructions to ensure satisfactory results. It is important not to overuse a product – not only is this wasteful (and not cost-

Product	Description
Gel (wet or dry look)	Used to mould and sculpt the hair and add definition to a style. Available in various forms including sprays and pump dispensers. Overuse may cause flatness, greasiness or a hard, stiff, unnatural texture. Usually have a stronger hold than mousses or sprays.
Mousses	Applied to wet hair prior to styling or setting. Will help to define curls prior to scrunch drying permed or naturally curly hair. Gives bounce and body to blow-dried hair. Use sparingly on very fine hair.
Blow-drying lotion and styling sprays	Used prior to drying the hair. Protects the hair against heat damage whilst giving some control and durability to the style. Many are thermo-active, requiring the addition of heat to make them work effectively.
Setting lotion	Available in different strengths, they are used on damp hair prior to setting with rollers to obtain a long-lasting shape or curl.
Curl activators	Used to maintain and define curly hair whilst adding shine.
Straightening products	Used in conjunction with hair straighteners or blow-drying to achieve a poker-straight finish and minimise the effect of humidity.
Wax	Used to hold the hair and add definition or texture to a finished style. Available in different forms; and softer versions are sometimes called 'putty' or 'hair gum'. Particularly useful for short hair.
Serum or gloss	Used to combat frizz and add shine to hair. Ideal for curly hair. Overuse may cause greasiness.
Dressing cream	Applied to dry hair in small amounts to smooth hair and add shine. Can make hair more manageable to sculpt and tease into shape.
Leave-in conditioner	Used sparingly can be an alternative to dressing cream.
Hairspray	Used to fix styles and finished dressing in place and protect the hair from environmental conditions, e.g. humidity. The best hairsprays are easily brushed out and leave an invisible coating on the hair surface. Available in different strengths. Can also be used when dressing long hair to help control and manage the hair.
Shine spray	Used to add shine to the hair. Many also offer UV protection. Can also reduce static in the hair.

Types of product for styling and dressing hair

effective) but it may also have an adverse effect on the finished hairstyle. Being aware of the product's features and benefits (see Chapter 6, page 109) will ensure you get the most out of the product and gain optimum results from the finished style.

REMEMBER

COSHH regulations will apply to all the products you use whilst styling and dressing the hair. Data sheets on all products are available from the manufacturer.

HANDS ON

Researching products

Choose a line of professional hair products (you can research different brands in magazines). Gather information about each of the styling and finishing products in the range and make a list of their features and benefits. Finally, suggest how and when the products may be used, for example to give volume to fine hair when blow-drying.

Shampooing and conditioning hair

The purpose of shampooing is to cleanse the hair and scalp. Where practical, shampooing and conditioning the hair prior to setting and styling is preferable, as dirt and debris on the hair's surface can act as a barrier and affect the finished result. The exception is dressing long hair, when freshly washed and conditioned hair can prove more difficult to handle. Most make-up studios will have a backwash basin as these are most comfortable for the client.

Occasionally, it may not be possible to use a backwash basin if there is a lack of facilities, if a client has a back or neck problem, or when washing children's hair. In these cases, a frontwash basin may be more appropriate. When using a frontwash, the client should be given a towel to hold over the eyes to protect them from water and chemicals.

There are several stages to shampooing a client.

Organise the work area

Prepare the client

Assess the condition, type and texture of the hair

Assess the condition of the scalp

Check for contra-indications

Choose products for the client

Shampoo the hair

Condition the hair

Organise the work area

As with all procedures for the make-up artist, it is important to be organised and professional. Preparing the work area prior to the arrival of the client will save time and appear professional. To perform a shampoo and conditioning treatment you will require the following:

* client gown
* towels
* butterfly clamp or sectioning clip to secure towel around the client
* range of shampoos and conditioning products
* clean wide-toothed (rake) comb
* clean hair brush.

Prepare the client

1 The client should be greeted and given a gown to protect the clothing or costume.

2 The client should be seated and the hair should be brushed through (from roots to tips) to remove any residual products whilst an assessment of the hair and scalp condition is carried out. Use this opportunity to check for contra-indications.

3 A towel is then draped around the client's shoulders, tucked into the gown around the neck and fixed at the front with a butterfly clamp or sectioning clip.

4 The client should then be seated at the backwash. It is important to ensure the client is seated correctly so that both a watertight seal is achieved and the client is comfortable. Guide the client back, adjusting the height of the basin as appropriate and ensuring there are no gaps between the client's neck and the basin.

5 Check the client is comfortable before turning the water on.

Assess the condition, type and texture of the hair

Begin by assessing the hair visually and by questioning the client. You are looking for indications of its porosity, density, texture, amount of curl and elasticity.

Assess the condition of the scalp

Is it normal, dry, greasy or affected by dandruff? Also check for signs of irritation or soreness.

Choose products for the client

Prior to applying any shampooing or conditioning product it is important to read the manufacturer's instructions. This will ensure the procedure is carried out safely and successfully. It is also vital to use the correct products on the client to achieve optimum results. There are a wide range of products for shampooing and conditioning the hair with numerous ingredients. Check the product label for suitability to the client's hair type. However, just as with skin care products, all hair products, whatever their individual properties, should be pH balanced. This will ensure the cuticle scales remain flat so the hair is protected against damage.

* **Shampoo**: The function of shampoo is to cleanse the hair from grease, dirt and product residue.

* **Conditioner**: There are two types of conditioning product – surface conditioners and penetrating conditioners. Both types of conditioner close and smooth the cuticle making the hair appear smooth and shiny. Penetrating conditioners have the added ability to treat the cortex as well, making them an excellent choice for damaged hair. Make-up artists are more likely to apply surface conditioners on a day-to-day basis as these are applied at the basin following shampooing.

KEY NOTE

The importance of using pH-balanced products is discussed in detail in Chapter 4, page 56.

Application techniques

The secret to a successful shampoo is keeping the client dry from the neck down and employing relaxing and comfortable application techniques. The application techniques are based on standard massage movements and should be carried out using the palms of your hands and the pads of your fingers. To ensure you do not scratch the client or cause discomfort it is important that your nails are kept short. The shampoo and conditioning procedure should take approximately ten minutes to complete.

Effleurage movements

Keeping one hand on your client at all times, use the palms of your hands, and apply slow, stroking movements over the client's head keeping a fairly firm pressure. Use this technique to apply shampoo and conditioner and relax the client. Effleurage movements down the length of longer hair will also spread the shampoo and cleanse without knotting the hair.

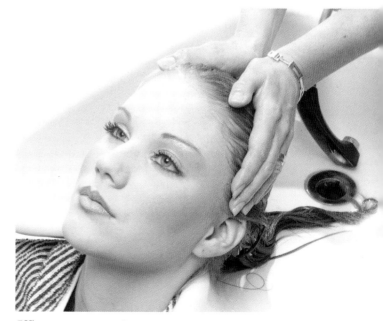

Effleurage movements

STEP-BY-STEP **Shampooing**

1 Turn on the cold tap first and then add the warm water. Test the temperature on the inside of your wrist. When happy, check the temperature on the client.

2 When the client is happy with the water temperature, thoroughly wet the hair and scalp. Protect the client's face from running water by using your hand as a barrier along the front hairline. Turn off the water.

3 Following the manufacturer's guidelines, pour the correct amount of shampoo into the palm of your hand and warm it between your palms.

4 Apply the shampoo from the front hairline to the nape and down the length of the hair using effleurage movements.

5 Begin rotary movements to the scalp, ensuring you cover the whole head. Continue until the shampoo has built up a good lather. Continue with effleurage movements down the length of the hair to ensure this part of the hair is also thoroughly cleansed.

6 Turn the water on and rinse thoroughly. Repeat the shampoo procedure, ensuring the final rinse leaves the hair squeaky clean. Turn off the water. Gently squeeze the hair to remove excess water.

7 Apply a surface conditioner using effleurage movements. Follow with slow, deep petrissage movements.

8 Comb through the hair with a wide-toothed comb to disentangle the hair and spread the conditioner down the length of the hair. Rinse thoroughly.

9 Gently squeeze the hair to remove excess water. Wrap a clean towel around the client's head and replace the towel around the client's neck if it is wet.

10 The client can now be seated at a workstation. The hair should be gently towel-dried to get rid of excess moisture and combed through using a wide-toothed (rake) comb to remove any tangles. The hair is now ready to be styled or set according to the design plan.

Rotary movements

Using the pads of your fingers, use circular movements over the client's head. This movement stimulates the scalp and deep cleanses, removing grease and dirt. Again the pressure should be fairly firm.

Petrissage movements

Similar to the rotary movement, petrissage movements are slower and deeper. They are used to apply conditioning products and release tension from the scalp whilst thoroughly relaxing the client.

Wet setting the hair

It is possible to temporarily change the shape of the hair by using many different methods. This section will look at:

* blow-drying
* rollering
* pin curling
* finger waving
* pin weaving.

It is possible to change the hair shape because of its natural structure and properties. Firstly it is hydroscopic, which means it is able to absorb water. Secondly, it is naturally elastic enabling it to stretch and then return to its original shape. When hair is wet, the water breaks down the hydrogen bonds allowing the hair to stretch. In this state it can be reshaped using one of the above methods. Heat is then applied, which dries the hair and reforms the bonds into the new shape. It is important that the hair is allowed to completely cool before any brushing or styling takes place. If the hair is still warm, some of the bonds may not be completely set and the new shape may be lost. This type of setting is also called **cohesive setting**.

The hair will stay in its new shape until it is physically made wet again or absorbs moisture from the air (humidity). This moisture breaks down the new temporary bonds that hold the shape in place; once these bonds are broken the polypeptide chains return to their original shape and the style will 'drop'. The more humidity in the atmosphere (for example a damp day whilst working on location), the more quickly this will happen. However, there is a simple measure you can take to reduce this effect. By using certain styling and finishing products you can reduce the amount of moisture absorbed by the hair and so help to increase the life of a set or blow-dry. These products coat the hair with a plasticiser, which creates a plastic film over the hair cuticle preventing atmospheric moisture from entering the hair shaft. The products are easily washed out with shampoo and warm water.

Blow-drying the hair

The usual critical influencing factors (see page 262) will affect the blow-drying process, so bear these in mind before beginning the procedure. It is also important to have a clear idea of the desired finished hairstyle in your mind as this will ultimately affect the choice of techniques, tools and products. As with most of the techniques in this book, practise is important if you are to become competent.

Tips for successful blow-drying

Ensure you create cleanly parted sections in the hair. The initial sections are best achieved using a tail comb; further sub-sections can then be created using the fingers. Sectioning keeps the hair under control whilst styling and allows an even tension to be maintained. Keep the sub-sections small as this will encourage root movement.

The most difficult aspect of blow-drying is handling the hair while at the same time working with sections, holding the drier and continuing to work in an unbroken rhythm at an acceptable speed. Each stylist will develop his or her own method of handling the hair whilst holding the drier. You may wish to try the following method when picking up sections, as once mastered it enables you to work quickly and continuously.

1   Place the brush *under* the hair, positioning it at the roots. Keeping the tension on the hair taut, continue down the length of the hair to the ends. Direct the airflow from the dryer so that it follows the movement of the brush. Keep the brush and dryer moving at all times.

2   Before releasing the ends of the hair from the brush, place the nozzle and front end of the drier under the section, near to the roots but not touching the scalp, to lift the section.

3   Release the hair from the brush so the section is resting on the drier. Move the brush back up to the roots, under the hair. Remove the dryer from under the hair and continue as Step 1. Repeat the action until the section is dried.

∗   When you are attempting to create a smooth, shiny finish to the hair, it is important to blow-dry the hair from roots to points (ends). This ensures the cuticle lies flat.

∗   Drying the hair from points to roots will ruffle the cuticle. This technique can be used to create:

   ∗   volume when drying curly hair with a diffuser

   ∗   a tousled, fuller hairstyle on wavy hair

   ∗   volume and body on fine hair by 'blasting' the hair with air

   ∗   texture on short hair during finger-drying.

∗   Always keep the hairdryer moving to prevent burning the scalp and hair. Be particularly careful around the neck and ears.

∗   Gently position the head downwards when working around the nape of the head.

* Remember to angle the brush in the direction you wish the hair to fall.

* Angle the brush upwards at the roots to achieve volume in this area. This works particularly well on fine, flat hair.

* Keep a taut, even tension as you work down the hair length.

* Feel free to use more than one type of brush when blow-drying a head of hair.

* Ensure each section is completely dry before moving onto the next, otherwise the style will not hold.

* Polishing the hair is a technique used to create a high shine and set a style. Hot air is used to dry the hair, quickly followed by a blast of cool hair, whilst the brush and drier are kept moving over the length of the hair. This seals the cuticle and helps to maintain the new shape.

* To create a particularly flat finish, the hair can be finished by blow-drying using a comb.

* Products will protect the hair from heat damage and can turn a good blow-dry into a great finished hairstyle. They will also help to maintain the style by protecting it from the effects of humidity.

* Keep checking the shape of the hairstyle in the mirror.

* Try to practise on as many different hair types and lengths as possible.

Whenever you prepare to blow-dry the hair, always remember the key areas that will affect the finished result.

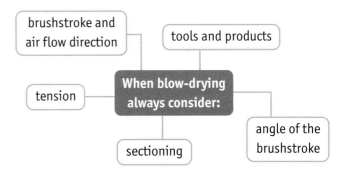

brushstroke and air flow direction

tools and products

tension

When blow-drying always consider:

sectioning

angle of the brushstroke

STEP-BY-STEP Blow-drying long hair

Equipment required

* Towel draped around the client's shoulders
* Styling products
* Wide-toothed (rake) comb
* Tail comb
* Selection of sectioning clips
* Selection of blow-drying brushes
* Hairdryer with nozzle or diffuser as appropriate
* Finishing products

1 Comb through towel-dried hair with a wide-toothed comb to remove any tangles. Apply a suitable styling product following the manufacturer's instructions.

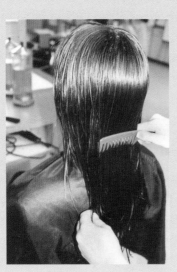

2 Using a high heat and speed setting, rough-dry the hair to remove excess moisture.

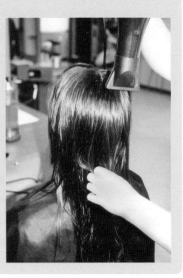

3 Section the hair into four: from ear to ear across the back of the crown and down the centre of the head from the front hairline to the nape. Secure the four sections using sectioning clips. Starting with the sections at the back of the head, create a sub-section by releasing some hair from each section nearest to the nape of the neck. Select a brush that is suitable for creating a smooth finish. Select a medium to hot setting on the dryer with a medium speed.

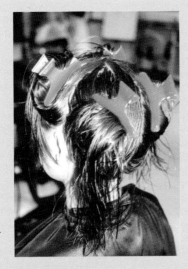

4 Place the brush under the hair, positioning it at the roots. Keeping the tension on the hair taut, lift the brush slightly upwards to achieve some root lift and continue down the length of the hair to the ends, directing the airflow from the dryer so that it follows the movement of the brush. Keep the brush and dryer moving at all times. As you reach the ends of the hair, curve the brush under. Repeat until the sub-section is completely dry.

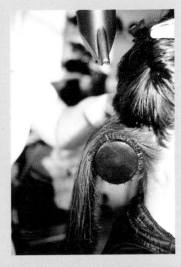

5 After finishing the first section, blow-dry several more sub-sections working your way up the head. Release a sub-section of hair from one of the top sections and dry it in the same way, working your way up towards the parting.

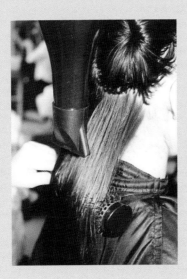

6 Continue in this manner until you have dried all the hair. If the client has a fringe, dry this last taking into account any strong natural growth patterns. Apply a finishing product according to the manufacturer's instructions.

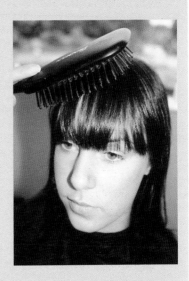

KEY NOTE

Sometimes it may be necessary to 'neutralise' strong hair growths such as cowlicks in the fringe. Alternatively, you may be required to change the direction of the hair growth because of the design plan. Blowing and brushing the hair in a variety of directions using the hot setting on the drier and concentrating on the root area will achieve this. Once the hair lies flat, finish by blowing the hair in the direction you wish it to fall using the cool setting on your drier.

Adapting the blow-drying technique for shorter, layered styles

The same basic techniques and principles are employed when blow-drying shorter, layered hairstyles. The differences lie in the selection of tools and products and the direction of the brushwork. These decisions, as always, will depend on the design plan.

STEP-BY-STEP Finger-drying

Finger-drying the hair is a simple way to create volume and texture on short hair. The best effects are achieved when this technique is combined with styling and finishing products.

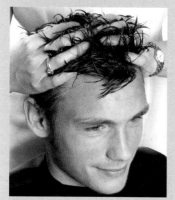 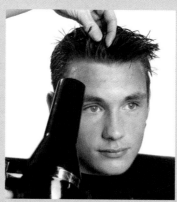 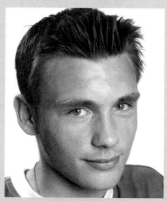

1 Comb through towel-dried hair with a wide-toothed comb to remove any tangles. Apply a suitable styling product following the manufacturer's instructions.

2 Using a medium heat and speed setting, begin to dry the hair by letting the airflow 'blast' at the roots whilst using your fingers or palms to tease the hair into the desired shape. Work through the hair working on each area from roots to points.

3 When the hair is completely dry, apply a suitable finishing product.

Scrunch-drying with a diffuser attachment on the hairdryer is an excellent method of drying curly hair without causing frizziness. Using the correct products is essential if you are to achieve maximum results.

STEP-BY-STEP Scrunch-drying curly hair using a diffuser

1 Apply product and section hair.
2 Beginning at the nape or the neck, take a section of hair and scrunch it in your hand with the diffuser.
3 Continue working each section in this way until all the hair is dry.
4 Even more volume can be created by asking the client to lean forwards and look downwards so the hair falls forward before you commence drying. Remember to give the client plenty of breaks from this position.

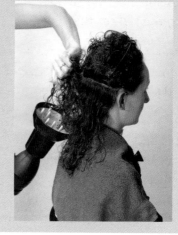

Scrunch-drying curly hair

Wet roller setting

Wet hair will take on the shape of whatever it is set on; in the case of rollers this is usually curls or waves. Whenever you prepare to set the hair using rollers, always remember the key areas that will affect the finished result.

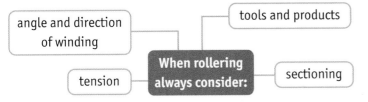

Tools and products

Rollers vary in diameter, length and the material from which they are made. Smooth rollers, i.e. without spikes or small bristles, will create a sleeker finish but are more difficult to put in than the 'spiky' kind that grip the hair well. Most rollers designed for use on wet hair are secured in place with pins and care should be taken to ensure they do not cause the client discomfort. The hair density and texture and the degree of curl required determine the roller size. The choice of roller will have a profound impact on the finished style, so choose carefully when preparing to set. The most important point to remember is: **the smaller the diameter of the roller, the tighter the curl.**

Naturally very curly hair can be turned into loose waves by setting on large rollers, whereas straight hair can form tight curls when set on rollers with a very small diameter.

As with most of the techniques discussed in this chapter, the finished result can be enhanced by the use of styling products. Setting lotions (available as soft or firm finishes) are ideal to apply to the hair prior to wet setting, but there are a number of alternatives available on the market. Products should be used as directed by the manufacturer.

Sectioning

Sectioning is a very important part of the rollering technique. It should be carried out giving due consideration to the following if successful results are to be achieved.

* **Size of the section:** This should be slightly shorter than the length of the roller and no deeper than the diameter of the roller. Sections that are too large will produce an uneven curl and will not dry evenly. If the sections are too small, you will have to use too many rollers. This will cause 'overcrowding' and the rollers will not lie appropriately on the head.

* **Creating cleanly parted sections:** The sections are best created using a tail comb. Sectioning keeps the hair under control whilst styling and allows an even tension to be maintained. Hair sections can be any shape providing they are cleanly parted.

Tension

Hair that is wound under tension will produce a superior and longer lasting style. It will also be distributed evenly around the roller achieving a regular and consistent curl.

Care should be taken not to overstretch the hair as this could cause damage. An elasticity test can be carried out prior to rollering to establish how resilient the hair will be to applied tension. Damaged hair that suffers from loss of elasticity should be handled carefully and the degree of tension should be adapted accordingly.

Angle and direction of winding

When winding the hair it is important to work in a methodical sequence. Always think ahead so that you do not run out of headspace, and give due consideration to the final effect you are trying to achieve.

* Winding should be a smooth, even action.

* To ensure a smooth wind, comb the section through, holding it at the angle you wish to wind. This will ensure good tension and avoid 'kinks' in the finished result.

* The ends (or points) of the hair should be neatly wound onto the roller to avoid distorted or 'fish hook' ends. A pin-tail comb can be used to tuck the ends smoothly around the roller. Alternatively, 'perming papers' can be wrapped around the ends to make them easier to control.

You can wind from **roots to point** (end) or from **point to roots**. The former, which is usually carried out on long thin rollers using a spiralling technique, produces an even, spiral-shaped curl. The latter, which is the more conventional style of winding, gives a looser curl at the roots (the diameter of the roller increases with each revolution of the roller because of the added thickness of the hair).

The angle

The angle at which you hold and wind the section of hair will ultimately determine the amount of root lift in the hairstyle. Root lift creates height and volume in a hairstyle. The angle of the wind can be varied over the client's head to achieve different effects, depending on the design plan for the hairstyle.

A section of hair held and wound at 90° to the scalp will create normal root lift. The base of the roller, once wound, will rest on the head.

If the hair is angled forward and wound at an obtuse angle to the scalp, but still able to sit partially on its base, increased root lift will be achieved.

If the hair is angled backward and wound at an acute angle to the scalp, with the roller sitting off its base, little root lift will be achieved. This technique can be used where the hairstyle requires less volume.

Direction

Using imaginative directive winding will produce interesting hairstyles that are easy to dress out and style. Roller direction must always be consistent with the desired effect.

Channel

Begin at the front hairline, directing the wind backwards away from the front hairline. Place a row of rollers down the centre of the head creating a channel. If there is a fringe, this can be left out to style later.

Move to the crown area, directing the wind downwards. Place a row of rollers each side of the centre channel to create a further two channels.

Complete the set by placing another set of rollers at the sides of the head, again winding downwards.

Brickwork

Begin at the centre of the front hairline. Wind one roller in a backward direction.

Take a second section from behind this first roller halfway along its length.

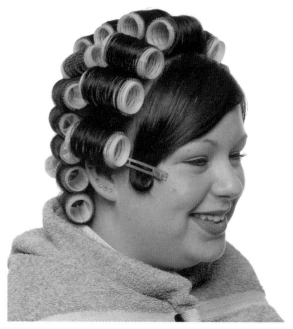

'Channel' rollering technique

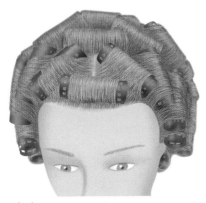

Brickwork technique

Continue in this way working down towards the nape. The finished result should resemble the brickwork of a wall. Some alterations in the rollering position may be required to account for different head shapes.

Directional

The hair is wound onto rollers and placed in the direction you desire the hair to be dressed. You can use any of the sectioning and winding techniques discussed in this chapter providing the hair is directed as appropriate according to the design plan. Different areas of the head may be rollered in different directions.

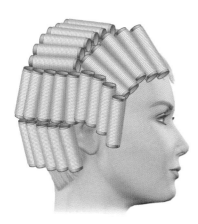

Directional winding

Advanced sectioning and winding techniques

Some conventional as well as more unusual techniques are described and illustrated below. Try them out and judge the finished effect for yourself.

Ringlets or spiral curls

This method is used to create spiral curls or ringlets. Long thin rollers are required.

1   Beginning at the nape, take a section of hair and wind either from roots to points, or from points to roots. Hold the roller vertically and rotate it ensuring the hair is evenly wound along the length of the roller. Try not to overlap the hair or leave large gaps as you continue to wind up or down the hair length. Some hairstylists like to twist the hair as it is being wound onto the rollers.

2   Using perming papers at the points will ensure the hair is held in place smoothly.

3   Work across the width of the head and then in an upward direction towards the front hairline. Around the hairline it is more flattering to rotate the roller towards the face.

4   The rollers are secured by bending.

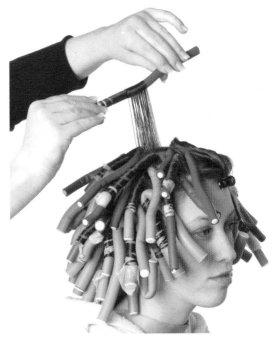

Spiral curls

Weaving

This technique will create different textures over the head.

1 The hair can be wound in any direction that suits the design plan.

2 Take a fine section of hair and wind it onto a smallish roller.

3 Take a further section of hair above the first roller and leave it out resting on the roller underneath.

4 Take a further section of hair above the section you have left out and wind it onto a roller. It should rest next to the roller beneath it.

Hopscotch

This technique produces curl going in different directions, creating a highly textured hairstyle.

1 Begin at the nape, working up towards the front hairline.

2 The hair is wound, leaving out a fine section of head between each roller. Place approximately four rollers at a time.

3 Pick up the hair that is left out and wind it together over the top of these rollers in a different direction.

4 Repeat until the entire head is rollered.

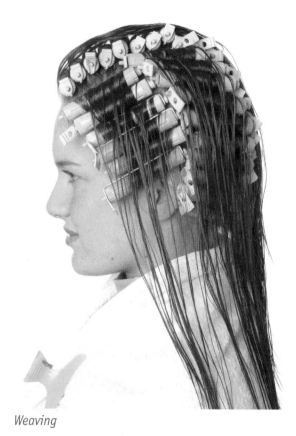

Weaving

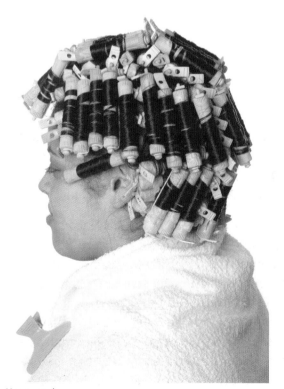

Hopscotch

Unconventional rollering techniques

Once you have mastered using rollers to set the hair, you may wish to begin experimenting with more unconventional setting tools to reshape the hair into more unusual shapes. The possibilities are only limited by your imagination, usability and consideration of health and safety issues such as the following.

* Is the tool flammable? It will have to be exposed to heat to dry the hair.

* Can the tool be secured to the head safely and securely?

* Will the tool conduct heat to ensure each section dries evenly?

* Does the tool have any sharp edges that may injure or be uncomfortable for the client?

The following technique is an example of an unconventional setting technique you may wish to try.

Pin weaving

This technique is best carried out on medium to long hair using geisha pins to reshape the hair. It will create a very full, tight zigzag effect (similar to crimping). It can be used to create high fashion or avant-garde effects.

1 Beginning at the nape, take a small section of hair. Hold the geisha pin with the closed end resting lightly on the scalp.

2 Pass the section of hair through the pin and weave the hair around the pin in a figure of eight, ensuring the hair is evenly wound along the length of the pin. Maintain a tight tension with no spaces between the winding. You could also try twisting the hair as it is being wound onto the pin.

3 Using perming papers at the points will ensure the hair is held in place smoothly.

4 Secure the ends of the hair to the pin using a double-pronged clip.

5 Work across the width of the head and then in an upward direction towards the front hairline.

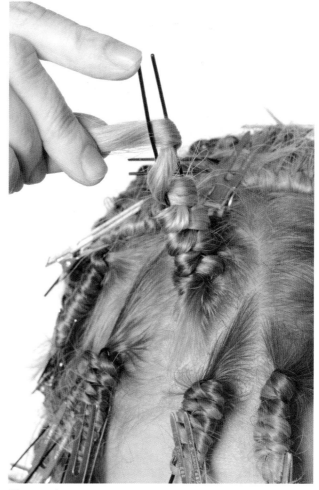

Pin weaving

Drying a wet set

Sets should preferably be dried under a 'hood dryer'. This type of dryer will dry the hair quickly and evenly without a strong airflow, which may disturb the hair. Portable hoods are available that attach onto the end of a hairdryer via a plastic hose. These are very useful when working on location.

The length of time the client spends under a dryer will depend on the hair density, texture, length and type of wind. It is important to make sure the sections are completely dry (not just surface dry) and cooled before the set is removed, or it will drop. Use a timer or check the time at regular intervals to ensure the client is not kept under the dryer for longer than necessary. Hair that is over-dried may become flyaway and difficult to dress out. Check that any pins or clips are not causing the client discomfort, particularly if they are made of metal and will retain heat. The ears, nape and front hairline can be protected with cotton wool or tissues if required.

When you are sure the set is dried, remove the client from the dryer and seat the client at a workstation with a mirror. Allow the hair to completely cool and then begin to remove the rollers from the nape, working upwards so the hair does not become tangled. The client's hair is now ready to be dressed out and styled.

Pin curling

Pin curling is the technique of using the fingers on hair to form curls, which are then secured with double-pronged clips. It is a very useful technique to learn and can produce a variety of effects when used either alone or in conjunction with roller setting. It is particularly useful for adding curl and wave to hair that is too short to be wound on rollers. The best results are achieved on healthy, medium length hair that has some natural wave. As with rollering, the hair must be wet and the application of a styling product such as setting lotion will enhance the finished result.

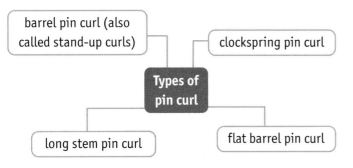

There are three parts to a curl:

* root or base – the immovable foundation of the curl

* stem – the part between the base and the first turn of the body or circle

* body or circle – the part that creates the full circle; it is the diameter of the body or circle that determines the size and tightness of the pin curl.

Type of pin curl	Description
Barrel pin curl	An open-centred curl, wound from roots to points around the fingers, or with a finger and tail comb. The point of the section is secured to the stem with a double-pronged clip. The curl stands away from the head. Gives lift and body.
Flat barrel pin curl	An open-centred curl that lies flat to the head. Wound around a finger from roots to points (the open-centre diameter should be about the size of a finger). The curl is secured flat to the head by a double-pronged clip across the centre. Creates even flat waves and movements.
Clockspring pin curl	A closed-centred curl that lies flat to the head. Wound from point to root, the diameter of the curl increases with each turn. The curl is secured flat to the head by a double-pronged clip across the centre. Creates a curly effect and is used mainly at the nape of the neck.
Long stem pin curl	Basically flat barrel curls with a long stem, giving a curl at the ends of the section only.

The size of the sections will depend on the length and texture of the hair and the effect required. Hair must be combed through thoroughly before winding to ensure there are no kinks in the final curl. Just as with rollering, give due consideration to the direction and placement of the curls. Barrel curls can be placed fully upright or half standing (useful around the front hairline, where the curls can be angled away from the face). Flat pin curls can be curled upwards, downwards, clockwise, anticlockwise and

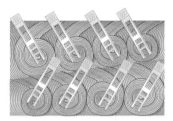

Reverse pin curls

laid to the left or right. An example of the importance of the direction when forming pin curls can be seen in the technique of deep waves using reverse pin curls.

Flat barrel pin curls are formed in one direction in the first row, and in the opposite direction in the next row. This pattern is repeated working up the head.

> **KEY NOTE**
>
> Make sure that when you wind the curls you do not twist the section of hair. If the hair is twisted, it will not lie in the correct direction once dressed.

Finger waving

Finger waving is a technique that can be used independently or in conjunction with reverse pin curling to produce deep waves in the hair without any root lift.

The technique involves sculpting the hair into 's' shapes using the fingers and a dressing out comb. It should be carried out on hair that is wet through but not dripping, and has had a generous application of styling product – gel works well. Try to follow the natural parting of the hair; this will make life much easier for you and will help to maintain the finished style. The technique works best on fine to medium textured, one-length hair with a slight natural wave. It is very difficult to achieve good results using this method on straight hair. Hair to shoulder length can be successfully finger waved; long hair can be reverse pin curled to achieve the same effect. It is important not to lean on the client's head when performing this technique. Use your outstretched fingers rather than your palms, which should remain off the head. Keeping your elbows high will encourage you to adopt the correct position.

STEP-BY-STEP **Finger waving**

1 Ensure the hair is wet through, tangle free and has plenty of firm-hold styling product applied. Find the natural parting on the client. The first wave should follow the hair's natural fall from the parting. Work on section widths about half a comb length at a time.

2 With your usual working hand, hold the comb with three fingers at the top and the thumb and little finger underneath. Check that the comb is in contact with the scalp at all times. The entire

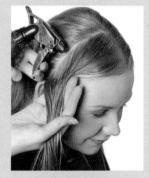

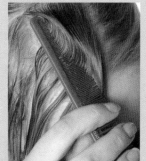

section of hair needs to move, not just the surface hair. Push the hair slightly up to form the crest of the first wave.

3 Leaving the comb in place, with the opposite hand place the index finger just below the crest you have just formed resting above the teeth of the comb and place your second finger just above the crest, holding it in place. Keep the elbow parallel to the hand to ensure a tight grip.

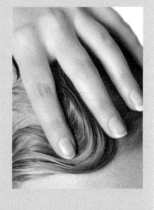

4 Checking the comb is in contact with the scalp, comb the hair in the opposite direction. Push the hair up slightly to form another crest.

5 Remove the index finger from the 'trough' of the first wave and place it to hold the new wave in position. Continue in this manner down the head until you reach the jaw line.

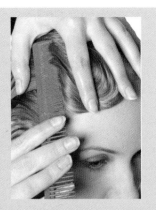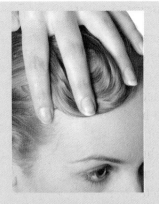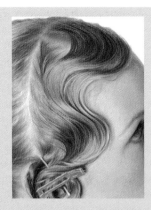

6 Any length of hair below the jaw can be pin curled in the opposite direction to the last finger wave, using flat barrel curls.

When finger waving a whole head, create your first wave on one side and continue to wave to the side of this first wave. Continue around the head so that you finish on the other side of the head at the front hairline. You can then start to form your next crest round the head. Alternatively, you may choose to wave both sides of the head first and then join them up around the back. It is best to avoid using clips to hold the waves in place as these will leave marks on the hair. Instead, use tape positioned in the trough part of the waves.

At the crown area the crest of the wave should be slightly flatter to make it look more natural. This is referred to as 'losing a wave' and is achieved by making the crest less raised.

Finger waves should be dried under a hood dryer to avoid disturbing the set. They are usually dressed out using a wide-toothed comb to avoid destroying the shape of the waves.

KEY NOTE

When setting hair, it is important it remains damp until it has been moulded into its new shape, for example with a roller, pin curls or waves. If the hydrogen bonds in the hair structure are allowed to re-form in their natural position before the hair is moulded into its new shape, the set will not take. Use a water spray to keep re-dampening the hair whilst you are working if it begins to dry out.

Dressing out sets

Dressing out refers to achieving the correct volume, balance and shape to the hairstyle. The direction of the hairstyle should already have been worked out during the setting stage, so the better the set, the easier it will be to dress out. When dressing out hair, always have the design plan to hand so that you are sure the finished result will reflect its requirements. Always work with a mirror and continually check your progress from all angles.

The techniques you use to dress out the hair will depend on the effect you wish to achieve, but in all cases you must ensure:

* the hair is completely dry and cooled before removing the set to dress out
* the direction you dress the hair is the direction it was set
* the finished hairstyle meets the requirements of the design plan
* the finished hairstyle suits the client's features and face shape (unless it is specifically designed not to).

The type of brushes and combs you use will depend on the style, texture and effect you wish to achieve. Begin by brushing the hair in the direction of the finished style, dressing the front and sides of the head first. Work around to the nape area building the style into its finished shape. Always check the finished result from all angles.

Backcombing and backbrushing

Backcombing is used to create lift and volume in a hairstyle. It can be carried out on the root area only to create support and height, or on the entire hair length with the surface hair smoothed over to create lots of volume in a hairstyle. It can also be applied to very fine or soft hair that is difficult to manage; in this case a light coating of fine hair spray will help the comb grip the cuticle surface. Some clients may be reluctant to have their hair backcombed, believing it will cause damage to the hair cuticle. However, if backcombing is carried out in the correct manner, it is easy to brush out and will leave the hair undamaged. The correct way to backcomb is described below.

1 If you are backcombing the entire head, always begin at the nape of the neck and work upwards. Otherwise take sections from the areas of the head that require lift or volume.

2 Take a section of hair and hold it at a 90° angle from the head.

3 Take a dressing-out comb or brush and position it about 5 cm from the base of the root. Push the comb towards the head. Depending on the comb tooth width, an amount of the hair will move with the comb. Remove the comb (do not drag the comb upwards through the hair or you will end up with a tangled mess!).

4 If more volume is required, place the comb approximately 5 cm above the previous position (i.e. 10 cm above the base of the root) and repeat the action described above. Continue in the same manner as far up the hair length as required by the design plan.

5 The top layers of the hair can be smoothed and styled using a dressing-out comb or brush. This will hide the backcombing beneath.

KEY NOTE

If you use a comb, you will work on smaller sections at a time but will achieve a strong effect. Using a brush will allow you to work on a larger area at a time and create a softer effect.

Teasing the hair

Teasing the hair refers to gentle backcombing or backbrushing of the top layers to blend sections and then finishing by encouraging the hair into its final shape, using the prongs on a dressing-out comb.

Using the fingers to dress the hair

When a softer effect is required the hair can simply be dressed by running your fingers through it. This is particularly useful when you do not want to break up the curl too much or when the hairstyle does not require any additional volume. Using an appropriate finishing product on the fingers can help to achieve the desired result.

Finishing products

The application of the correct type of finishing product can greatly enhance the final effect and complete a truly professional hairstyle. It can also help to control the hair when dressing out. The secret to the successful use of finishing products is knowing which product to use to achieve the desired effect and following the manufacturer's instructions.

Wax	Used to hold the hair and add definition or texture to a finished style. Available in different forms and sometimes called 'putty' or 'hair gum'. Particularly useful for short hair.
Serum or gloss	Used to combat frizz and add shine to hair. Ideal for curly hair. Overuse may cause greasiness.
Dressing cream	Applied to dry hair in small amounts to smooth the hair and add shine. Can make hair more manageable to sculpt and tease into shape or to add definition to curls.
Leave-in conditioner	Used sparingly can be an alternative to dressing cream.
Hairspray	Used to fix styles and the finished dressing in place and to protect the hair from environmental conditions, e.g. humidity. The best hairsprays are easily brushed out and leave an invisible coating on the hair surface.

	Available in different strengths. Can also be used when dressing long hair to help control and manage the hair.
Shine spray	Used to add shine to the hair. Many also offer UV protection. Can also reduce static in the hair.

Troubleshooting common problems when wet setting the hair

Problem	Likely cause	Troubleshooting
Set has not taken	Hair not left to dry and cool sufficiently	Remove one roller or hair section to check the hair is dry and cooled before removing the entire set.
Fish hook (buckled) ends on hair	Hair points not wrapped properly when the hair was set	Try using a hot tong to reshape the ends. Ensure you are more careful when setting hair next time and consider using 'perming papers'.
Hair too curly	Incorrect size of rollers or barrel used (too small)	Blow-dry the hair to relax the curl.
Curls too loose	Incorrect size of rollers or barrel used (too large)	Use hot tongs to increase the curl.
Hair going in wrong direction	Incorrect placement of rollers when setting hair	Try to redirect the hair by blow-drying. Give due consideration to the finished style next time.
Hair is difficult to manage	Hair has just been shampooed, or may be a natural characteristic of the hair type	Consider using a suitable product to help control the hair.
Hair is greasy and lifeless	Hair has had too much styling or finishing product applied	No solution other than to re-wash and set the hair.

Dry styling using heat

Hair can also be reshaped using a variety of heated equipment to produce a range of temporary effects. Even when the hair is dry, some moisture is retained within its structure. When heated equipment is applied to the hair the small amount of moisture evaporates, breaking some of the bonds. This effect is increased if styling products are applied. The hair is then 'baked' into its new shape. Dry setting the hair is less durable than wet setting.

Dry styling is useful because it is quick to undertake and many different effects can be achieved. It is particularly suited for fashion work, where time and facilities are limited and wet setting would prove impractical. However, because of the evaporation of the natural moisture within the hair when using heated styling equipment, repeated use will cause the hair to become dehydrated and brittle.

REMEMBER

Prior to using any piece of electrical equipment, you must ensure it is safe to use and complies with current legislation. You must always work in a safe and responsible manner to avoid injuring the client or yourself. Ensure you are fully acquainted with the section on electrical safety precautions (Chapter 2, page 16).

Working with electrical equipment

* Ensure the hair is completely dry.
* Always follow health and safety precautions when using heated electrical appliances.

* Ensure the client is comfortable and you are able to work in a safe and comfortable position that allows you to reach all areas of the head without increasing the risk of burning.

* Always pre-heat electrical appliances prior to use to save time.

* Avoid using mousse and gels as styling products. These may cause the hair to stick to the heated surface of the equipment, increasing the risk of damage to the hair and making the appliance less effective. Stick to thermo-active styling sprays.

* Work with cleanly parted, suitable sized sections The sections are best achieved using a tail comb. Sectioning keeps the hair under control whilst styling and allows an even tension to be maintained. Hair sections can be any shape providing they are cleanly parted.

* To achieve lift at the roots, place the appliance at 90° to the head.

* Always consider the direction of the hairstyle when using the equipment.

* Always protect the client's skin (paying particular attention to the scalp, neck and ears) from accidental burning. Never allow the heated appliances to touch the skin.

* The heated equipment should be applied to the hair for the minimum time necessary to achieve the desired result.

* Allow the hair to cool before dressing out.

* Clean heated electrical equipment with surgical spirit, not water.

* Always allow the equipment to cool before storing.

The equipment you should become familiar with includes:

* heated rollers

* heated flexi-shapers

* tongs

* hot brush

* straightening irons

* crimping and waving irons.

Heated rollers

Heated rollers are available as sets that usually contain about twenty rollers of varying sizes. The more conventional types are secured with pins that are usually colour coded. Rollers usually take between 10 and 15 minutes to heat up, so make sure you turn them on ahead of when you plan to use them. They take about 30 minutes to completely cool down. Heated rollers are ideal for quick sets to give curl and body to hair. They are also useful for preparing long hair prior to dressing.

A basic set using heated rollers

1 Heat the rollers according to the manufacturer's instructions. Brush the hair through thoroughly to remove any tangles.

2 Take a section, hold it at a 90° angle from the head and spray it lightly with styling product. The width of each section should be just short of the width of the rollers. Ensure the sections are not too deep or the heat may not penetrate through to all the hair once it is wound on the roller. Use medium and smaller rollers at the sides and front of the head, and larger rollers around the crown and back. Place the rollers in the direction the hair is to be styled.

3 Keeping a good even tension, wind the hair downwards, making sure the ends are tucked under smoothly. Secure each roller. When the entire head is 'rollered', give the hair a final light spray of styling product.

4 Allow the rollers to completely cool and then gently remove them, beginning at the nape of the neck. Try not to pull on the curl as you unwind each roller.

5 For a loose, soft finish, apply a little finishing product on your hands and dress with your fingers.

Heated flexi-shapers

STEP-BY-STEP **Using heated flexi-shapers**

This type of heated appliance can create various effects. It works particularly well on medium to long layered hair.

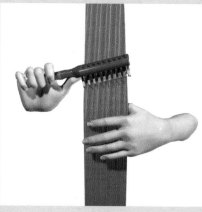

1 Heat the rollers according to the manufacturer's instructions. Take a section and comb it through, holding it taut with one hand. Spray lightly with styling product.

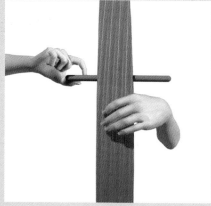

2 Hold a heated flexi-shaper about 5 cm from the root of the first section. The width of each section should be about one-third of the length of the flexi-shaper. Ensure the sections are not too deep or the heat may not penetrate through to all the hair. Angle and direct the winding according to the desired effect.

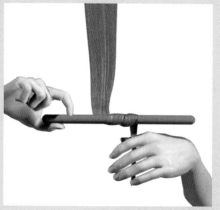

3 Keeping a good even tension, wind the hair below the flexi-shaper around it, making sure the ends lie smoothly.

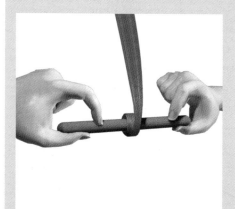

4 Holding the ends of the flexi-shaper, unwind a little way and then rewind to trap the ends of the hair. Continue to wind up to the roots, or as far as the hairstyle dictates.

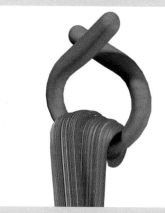

5 Secure by folding the ends of the flexi-shaper as illustrated. Continue winding the rest of the head and give the hair a final light spray of styling product.

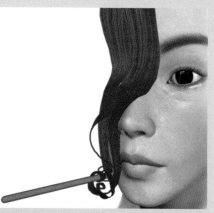

6 Allow the flexi-shapers to completely cool and then gently remove them, beginning at the nape of the neck. Try not to pull on the curl as you unwind each shaper. For a loose, soft finish, apply a little finishing product on your hands and dress with your fingers, separating the curls as desired.

How to create different effects using flexi-shapers

Veronica Lake waves

* This style works best with a side parting.
* Take care to create neat sections.
* Drag the hair downwards so it lies flat on the head.
* Position the flexi-shapers as illustrated.
* Leave the flexi-shapers until completely cool, then remove.
* Smooth the hair with a dressing out brush.
* Apply finishing products to create a sleek, shiny head of hair.

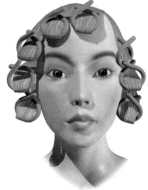

Positioning for Veronica Lake waves

Tight curls

* Begin at the front hairline.
* Divide the hair into small sections (approximately 2–3cm wide).
* Position the flexi-shapers as illustrated.
* Leave until completely cool, then remove.

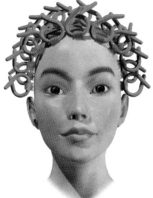

Positioning for tight curls

* Use your fingers or a wide-toothed (rake) comb to gently separate each curl.
* Apply a little dressing cream to separate and define each curl.

Loose curls

* Begin at the front hairline.
* Divide the hair into medium sections (approximately 4–5 cm wide).
* Position the flexi-shapers as illustrated.

* Leave until completely cool, then remove.
* Use your fingers or a wide-toothed (rake) comb to gently separate the hair.
* Apply a finishing product to promote shine and give a soft hold.

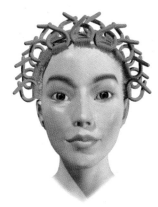

Positioning for loose curls

Tongs

Tongs consist of a round heated barrel and a clamp, which fits around the barrel when closed and traps the hair in position. They are used to create curls and ringlets without root lift.

1 Ensure the hair is completely dry.
2 Turn the tongs on and allow them to heat up in a safe position. Do not let the heated barrel rest on a surface that may scorch or burn.
3 Decide on the size of the curl and the direction it should go. Section accordingly. Begin at the nape of the neck.
4 Comb through each section to remove any tangles. Spray each section lightly with a thermo-active styling product.
5 Position the tongs near to the roots but not touching the scalp. Open the clamp and wind the section around the barrel, taking care not to bend the ends. Make sure you are winding in the right direction for the hairstyle – hair around the face is more flattering wound forwards.
6 Close the clamp and hold the tongs in place for a minute or so, or for the minimum amount of time required to achieve the desired result.
7 Open the clamp and gently remove the barrel from the hair without pulling the hair

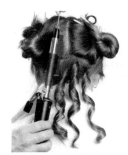

Placing a comb between the tongs and the scalp to prevent accidental burning of the skin

downwards. Continue working up and around the head. Leave the curls to cool before styling.

8   Depending on the desired effect, either leave the released curls (these will resemble ringlets) or separate and soften them with your fingers or a wide-toothed (rake) comb. Apply a suitable finishing product.

> **KEY NOTE**
>
> Be careful when tonging bleached or white hair as it may cause discolouration.

Hot brushes

Available in different sizes, hot brushes are used to give root lift, curl and body to the hair. Cordless hot brushes, which run on butane gas cartridges or batteries, are very useful when working on location. Air styling brushes are a combination of a hairdryer and a hot brush: warm air is blown through a brush attachment and can be used on damp or dry hair. Hot brushes usually come with a variety of brush and tong attachments. They are a good choice for giving curl and volume to short to medium length hair.

1   Ensure the hair is completely dry.

2   Take a section of hair appropriate to the amount of curl you wish to achieve and apply a light coating of thermo-active styling spray.

3   Using the brush, smooth the hair from roots to ends and remove any tangles from the section.

4   Hold the section at a 90° angle to the head and place the brush near to the roots. Use your free hand to wind the hair around the hot brush. Wind the brush to the roots, trapping the ends of the hair.

5   Hold for a minute or so, or for the minimum amount of time required to achieve the desired result. Gently unwind the section without pulling the curl out.

6   Continue working around the head. Allow the hair to cool completely before styling. Apply a suitable finish product.

A tighter curl can be achieved if you pin each section into a barrel pin curl immediately after unwinding it from the hot brush. Large-barrelled hot brushes are useful for adding volume to the crown area on shorter hair.

Straightening or flat irons

Straightening or flat irons are used to create a poker-straight finish to hair by removing frizz and waves. They work at very high temperatures and are designed for occasional rather than daily use to prevent dehydration and damage to the hair.

1   Ensure the hair is completely dry. Brush the hair through to remove any tangles.

2   Beginning at the nape, work on a section of hair at a time (not too big).

3   Apply a light mist of thermo-active styling or straightening product to the section. Beginning at the roots, slowly slide the irons down the hair to the ends. Do not let go of the hair.

4   Comb through the section and repeat the action with the irons once again. Repeat until the section is completely straight and then move onto the next section.

5   Apply a few drops of shine serum to prevent static and to create a sleek, shiny finish.

You can also create flicked-up ends to the hair using straightening irons. As you reach the end of each section turn the irons upwards and hold for a few seconds. The ends of the hair can then be defined using a small amount of wax or other similar product.

Crimping and waving irons

Crimping and waving irons are applied in exactly the same manner as straightening irons. A variety of different effects can be created depending on the shape and pattern of the plates that clamp the hair. For a professional finish the hair should be straightened first by blow-drying or using straightening irons. To create more volume on crimped hair, comb or brush through after the hair has cooled.

Dressing long hair

Numerous techniques are used to dress long hair, which used alone or in combination with each other can create an endless number of different looks. This section looks at the main techniques that form the basis for many of the hairstyles you may be required to create. Once you have mastered these techniques you can begin to design your own hairstyles and to break down and create any given hairstyle.

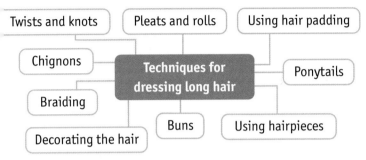

In addition to the usual critical influencing factors, you should give consideration to the following.

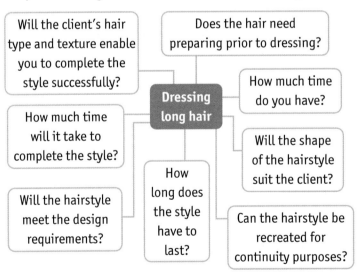

Equipment required to dress long hair

When styling and dressing long hair, it is very important that you are organised and have all the equipment you require to hand. You may also find it useful to have an assistant working with you who can pass grips and pins and hold sections of hair for you whilst you are working. Many make-up artists keep hair pins and grips, etc. in a container with different compartments so it is easy to locate the different sizes and types. There is

nothing worse that taking the time to create a beautiful shape with a section of hair and then realising you have run out of or cannot put your hands on the correct pin or grip.

To dress long hair you will need:

* plenty of hair grips
* plenty of hair pins in different sizes and strengths: geisha pins, straight pins, wavy pins, fine pins
* dressing-out and styling combs and brushes, and tail combs for sectioning
* covered bands
* hair nets in various colours
* lengths of crepe hair (to create hair padding)
* bun rings
* a range of finishing products
* hair decorations.

Preparing the hair for dressing

The way long hair is prepared prior to dressing is dependent on the style requirements and the hair type of the client. The hair may be wet or dry set, although many hairstylists prefer not to work on hair that has been freshly washed as the hair becomes very soft and difficult to manage. If it has just been washed, the hair can be gently backbrushed and lightly misted with hairspray to make the cuticle slightly ruffled and the texture more manageable. Remember to ask your client to wash the hair the night before it is being styled to avoid this problem. When rollering hair that is to be dressed, always

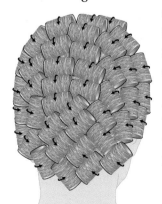

consider the direction of the set, which should reflect the requirements of the hairstyle.

Any of the dry setting techniques can also be used to prepare the hair for being dressed.

Rollers positioned for vertical roll

Securing and controlling long hair

Faced with a mane of long hair and being asked to create a hairstyle with it can be daunting. However, success can be achieved through:

* clean sections
* consideration of the direction and angles when positioning sections
* correct tools
* correct products
* securing the hairstyle
* balance in the finished style.

When dealing with a lot of hair, section it carefully and secure any hair you are not working on out of the way.

Pins and grips (unless they are decorative) should be placed out of sight and should not cause the client any discomfort. Each pin you insert should have a purpose – do not insert lots of pins or grips for the sake of it. A few firmly placed, well-positioned pins or grips will be more effective than lots of loose, poorly placed ones.

All of the above pins and grips are available in a variety of colours to match the client's hair.

Using grips

Type of pin or grip	Description
Geisha pin	Heavy duty hairpin used to secure upswept styles. Particularly useful when dealing with lots of hair.
Straight pins	Used to secure upswept styles. Available in various sizes and weights.
Fine pins	Used to secure and hide the ends of hair, creating a smooth, tidy finish to a hairstyle.
Grips	Used to hold styles in position. Are often 'cross gripped' for added security when pinning up hair. Can also be used to attach decorations to the hairstyle.

Types of pins and grips

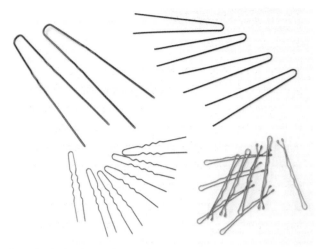

Pins clockwise from the top left: Geisha, straight, grips, fine

Grips should be parted slightly to ensure they slide over enough hair to establish a firm grip. It is important to use your fingers rather than your teeth to open the grips. Not only is it very unhygienic to put grips in your mouth, but you may also damage your teeth.

Using pins

To obtain a firm grip with hair pins it is necessary to anchor them by pushing them back on themselves when sliding them into the hair. Take a pin, pick up a small amount of hair and slide the pin in the opposite direction to that in which it will finally be placed. Then turn the pin so it has reversed direction and push it back firmly into the hair until it is hidden.

Using hair nets

Hair nets can be used to secure and smooth the hair and can be particularly useful when creating rolls in the hair. They are available in various colours to match the client's hair colour and the finest nets can be virtually invisible to the naked eye.

Creating ponytails

Several types of hair bands can be used to create ponytails in the hair. Whichever type you use, it should be covered or snag-free to protect the hair from damage. Never use household elastic bands; lengths of elastic that have hooks at either end are ideal. These allow you to secure the hair while maintaining a firm grip on the hair with the other hand. It is easy to make your own economical version of these hooked elastics: take a length of hat elastic and tie it into a circle. Slide two hair grips onto the elastic, one at either end of its length.

1 Decide what position you want your ponytail to have. Spray a little hairspray onto a dressing-out or finishing brush. This helps to control the hair without overloading it with product.

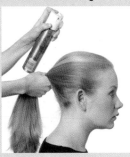

2 Brush the hair back and gather it firmly in the opposite hand in the correct position.

3 Fasten the ponytail with a covered hair elastic. Push the hook or grip flat to the head at the base of the ponytail and wrap elastic tightly around the hair until it is pulled taut. Now position the second hook or grip under the hair towards the scalp to secure. Brush the pony tail and smooth with a suitable finishing product.

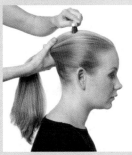

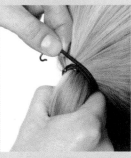

4 If the hair elastic is visible you may wish to cover it with a piece of hair for a more attractive finish. Take a small section of hair from the

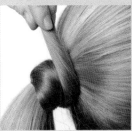

Covering the hair elastic

underneath of the ponytail and wrap it around the base, covering the elastic. Secure with a grip on the underside that is pushed upwards into the base.

Creating pleats and rolls

Creating a vertical roll

The vertical roll (also called a pleat) is a useful technique to learn. Once you have mastered the technique you can try various adaptations of this style, such as the double roll. Practising the technique will improve your manual dexterity and sense of balance in a hairstyle. Hair can be prepared by setting the hair on rollers and winding in the direction of the roll (see illustration on page 00). If the front of the hair is shorter but the back can be dressed up, then section the hair appropriately and work in a logical way, thinking all the time about the desired result. If the hair is very fine or lacks density, hair padding may be used to create extra volume and fullness to the roll.

1 Beginning at the nape of the neck, gently backbrush the hair section by section to create bulk and volume. The amount of backbrushing required will depend on the hair

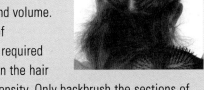

texture and density. Only backbrush the sections of hair that will be included in the roll.

2 Smooth the hair to be included in the roll over to one side using a dressing or finishing brush that has been sprayed lightly with hairspray to help control the hair. Secure the hair slightly off centre with crossed grips for an extra firm hold.

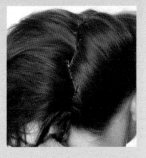

3 Smooth the top layers of hair on the opposite side. Hold the hair with your working hand, and sweep the hair over the line of grips. Check the position of the roll: is it central and straight? Tuck the ends of the hair into the roll using a tail comb. Check the positioning once more.

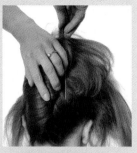
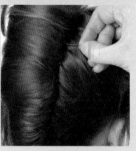

4 Secure the roll firmly using pins or grips. Ensure they are hidden from view.

5 Any shorter layers can be blended into the roll by smoothing and securing them with pins. Fine pins can be used to tuck any stray hair ends out of sight.

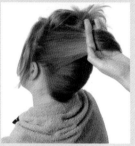

6 The ends of the hair at the top of the roll can be tucked in for a formal style. Alternatively, they can be left out and styled using tongs or crimping irons, or dressed into pin purls, etc. Complete the hairstyle by applying a finishing product that will add shine and hold.

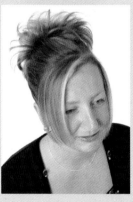

Creating a horizontal roll

1 Beginning at the nape of the neck, gently backbrush the hair all over to create plenty of volume. The amount of backbrushing required will depend on the hair texture and density.

2 Smooth the hair, flat to the head, from the front hairline to the back of the head using a dressing or finishing brush that has been sprayed lightly with hairspray to help control the hair. Secure the hair with a row of crossed grips across the back of the head.

3 Divide the hair below the crossed grips into three equal sections. Take one section and smooth the underside of the section – this is the hair that will be visible once the section is rolled over. Roll the section over your hand until a large loop is formed.

4 Tuck the ends of the hair into the roll and secure them firmly using pins or grips. Ensure they are hidden from view.

5 Repeat on the opposite side, leaving a 3–5 cm gap in the centre between the crossed grips. Complete the roll by taking the centre section and folding it upwards. Pin to secure. Use the prongs on a dressing-out comb to blend the three sections of the roll.

6 Complete the hairstyle by applying a finishing product that will add shine and hold. Ornamentation can be added to decorate the inner edge of the roll.

Once you have mastered this technique, try a double vertical roll. This is when the hair is parted down the centre of the back of the head and a roll is created either side, meeting at the centre parting.

Creating a bun

The easiest and quickest way to create a bun is using a bun ring (see illustrations below). Buns have been around for a very long time and their position on the head will depend on the period when working on historical hairstyles.

1 Decide on the position of the bun on the head. Style the hair into a ponytail. Place a bun ring around the base of the ponytail and pull through the tail of hair. Ask the client to bend the head forward.

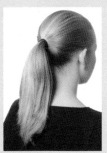

2 Using a dressing comb, spread the ponytail around the bun ring until it is entirely covered by hair. Apply some dressing cream onto the hair to help control and smooth the hair as you work. Place a no-snag hair band over and around the outside of the bun ring, trapping the hair tightly around the ring.

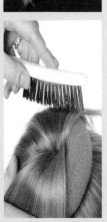

3 The ends of the hair can now be tucked under the ring by wrapping the hair around the ring and pinning it securely. Alternatively, it can be dressed in pin curls or finished in the desired style. Apply a finishing product to help smooth and tame the hair.

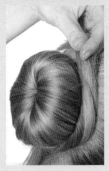

Creating a chignon

Creating a smooth finish is very important for this style. Use a little dressing cream on your hands as you work to help smooth and mould the hair into shape. You may find it easier to create the chignon if you ask the client to tilt the head forwards.

1 Style the hair into a low ponytail (see page 290) and gently backbrush the tail to increase its volume.

2 Smooth the top layers of the hair with a dressing or finishing brush. Standing to the side of the client, hold the hair to one side between the fingers and thumb (as shown). Hold the ends of the hair with the other hand.

3 Twist the hair upwards and over to the opposite side, gently pulling the remainder of the tail downwards.

4 Secure the hair with pins and grips, making sure they are hidden.

5 Stand on the opposite side of the client. Take the remainder of the hair, roll it downwards and secure it under the chignon. Make sure the ends of the hair are tucked away out of sight.

6 Complete the hairstyle by applying a finishing product that will add shine and hold. Ornamentation can be added to decorate the hair.

Twists and knots

This technique is quick and easy to achieve and can be carried out on wet or dry hair. The hair may be twisted tightly to the scalp or left looser depending on the effect you wish to achieve. Likewise, the hair may be twisted tightly to the ends and coiled back on itself to achieve 'knots', or the ends of the hair may be left free and styled according to the design plan. Once again, the size and direction of each section of hair that you twist will ultimately determine the finished result. The hair should be secured with grips (cross gripping is useful when handling large sections of hair), which should be hidden unless required to be exposed by the design plan.

One of the most common forms of braiding is the three-stem scalp plait, also called a French plait, where the hair is kept close to the scalp.

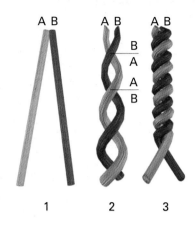

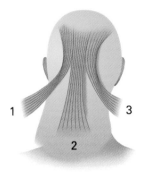

Beginning at the front of the head, take a small triangle of hair and split into three equal strands.

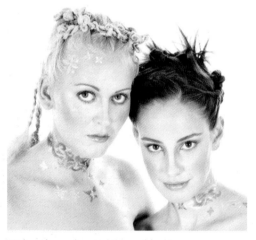

Hairstyles using twists and knots

Braiding the hair

Braiding the hair is a versatile skill that should be learnt by the make-up and hair artist to achieve a variety of looks both in contemporary and historical hairstyling. Different looks can be achieved by varying the number of stems, varying the width of the stems, varying the direction of braiding, over or under laying the hair and incorporating decoration such as ribbons and added hairpieces. Effects can range from the simple to the elaborate. Working with smooth stems of hair is very important for this technique. If you are working on dry hair, use a little dressing cream on your hands to help smooth the hair as you work. It is often easier to work on damp hair when tight braids are required.

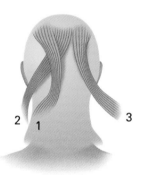

Cross the left strand (1) over the centre one (2) so that the left strand becomes the new centre strand.

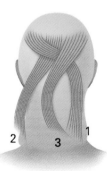

Cross the right strand (3) over the centre strand (1). It is important to keep the tension equal in each strand so that the finished braid will be even

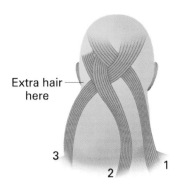

Holding the braid with the right hand, gather extra hair from the left front hairline, about half the thickness of one strand, and add it to the left strand (2). Cross this increased strand over the centre strand (3).

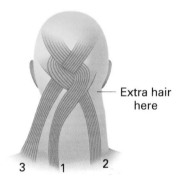

Repeat the previous step but hold the braid with the left hand and gather the extra hair from the right. Add it to the right strand (1) and pass this new increased strand over the centre strand (2).

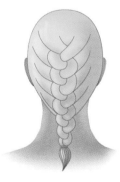

Repeat these two steps until there is no loose hair at the hairline. Plait the remainder of the three strands and secure the ends with a clip or band.

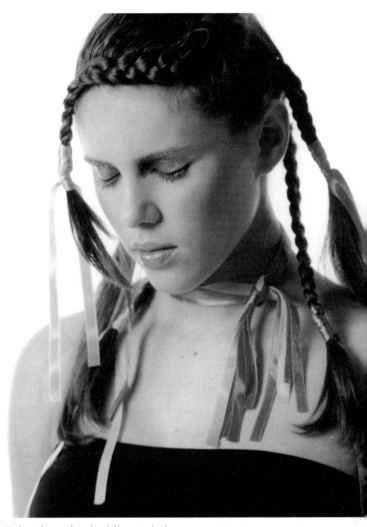

Hairstyles using braiding techniques

The four-stem variation (fishtail plait) is a useful plait for historical hairstyling.

Begin by taking the stems from left to right, passing over and under and over until you reach the opposite side, picking up extra sections of hair from each side as you continue down the length of the braid. The finished result should resemble a herringbone pattern.

Using hair padding

Padding may sometimes be required to give extra fullness, volume and shape to the natural hair. It is particularly useful when creating period or avant-garde hairstyles. It is easy to customise your own hair padding to suit the specific requirements with regard to colour and size. Crepe hair or synthetic hair can be used to create padding; the choice will depend on personal preference and budget.

* **Crepe hair** is supplied in lengths and is braided around string. Begin by selecting the appropriate colours for your model, cut the strings of the braid and gently unbraid the hair. Do not cut the hair but gently pull from the ends. The hair should break away in approximately 12 cm lengths. Gather together as much hair as you need and tease it to create fullness and volume. Mould the crepe hair into the desired shape and wrap a hair net around it, pinning to secure it.

* Alternatively, take a ponytail hairpiece made from **synthetic fibres** (it may be cut in half if very long). Fold the length in half and tie a hair band around the halfway point. Backcomb the hair into a large ball and lightly coat it with hairspray. Mould the hair into the desired shape (ensuring the band is in the centre) and wrap a hair net around it, pinning to secure it.

Adding hairpieces

You may wish to add hairpieces to the design for a number of reasons. Hairpieces can:

* give extra volume to the style
* extend the length of the hair
* add colour to the hair
* create avant-garde hairstyles.

Hairpieces are available in a variety of lengths, textures and styles and are sold as wefts, switches, coloured slices or loose bundles. They are made from either synthetic fibres or human hair.

It is important to ensure the hairpiece is securely attached to the head, particularly if the model is required to move around (as on a catwalk). If the model does not feel confident that the hair will stay in place, it will affect posture and movement. If the piece has a base or fixing point, this must be well hidden. If the piece has a comb attachment, grips can be used to provide extra security.

All hairpieces should be chosen and applied with great care to ensure the design plan is achieved. If the piece is supposed to look natural, it is vitally important that it is perfectly blended with the natural hair and due consideration is given to the shape and balance of the final hairstyle.

Hair type	Advantages	Disadvantages
Synthetic	* Cheaper option * Available in a wide range of colours * Available in a wide range of styles	* Looks artificially shiny under certain lighting * Great care must be taken when using heated equipment on this type of hairpiece as hot temperatures will melt the hair fibres
Human hair	* Will blend with the natural hair to look completely natural * Can be coloured or permed to match the natural hair * Can be styled using heated equipment	* Require specialist finishing products * Expensive option * Limited range of colours

Decorating the hair

Many items can be used to decorate the hair and enhance its dressing, ranging from the conventional to the more unusual. Providing the attachment can be secured safely, almost anything can be used – so be creative and use your imagination. Below is a list of some items you may wish to experiment with:

* ribbons and other haberdashery items:
* combs and slides
* hats and scarves
* jewellery
* feathers
* flowers.

When choosing hair ornaments, consideration should be given to the following.

* Does it meet the requirements of the occasion or design brief?
* Does it match or contrast with the clothes and hair?
* Does the decoration enhance the hair design or detract from it?

Temporary colours

The addition of temporary colour to the hair may sometimes be required. Temporary colours work by coating the cuticle with large molecules that cannot penetrate the cuticle but stain the hair.

Temporary colours come in a variety of forms including mousses, hair mascaras and sprays. Because of the staining action of these products, it is important to protect the client's skin and clothes and your own hands whilst applying them. Ensure you follow the manufacturer's instructions during the application and removal of colour products so the process is both safe and successful.

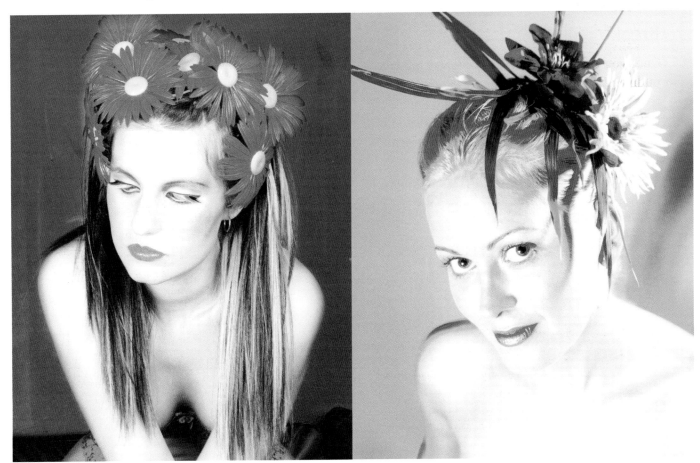

Hairstyles enhanced with decoration

REMEMBER

Always use spray products in a well-ventilated area away from naked flames and sources of heat.

For period productions it may be necessary to cover a performer's highlights for authenticity. For lengthy period productions the performer will probably be asked to permanently cover highlights, but for shorter productions or when working with extras, etc. this may be unrealistic. In this case, silicone paints can be applied to the affected strands of hair to cover any unsuitable colouring. Reel Creations, Temptu Pro and Premiere Products (Skin Illustrator) manufacture a number of palettes.

Airbrush paints can also be applied to the hair to create colourful fantasy effects (see Chapter 16, page 368, for more information).

Breaking down hairstyles

Once you have mastered the various techniques outlined in this chapter, you should be able to recreate any hairstyle (within reason) using these skills. If you are asked to recreate a particular hairstyle, you will begin by 'breaking it down'. This term refers to taking a style and reducing it to its fundamental elements, so that you are able to recreate it successfully and accurately. Most styles will be derived from a combination of styling techniques.

HANDS ON

Breaking down a hairstyle

1 Research and choose a hairstyle suitable for your model's length of hair. You may have to make adaptations for fringes, layers, hair type, etc. You may also have to consider using added hairpieces or padding to recreate the desired effect.
2 Study the hairstyle and consider any equipment and products you will require for its recreation. Make sure they are ready to hand.
3 Begin by considering any partings in the hairstyle. The placement of partings is particularly critical when recreating period hairstyles.
4 Then consider the shape and structure of the hairstyle. Is the front styled differently from the sides and back or crown of the head? This will determine how the hair is sectioned for setting or styling.
5 Next study the direction of the hair in each section. This will determine the direction of winding or styling.
6 Consider the movement of the hair for each section – is the hair tightly curled, loosely waved, straight, braided, twisted, etc.? This will determine your choice of setting and dressing method.
7 Is the hair decorated?

Have a close look at some period and contemporary hair designs and think about how you would achieve the same look. Ideally your portfolio should contain evidence of accomplishing the following:

* classic hairstyles
* period hairstyles
* high fashion hairstyles
* avant-garde hairstyles.

Knowledge Check

1. Describe the difference between hair texture and hair density.

2. Which bonds are broken when carrying out a cohesive or wet set?

3. Name three contra-indications specific to hairstyling.

4. How should the hair be styled for a client with a round face shape?

5. When using heated styling equipment should the hair be wet or dry?

6. When may you use serum or gloss on the hair?

7. Describe the three types of massage movements used when shampooing the hair.

8. To achieve root lift when blow-drying the hair, at what angle should the brush be held to the scalp?

9. Why do we normally blow-dry from roots to points?

10. Why should the hair dryer be kept moving?

11. When rollering the hair, what type of curl would rollers with a small diameter create?

12. Why is it important to maintain an even tension when rollering the hair?

13. When may you be required to create reverse pin curls on a client?

14. Describe the correct method of backcombing the hair.

15. List three safety precautions when using electrical equipment.

16. How can you prevent burning the scalp when using heated tongs?

17. Why do we use no-snag or covered bands on hair?

18. Describe the advantages and disadvantages of using synthetic hairpieces.

19. How do temporary colours work?

20. Describe what is meant by 'breaking down' a hairstyle.

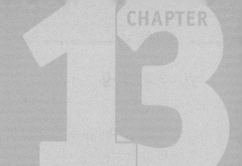

Maintaining wigs and hairpieces

Maintenance of wigs can be divided into four areas: cleaning, blocking, setting and dressing. Wigs and hairpieces are used to:

* create a character
* create historical hairstyles
* create a fantasy or high fashion effect
* change the length, colour or texture of the hair
* maintain continuity
* achieve hairstyles which when dressing the natural hair would prove impractical.

Aim and objectives

Aim of this chapter: to provide you with the knowledge of maintaining wigs and hairpieces. You should achieve the following **objectives:**

* Recognise various wig types and evaluate their uses
* Take measurements of a head for a wig fitting
* Complete a postiche order form
* Prepare a malleable block and 'block' a wig in preparation for washing, setting or dressing
* Set and dress wigs according to design requirements
* Store and protect wigs
* Fit a lace-fronted wig to a model
* Remove a lace-fronted wig from a model
* Clean various types of wigs safely and effectively.

Types of wig

Weft wigs

These mass-produced wigs vary in price and quality, but tend to be significantly cheaper than knotted wigs. The wig foundation is often made from elastic net. The hair is usually made of synthetic fibres but can also be made of human hair. These wigs are pre-set, so after washing they only require shaking and they should be left to dry naturally. They cannot be restyled. They are hot to wear and are not as durable as custom-made knotted wigs. Because the hair is synthetic, they tend to reflect the light. This makes them look unnaturally shiny on stage and television, although matt synthetic fibres are now available to reduce this effect. Heated equipment should be used with extreme caution on this type of wig as heat can melt the synthetic fibres. They are available in a wide range of colours and styles and are easy to maintain.

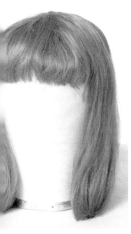

Synthetic weft wig

Knotted wigs

Knotted wigs are usually made to measure and are therefore expensive. Price will vary according to quality and hair type (wigs made from blonde hair tend to be more expensive than brown or black hair). The wig foundation is made from hand- or machine-sewn vegetable netting, with a galloon base. Real human hair is then knotted onto the base. If well maintained, these wigs can last for many years (the foundation often wears out first, but can be repaired up to a point). Because the hair is human, the wigs can be washed, styled and re-styled, permed or coloured. They are comfortable and cool to wear.

Lace-fronted knotted wigs

Designed specifically for media and theatrical use, the lace-fronted knotted wig has a piece of net sewn across the front hairline that allows a front hairline to be knotted. This creates a very natural hairline on the wearer. The lace is glued to the wearer's skin on the forehead and disguised with make-up. The texture of the lace can vary from very fine (suitable for film and television) to coarse (suitable for theatre): the finer the lace, the more expensive the wig. This type of wig requires 'blocking' to a malleable block prior to washing, setting and dressing (see page 302).

Wigs and their application

When working on a big budget production, any principal performers requiring wigs will usually have made-to-measure knotted wigs that fit them perfectly. At the end of the production schedule, these wigs may be stored or altered for reuse on a new production. For lower budget productions, wigs will often be hired. Although these will not be made to measure, a good fit can be assured by sending the wig company details of the size, colour and style that is required. For extras, mass-produced weft wigs made of human hair are often used. Synthetic weft wigs are usually only used when fantasy effects are required or when the hairstyle does not need to look completely natural, for example in pantomime or for avant-garde fashion shoots.

> **REMEMBER**
>
> If is very important to observe safe working practices and hygienic procedures whilst performing techniques described in this chapter.

Measuring for a wig

When ordering wigs from a wig-making company it is important to supply accurate information with regard to size, colour and style required. This is usually the responsibility of the make-up supervisor on a production. The head measurements are taken by the make-up artist, recorded for future reference and sent to the wig company. Sufficient information should be given to the wigmaker so that a foundational postiche can be made for a personalised fit.

STEP-BY-STEP | Taking wig measurements

Equipment required

* Tape measure (ensure it has not stretched over time by checking against a ruler)
* Pen to complete order form
* Postiche order form
* Brush and hair band to secure hair away from the front hairline
* Sheet of tracing paper
* Marker pen
* Pins

1 Ensure you have the order form, pen and tape measure to hand.
2 Sit the client in a chair in front of a mirror.
3 Discuss with the client his or her requirements, making reference to style, length, density and texture of hair and degree of curl.
4 Prepare the client with a protective gown.
5 Record the following measurements:

   a circumference: the total distance around the head (starting the measurement approximately 2 cm back from the front hairline)

   b from centre of front hairline to nape: this is taken from the centre of the front hairline, over the crown of the head to the centre of the nape

   c across the front hairline from ear point to ear point

   d over the top of the head from ear arch to ear arch

   e from temple to temple around the back of the head (making sure the tape measure passes over the bony prominence at the back of the head)

   f the nape of the neck (across the back of the neck)

   g from ear arch to nape.

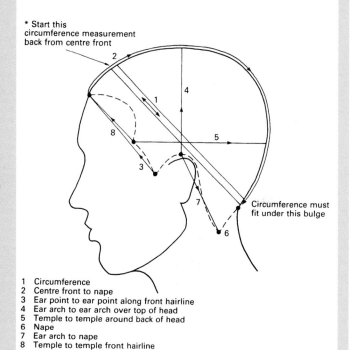

1 Circumference
2 Centre front to nape
3 Ear point to ear point along front hairline
4 Ear arch to ear arch over top of head
5 Temple to temple around back of head
6 Nape
7 Ear arch to nape
8 Temple to temple front hairline

Measurements for a wig

6 Identify any abnormalities of the scalp (any large prominences, etc).
7 Record the length and position of the parting if required.
8 If the wig is to be styled, state the style required and attach a picture if possible.
9 Indicate or attach a colour sample.
10 Complete the postiche order form.

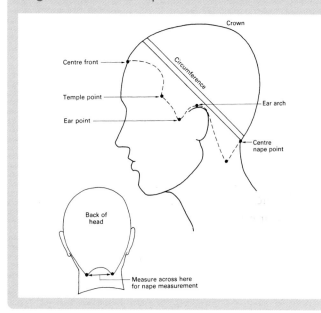

Head measurement terminology

Tracing the front hairline for a lace-fronted wig

1 Cut a sheet of tracing paper to approximately 30 cm deep by 70 cm wide.

2 Fold the paper in half along its length and depth to find its centre point.

3 Prepare the client with a protective gown and secure the hair clear of the hairline.

4 Place the centre point of the tracing paper on the centre of the front hairline and slide it back 2 cm so the point now lies on the circumference line at the centre of the front hairline.

5 Wrap the tracing paper around the head and secure it by pinning at the nape. Check the centre point is still in the correct place.

6 Make a tracing of the natural hairline of the client using a marker pen on the tracing paper. Continue until you reach just past each ear.

7 Remove the paper.

8 Cut out the pattern of the hairline.

9 Place the pattern on the client to check the accuracy of the hairline.

10 Restore the client's hairstyle.

11 The pattern should be attached to the postiche order form.

A pattern can also be made of the nape hairline using the same technique.

It is important to confirm the estimated cost and delivery date with the supplier before processing any orders.

Clients's name ....

Address ....

....

Telephone: home .... work ....

Order for: 1 wig ☐ 2 wigs ☐ Hand-made ☐ Acrylic ☐ Hair-lace front ☐

Measurements
Circumference (1 cm back centre front)
Front to nape
Ear to ear (front)
Ear to ear (top)
Temple to temple (back)
Nape of neck (width of nape)
Parting length
Parting: left ☐ centre ☐ right ☐
    Distance from centre ....

Measurements	Notes

Natural break: left ☐ centre ☐ right ☐ crown ☐ ....

Abnormalities: scalp ☐ bumps ☐ other ☐ ....

Details of hair
A Length: front ....
        temples ....
        crown ....
        nape ....
B Exact colour: pattern ....
    Enclosed samples

C Straight ☐ waved ☐
    Curly ☐ loose ☐ medium ☐ strong ☐
D Full fringe
E Weight of wig: light ☐ normal ☐ heavy ☐

Drawings, picture or photo
Front   Back   Side

Cost .... Client signature ....

Deposit .... Date ....

Wig to be completed by .... Date ....

Made by ....

Checked by ....

Dressed by ....

Postiche order form

Blocking a lace-fronted wig

Lace-fronted wigs must be 'blocked' prior to washing or setting and dressing. Blocking a wig refers to attaching it to a malleable head block.

Malleable blocks are available in various sizes: the size relates to the head circumference that is indicated on the base of the block. It is important to use a block with the same circumference as the wig so the wig is not damaged. The average block size is 54 cm. The bases of malleable blocks have a pointed shape on one side to indicate the back of the block when the wig is in position. As the block has no ears, you should ensure the wig is straight when you attach it, otherwise the hairstyle will be unbalanced and wonky when it is placed on the performer.

STEP-BY-STEP **Preparing the malleable block**

Equipment required

* Malleable block in appropriate size
* Wig stand
* Cling film
* Sellotape

1 Place the malleable block on a floor-standing block holder (wig stand).
2 Wrap the entire surface of the block with cling film (plastic wrap), making the surface as smooth as possible.

3 Apply strips of sellotape to hold the cling film in place. This protects the canvas of the block and makes it water resistant.

STEP-BY-STEP **Attaching the wig to the malleable block**

Equipment required

* Wig
* Prepared malleable block with the same head circumference as the wig
* Padding (may be required)
* Box of blocking-up pins (approximately 3 cm long)
* Box of fine pins
* Blocking tape
* Brush (to knock pins into the block)

1 Turn the wig inside out.
2 Locate the centre point of the front hairline (not the lace edge) and place it on the centre seam of the block.
3 Turn the wig back on itself to bring it over the crown of the block and pull down each side. Then pull the nape of the wig down the nape of the block (pointed side).
4 Check the wig is correctly positioned: use the centre point of the front hairline and check the ear points are level. Correct any discrepancies.
5 The wig foundation should fit the block snugly across its entire surface. Padding can be applied under any loose areas of the wig.
6 Apply blocking tape along the edge of the lace, and keeping the lace taut, place a blocking pin at the following points:
   * at the centre point of the front hairline
   * at the temples
   * at the ear points.

7 The pins must be pushed right in, otherwise hair will get caught in them: use the back of a brush to bang them into the block.
8 Pull the nape of the wig downwards removing any slack and place a blocking pin at either side of the nape, keeping tension between the points.
9 If you are happy with the overall placement of the wig on the block (check there are no slack areas and that it is straight on the block), continue by placing fine pins at 1 cm intervals along the lace edge between the blocking pins. Do not use fine pins around the nape of the wig as these could be easily missed when removing it from the block and may present a hazard to the performer.
10 The wig can be removed from the block by lifting the tape, which will loosen and lift the pins for ease of removal.

The wig needs to fit snug to the block to avoid damage during the washing, setting and dressing process. Any slack areas may be torn when you brush or comb the wig. A snug fit will also prevent the knotted hair from working loose when the wig is wet.

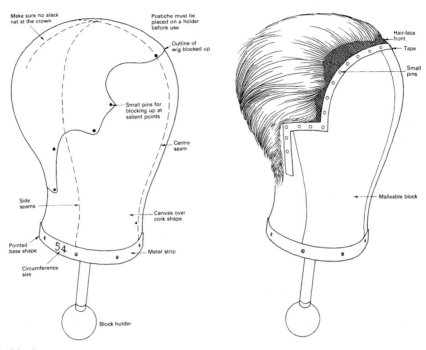

Blocking up a malleable block

Setting and dressing wigs

You will often be required to set and dress the hair on wigs to achieve a desired style as set out in the design plan or production brief. Setting and dressing techniques are the same as those described in Chapter 12 (Hairstyling for the make-up artist), the only difference being how the set or style is secured in the hair and dried.

STEP-BY-STEP | **Preparing the wig for setting and dressing**

Before the wig can be set or dressed it needs to be combed through to remove any tangles. The most important thing to remember is that the hair must be brushed from the points (ends) up to the roots. You should work carefully and methodically to avoid damaging the wig.

Equipment required

* Blocked wig
* Large dressing comb

1 Start at the nape and work your way up to the crown.
2 Start at the ear point and work up to the temple point on each side.
3 Start at the crown and work towards the front hairline, combing the hair forward. Finish by combing the hair back towards the nape.

STEP-BY-STEP Setting wigs

(Refer to Chapter 12 for setting techniques.)

Equipment required

* Wig which has been blocked and combed through
* Water spray
* Combs and brushes (clean and sterilised)
* Setting lotion
* Hair nets
* Rollers, clips and wooden doweling (to create ringlets) as required
* Postiche pins
* Tape for setting
* Postiche oven, hood dryer or hair dryer

1 Decide on appropriate technique to achieve the planned style.
2 Select the correct equipment and styling tools to create the desired effect.
3 If the hair is dry, you will need to wet it to perform a wet-set. A water-spray is useful for this. Make sure the foundation of the wig remains as dry as possible.
4 Apply setting lotion if required (this will make the hair more manageable and help the set last longer).
5 Make appropriate sections, ensuring they are neat and clean.
6 Set the hair using appropriate techniques, for example rollering, pin curling, finger waving, creating ringlets, etc. Secure the set without causing distortion to the roots, marking the hair or damaging the foundation. Use postiche pins to secure rollers and pins as they can be easily placed into the malleable block without marking the hair. Use tape to secure the weight of the hair whilst the ends of the hair are set.
7 Cover the set with a hair net.

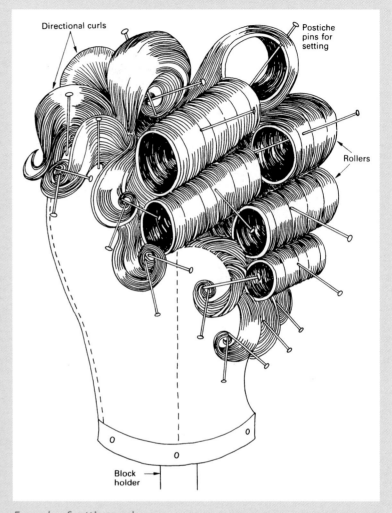

Example of setting a wig

8 Dry the wig. Using a postiche oven is the preferable method of drying wigs (the oven will slowly 'bake' the wig, giving a strong set). However, postiche ovens are very expensive and may not always be available. Alternatively, a hood dryer could be used, or if the wig is not required for a couple of days it could be air-dried at room temperature or placed in an airing cupboard.
9 The wig should be allowed to completely cool before the set is removed.

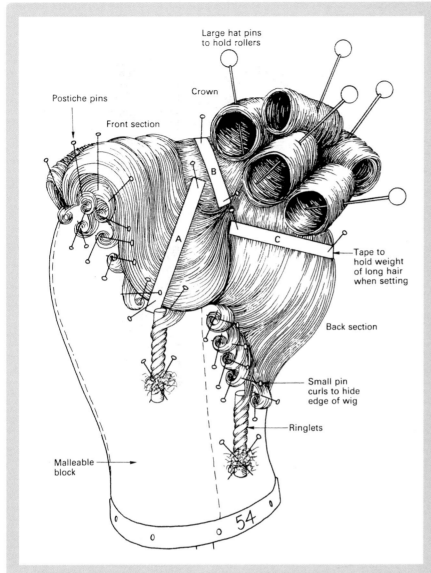

Large hat pins to hold rollers

Crown

Postiche pins

Front section

B

A

C

Tape to hold weight of long hair when setting

Back section

Small pin curls to hide edge of wig

Ringlets

Malleable block

54

Example of setting a wig

Creating ringlets

Ringlets can be created on wigs using wooden dowels cut to length. The diameter of the dowel will determine the size of the ringlet. The hair needs to be very wet. Starting at the end of the dowel, trap the end of the hair and wind it up the dowel smoothly. The hair should not overlap but there should be no gaps between each rotation of hair. The doweling should be secured with a postiche pin at the top and bottom. The sides of the head should be symmetrical. Ringlets around the face should be rolled forward as this is more flattering for the wearer.

KEY NOTE

Hard fronted wigs, i.e. those without a lace edge at the front hairline, should be set and dressed in hairstyles that conceal the edge of the wig so a natural hairline is created.

White or pale wigs should be handled with great care. When drying these wigs, they should be covered with tissue paper and the temperature of the dryer should be reduced. If the hair has yellowed, a neutralising rinse can be added when the wig is washed.

STEP-BY-STEP | **Dressing wigs**

(Refer to Chapter 12 for dressing techniques.)

Equipment required

* Selection of combs and brushes
* Dressing cream and other finishing products
* Hair spray or plastic spray to maintain the style

1 Brush through the hair to remove all roller and pin marks (some setting styles such as finger waving and ringlets should not be brushed through).
2 Brush the hair into the desired shape and style.
3 Backbrush or backcomb the hair, or tease it into position where necessary.
4 Dress the hair to give the desired effect. Any hair grips used should be matt, to avoid reflecting light. Hair pins and grips should be hidden from view.
5 Finish the style with a light coating of hair spray or plastic spray for a longer hold.

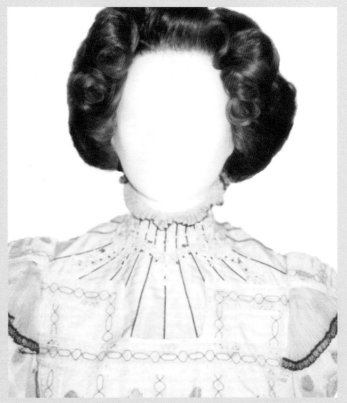

Wig dressed in an Edwardian hairstyle

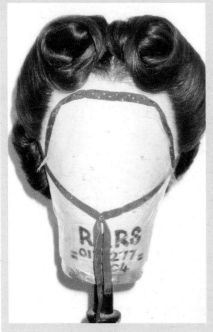

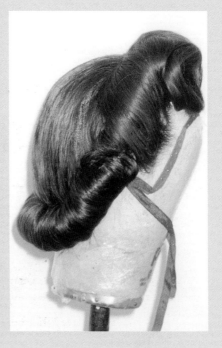

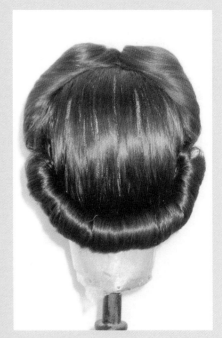

Wig dressed in a 1940s hairstyle

Protecting and storing wigs

Once a wig has been dressed it can be left on the malleable block and stored until required. It is useful to label the block with the performer's name and character name and the title of the production. Alternatively, the wig may be removed from the block, padded out with tissue paper and stored in a labelled box.

STEP-BY-STEP **Applying a lace-fronted wig**

The natural hair should be prepared for a wig application by one of the following methods.

* **Long hair:** You should not create height when preparing the natural hair. Place a large pin curl on the crown and on each side of the head and secure them by cross gripping (the hairgrips should face back so they do not catch the wig). Section the rest of the hair in two and wrap the sections around the head in opposite directions to lie as flat as possible.

* **Medium length hair:** Pin curl the hair all over.
* **Short hair:** Cross grip all over the hair.
* **Very short hair:** Section the hair and tie it in 'tufts' with rubber bands.
* **Men with short hair:** Apply hair grips at anchor points on the crown and sides. A hair net or stocking could also be used.

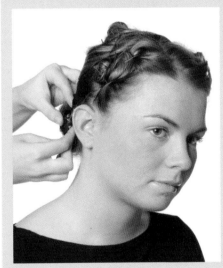

1 Prepare the natural hair.

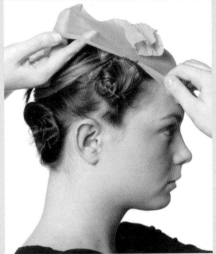

2 Cover the hair with a hair net or stocking. Ask the client to hold the front of the net or stocking (the edge should be a little back from the hairline), put your hands inside the net or stocking and pull it over the head. Pin the net to the head using hair pins, turning them in on themselves. Do not place them too near the hairline; put a couple in the crown. Do not place around the back of the neck or up into the fleshy part behind the ears as this will be painful for the performer.

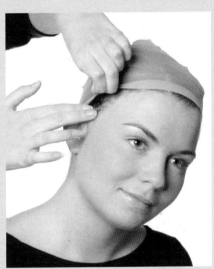

3 Gel or soap short hairs around the hairline. Take the wig from the block (the wig should be unblocked well before it goes on the performer so you do not keep the performer waiting).

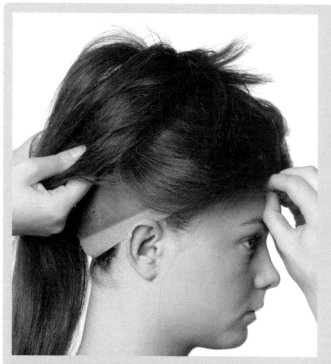

4 Ask the performer to hold the wig by the wig lace, half way down the forehead (the fingers should be placed over the lace, not under it).

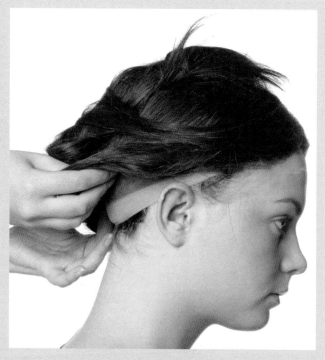

5 With hands inside the wig the 'wigger' pulls the wig over the net or stocking into place. Once the wig is on it cannot be pulled forward, but can only be 'jiggled' into position.

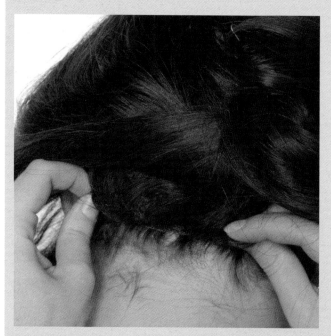

6 Pull back the wig into the correct position, checking at the nape of the neck.

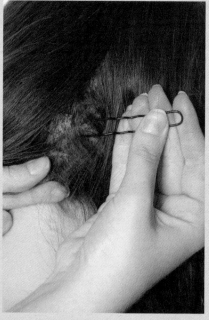

7 Pin the wig to secure it. Use pins and grips that are matt and match the colour of the wig.

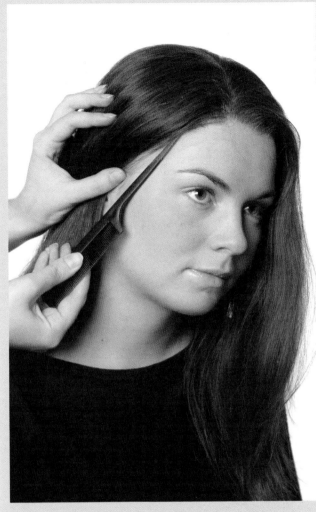

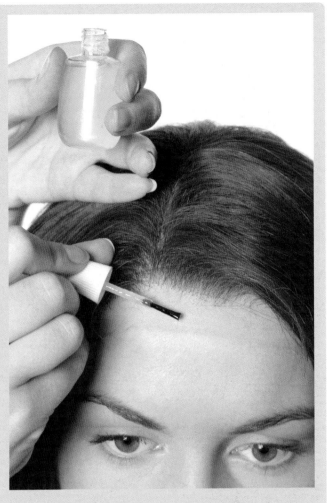

8 Make sure natural hair is not visible under the lace. Any stray hairs can be pushed away with a pin tail comb.

9 Glue the lace into place using matt mastix glue (be aware of COSHH regulations and keep the lid on when not in use). Roll back the lace and place three to four blobs of glue on each side. Wait for the adhesive to become tacky and pull the lace into position with tension. Use a damp cloth free of lint (muslin or silk) to spread the glue. For the centre of the lace, place a few blobs of glue over the lace and use the cloth to spread it to the sides. If all the lace is glued firmly down the performer has difficulty with facial expressions.

KEY NOTE

If the wig falls short at the nape and matches the natural hair colour, you could leave out a section of natural hair at the nape. This can be used to dress and blend in with the wig to create a natural hairline here.

KEY NOTE

You may not always be required to create beautiful hairstyles. Occasionally you may be asked to 'dirty down' a wig, which refers to making the hair look unkempt or dirty.

Removing a lace-fronted wig

The procedure should be carried out carefully and gently.

1 Using a brush, apply mastix remover (MME) to the lace, working from the edges inwards, until the lace begins to lift from the skin. Ask the client to hold a tissue below the lace, so that any drops of adhesive remover are caught before they enter the client's eyes.

2 Once the lace is completely lifted from the skin, check for any sticky areas and gently remove them with mastix remover. Tone and blot the skin dry.

3 Remove the hair pins attaching the wig to the head.

4 Lift the wig off from behind, holding it carefully by the foundation at the sides of the nape. Pull the wig gently forward and off the head.

5 Detach the hair net or stocking and hair grips from the hair.

6 Restore the natural hairstyle.

Fixing a hairpiece to the head

The area of the head to which the piece is to be attached should be sectioned off and pin curled with plenty of hairgrips. If the hairpiece has a slide attached, this should be inserted into the pin curled area and secured with more grips. Check the piece is securely attached and dress the natural hair to blend with the hairpiece.

Cleaning wigs

Cleaning the hair lace on a lace-fronted real hair wig

Once the wig has been removed the lace will need cleaning of adhesive and make-up. You must never give a dirty wig to a performer.

1 Ensure the room is well ventilated and protect your hands with fine rubber gloves.

2 Pour some acetone into a small glass bowl – you will need to work quickly as the acetone will evaporate.

3 Place a towel covered with a sheet of paper roll on a table. Place the hair lace of the wig on the paper.

4 Dab the acetone onto the lace with a brush (do not use cotton wool) and rub gently until the dirt and glue comes off on the paper, which is then thrown away.

5 Once the lace is clean, place the wig on the block ready for blocking.

6 Always wash your hands after cleaning wigs to remove traces of acetone.

Washing real hair wigs

This procedure must only be performed on a wig that has been firmly blocked onto a malleable block which has been covered in cling film.

1 Comb the wig thoroughly and ensure the hair is tangle free.

2 Fill the sink with water – make sure it is not too hot as this can shrink wigs.

3 Add some shampoo (one specifically designed to remove product build-up is useful) to the water.

4 Holding the end of the malleable block, take the blocked wig and dip the hair into the water (try not to get the block wet). If the hair is long it can be loosely braided as this helps to prevent tangling.

5 Swish the hair around in the water. Do not rub, as this will unknot the hair!

6 Rinse the hair with fresh water several times in the same manner.

7 For the final rinse, use fresh water with a small amount of fabric conditioner. Do not rinse this out.

8 Pat the wig dry in a towel. Set, blow dry or leave it to dry naturally.

Some examination schemes still refer to the method of dry cleaning human hair wigs. For this reason the procedure is described below. The cleaning fluids used are based on trichlorethylene and should only be used in a well-ventilated area and according to good health and safety practice. Contact with the skin should be avoided.

1 Comb the wig thoroughly and ensure the hair is tangle free.

2 Pour enough cleaning fluid into a bowl to cover the wig.

3 Turn the foundation inside out.

4 Immerse the wig in the fluid and leave to stand for a few minutes.

5 Draw the postiche through the fluid, making sure the fluid runs from roots to points. Continue until the wig is clean.

6 Remove the wig from the fluid and place it on a towel, pressing out surplus moisture.

7 Hang the wig by the nape on a clothes line (or similar) in the open air to allow the cleaning fluid to evaporate. This may take several hours.

Cleaning synthetic wigs and hairpieces

1 Prepare a bowl of shampoo and lukewarm water.

2 Turn the postiche inside out.

3 Immerse the wig in the bowl.

4 Squeeze the wig gently.

5 Rinse the wig thoroughly in lukewarm water.

6 Gently squeeze out excess water.

7 Allow the wig to dry naturally.

8 Shake or lightly brush the wig into shape.

Knowledge Check

1 What type of wig is predominantly used in theatre, television and film?

2 What are the disadvantages of using synthetic weft wigs?

3 Explain how you would measure the circumference of the head.

4 How should the malleable block be prepared for having a wig blocked to it?

5 In which direction should a human hair knotted wig be combed through prior to setting or styling?

6 How are rollers and pin curls secured when setting a wig?

7 How should a client with natural long hair be prepared for a wig application?

8 Describe the procedure for cleaning the lace on a lace-fronted wig.

9 How should a wig be stored and protected once it has been dressed?

10 Describe the procedure for washing synthetic wigs.

Characterisation

In the context of make-up artistry, a character can be described as a person who appears in a script. A characteristic is a distinctive or typical feature of that person. Characterisation is the means through which the character is portrayed. The successful characterisation of a performer is reliant on many elements in a production – the actor's skills, the direction, the costume, make-up and hair design. The make-up artist is often required to assist performers and directors in defining characters by changing or enhancing their appearance.

Aim and objectives

Aim of this chapter: to look at the fundamentals of characterisation and the processes involved in some common examples.

You should achieve the following **objectives:**

* Discuss the elements of appearance that suggest character
* Appreciate the role of 'stereotypes' when presenting characters to an audience
* Recall the importance of researching and creating a reference file
* Create a variety of characters using a range of make-up techniques
* Create the stages of ageing, using make-up, for film and stage
* Temporarily age the skin using latex.

Responding to appearance

Each individual is made up of a unique and distinctive set of characteristics that determine his or her persona. This persona is projected to other individuals via external appearance and behaviour. Make-up artists are concerned with the former – the external appearance.

We consistently judge, and are judged by, appearance, both on a conscious and subconscious level. These judgements are based on instinct (shaped by evolution) and learned responses (shaped by culture and experience).

Instinctive responses

Charles Darwin, a nineteenth-century biologist famed for his theories of evolution, noticed that some animals shared the same facial expressions as humans. This led him to believe that basic expressions were an instinctive response rather than a learned response. He concluded that expressions represented the same emotions all over the world – the smile suggests happiness, the frown anger and a wide-eyed expression fear. Recent research showing detailed images of smiling babies still in the womb seems to correspond with this theory. There are seven universally accepted facial expressions – anger, fear, happiness, sadness, disgust, surprise and contempt. These expressions allow us to read the emotions of the wearer and are an indication of the inner state of the individual. Repeated emotions result in repeated expressions becoming etched on the wearer's face over a period of time and these say something about that individual's character. How this understanding of expression and emotion can help the make-up artist in the characterisation process is discussed on the next page.

As human beings we are instinctively drawn towards beauty. Although the perception of 'beauty' varies from person to person and is affected by cultural and social contexts, research has shown that ultimately, all over the world,

people share opinions on faces they consider beautiful. Traits of the commonly accepted beautiful face include:

* smooth, unblemished skin
* big eyes
* plump lips
* even, symmetrical features
* strong, square jawline on men.

Scientists have suggested that symmetrical bodies are an indication of healthy genes and that our attraction to symmetrical faces is an instinctive response to years of evolutionary development.

Babies' features are designed to bring out a nurturing and protecting instinct in us, to ensure the survival of the human race. Big eyes, round cheeks, a high forehead, a small nose and rose-bud lips are typical characteristics of a baby. When a person's face retains an essence of these traits into adulthood, psychologists have suggested that it will evoke a similar response towards that person. It is also closely linked to our idea of beauty in the Western world. Again, this is useful knowledge when attempting to induce a particular response from an audience towards a character and it has been repeatedly exploited in the media.

Learned responses

Although many of our responses to appearance are instinctive, others are undoubtedly learned through experience and behaviour. These learned responses will vary according to social and cultural contexts and may adapt through periods of time. Below are some typical examples of learned responses to appearance found in twentieth-century Western culture.

Appearance	Response
Wearing glasses	Sign of intelligence
Blonde hair	Sign of sexiness, flirting Lack of intelligence

Shaven heads	Sign of aggression (though this has begun to change recently as it has become fashionable for balding men to shave their hair). The style of dress would help to distinguish between fashion and other intended statements of the individual.
Sun tan	A good example of how our learned responses change according to social context. In 1950s and 1960s Britain, the sun tan was a sign of wealth because only wealthy people could afford to travel abroad to hotter climates. In today's social climate, most people can afford a holiday abroad, and concerns about the connection between exposure to sunlight and skin cancer have taken precedence. The sun tan is now slowly beginning to gain a new learned response – a suggestion of ill health and risk.

These learned responses result in a series of 'stereotypes', and although we realise they are just that – not everyone who wears glasses is intelligent, nor are all blonde women flirtatious – we are able to 'tap' into and understand the messages within them.

Projection of character through appearance

In the same way, the presentation of our appearance to others is two-fold – we both have control and have no control over how others see us. We are all born with a unique set of features that constitute our external appearance – these are determined by our genes and we have little control over them (unless we opt for cosmetic surgery). Yet, a person's appearance is much more than a pattern of features; a lifetime of experience will inevitably become etched on a face, suggesting something of the character of the individual. Occupation, emotion and lifestyle will all leave their mark that will be visible to others. Again, we have little control over this without resorting to cosmetic surgery.

However, the presentation of our character is not entirely out of our hands. We all make conscious choices about our appearance that reveal much of our inner character. For most of us, these choices are as much about making an impact on others as they are about pleasing ourselves. They may be about:

* clothes
* hairstyle
* whether men wear facial hair
* decisions to wear tattoos
* body-piercing
* glasses
* the choice to have cosmetic surgery.

Within these conscious statements are 'hidden' messages that exist within a cultural context.

The use of stereotypes in characterisation

It is the processes of projection and response that a production team, including the make-up artist, exploit when exploring characterisation. Casting agents are specifically employed to ensure the correct-looking model or actor is selected to suit the requirements of the production (or photo-shoot) and that the actor will evoke a particular response from the audience. It is then up to the make-up artist to ensure this characterisation is conveyed through the hair and make-up design.

Characterisation often relies on the audience identifying with stereotypes (stereotypes evoke a similar response in many people sharing a similar cultural bias) and therefore relating to the character immediately. You can see examples of this every time you turn on the television or go to the cinema. Advertisements are packed full of stereotypes and companies will often pay huge amounts of money to ensure the 'right face' is promoting their particular brand or product, for example the high-profile, glamorous celebrities used in the L'Oréal commercials. But a 'glamorous' face will not promote all products. Commercials for household products and DIY stores, for example, tend to use more ordinary-looking people that we feel comfortable with and can relate to, rather than the glamorous celebrities of the L'Oréal commercials that we might aspire to. 'Serious' products such as pensions, insurance, etc. tend to use serious, reliable-looking people in their commercials.

When selling products associated with appearance, advertisers will use beautiful and glamorous models. However, not every job will require you to make the performer or model look glamorous; sometimes you will be asked to do just the opposite and make someone look suitably unglamorous.

Characterisation also relies heavily on audience projection. In the case of the L'Oréal commercials the audience relates to the very beautiful, glamorous, sexy characters in an aspirational sense – in using the product people aspire to become more like these characters. The fashion industry consistently receives criticism over its choice of models for this very reason. Magazines, full of pictures of beautiful but underweight models, lead young girls to attempt to emulate this unrealistic portrayal of the female body.

In television and film, we often recognise in lead characters qualities that we would like to possess ourselves. Projection in this positive way can lead to a form of hero-worship where the audience's fantasies and dreams can be lived through the character in question. In order for this to work, the character must live up to our expectations in terms of his or her appearance. The action hero should have rugged good looks; the sensitive, funny guy should have boyish good looks (think of Hugh Grant's characters). Heroes and heroines invariably possess many of the characteristics that will promote instinctive and learned positive responses from us.

Anti-heroes or villains can expect similar treatment, but in this case negative projection

plays its part – we project traits and qualities that we would like to disassociate ourselves from onto our villains. In terms of appearance, anti-heroes tend to share common characteristics – they often wear black, have scars, wear tattoos and possess uneven features. Caricatures of 'baddies', in which these characteristics are exaggerated, can be seen in cartoons and children's films, where 'pointy' features and faces, big noses, large jaws and close-set eyes are frequently associated with this type of character. Charles Bell in his *Essays on the Anatomy of Expression in Painting* (London, 1806) suggests that 'to brutify a human countenance, we only have to diminish the forehead, bring the eyes nearer, lengthen the jaws, shorten the nose and depress the mouth.' Again, directors and designers on a production will often refer back to characteristics that promote both instinctive and learned negative responses when casting and creating anti-heroes.

It is the job of the make-up artist to draw out and relate the character to the audience through the use of make-up and hairstyles and it is important to fully understand the psychological factors that influence characterisation. Why do all witch characters look similar? How is it possible we can all recognise faerie characters when none of us have seen a real one? How can we imply a character is sinister by the make-up design? A thorough understanding of human responses and cultural stereotypes can help us answer these questions.

Realism versus acceptance

Sometimes the make-up artist needs to modify the make-up and hair design to ensure that creating an accurate and realistic portrayal of a character does not alienate the character from the audience. For example, the lead lady or man in a period production, set in the Restoration age, would be unlikely to wear realistic make-up and appear true to the period, as the audience would not be able to relate to the performers as attractive and appealing

Drawing a wizard

Get together with a group of friends. Without discussing the exercise give each person a sheet of paper, pencil and coloured pencils and ask them to draw a wizard. *You must not look at or talk about each other's drawing.* Give yourselves a maximum of fifteen minutes to complete the exercise. When everyone has finished, compare your drawings. You will probably find they look amazingly similar. Spend some time comparing the drawings and discussing their similarities and differences. Why do you think they look so alike? Discuss each person's influences – think about television, books, childhood memories, etc. As a make-up artist and designer it is important to acknowledge the influences from the world around us that we share with others.

heroes or heroines. Instead, the make-up and hair design would suggest something of the period in question but would be modified so that the performer did not appear too far removed from today's accepted notion of beauty. You can see numerous examples of this in both film and television, for example the portrayal of Glenn Close's character in *Dangerous Liaisons* (1988) is far removed from the reality of the time. Rotting teeth and skin, thick white make-up, patches and an enormous insect-infested wig are replaced by a hint of the period – pale skin tone, red lips and beauty spots – allowing Glenn Close to retain a beautiful appearance that will appeal to the audience in 1988. Sometimes the opposite technique is employed and a more realistic appearance is used to portray the anti-hero or comic character.

Researching characters

In order to help you create specific characters, it will be useful to recall the information in 'Keeping a reference file' (Chapter 5, Developing the artistic eye, page 70).

You may find it useful to categorise your collection into sub-sections, for example:

* dance and ballet
* rough characters ('dirtying down')
* characters of different ethnic origins
* historical characters
* transgender characters
* fantasy characters
* fairytale characters
* pantomime characters
* aged characters.

In order to show examiners and prospective clients the full breadth of your skill, you should consider creating and displaying in your portfolio an example of a make-up from each of these sections.

Ageing make-up

Visual patterns of ageing

Ageing a performer past his or her years is a frequent but difficult challenge for the make-up artist. One of the major problems is that no two people will age in the same way, hence there is no single set of instructions that will accommodate all. The effects you choose to create will depend on a number of factors:

* the actual age of the performer
* the age you are transforming the performer to
* the bone structure, muscle and skin condition of the performer
* the state of the character's health
* the ethnicity of the character
* the lifestyle of the character
* the type of character, for example emotions that are etched on the face.

Even though ageing is an individual process, there are some external features that are common in most people due to the biological process of ageing.

When designing an ageing make-up it is important to consider the character being portrayed. Some

HANDS ON

Creating a reference file for ageing make-ups

Plenty of reference material will play an essential part in creating a realistic ageing make-up. In your file you should have pictures of faces of all ages and all ethnicities. If you can get hold of images showing progressive ageing, for example the same person at various stages of his or her life, all the better. Remember, the most accessible material is the people you meet on a day-to-day basis. What makes people look their age? It is important to study faces to really understand ageing. You will learn to adapt and interpret this material, taking elements from it that apply to your make-up and performer.

KEY NOTE

In order to complete an ageing make-up you will require skills and knowledge learnt in earlier chapters. Take a moment to look over the following sections:
Bones of the skull (Chapter 4, page 46)
Muscles of the head and neck (Chapter 4, page 47)
The skin and the ageing process (Chapter 4, page 56)
Mixing highlights and shadows for skin tones (Chapter 5, page 69)

Male patterns of ageing	Female patterns of ageing
The beard line gets stronger, eventually turning grey.	Facial hair may increase.
Baldness or receding hairline. Exposed skin becomes prone to age spots and hyper-pigmentation	Hair thins on the head.
Hair greys, starting at the temples.	Hair greys, but the majority of women will dye their hair until old age.
Brows get bushier and coarser, and will go grey.	Brows and lashes become sparse and will eventually go grey.
The neck loses tone, and often thins making the Adam's apple more pronounced.	The neck loses tone and thins.

Wrinkles (lines) appear on the skin surface. A deep wrinkle usually appears along the nasolabial fold (from nose to mouth). Frown lines are also common (between the brows) and heavy wrinkling around the eyes is often apparent.
Loss of tone in the skin leading to eye bags, deep nasolabial-folds, sagging jaw lines.
Cheekbones recede on thinner faces (beginning to resemble the skull underneath). On heavier faces cheeks, jowls, jaw line and neck gain weight.
Skin becomes discoloured with hyperpigmentation. Skin tone may change.
Lips become thinner, particularly the upper lip, and lose colour.
The back of the hands usually become hyperpigmented. Veins are more pronounced and the skin becomes loose and 'leathery'. Fingers become thinner and joints are more pronounced. Palms change very little.
The ears and nose look big on old people, not because they grow but because the rest of the body shrinks.

people will show these signs of ageing more than others because of environment and lifestyle differences. People who have spent much of their life outside may appear ruddier and exhibit more hyperpigmentation than those with a more sedentary lifestyle. Those with a history of heavy drinking will often have more dilated capillaries across the cheeks and nose, and certain underlying medical conditions will affect an ageing face, particularly its base colour. People will also age faster if they suffer poor diet and living conditions.

A person living some centuries ago would have had a much shorter life expectancy than today and so aged much sooner. Social conditioning also has an impact on the age people are perceived. Factors like life expectancy, medical advances, improved living conditions, cosmetic surgery and social changes all mean the 'older generation' is becoming 'younger'. Hairstyles, clothing, glasses and facial hair all suggest the age of the wearer. It is common to see older women wearing make-up and hairstyles that were in fashion when they were more youthful. An excellent example is that of Wallis Simpson the late Duchess of Windsor.

Facial hair can also age men significantly. It is possible to age a male performer by simply darkening his beard line. Adding a moustache or beard will add even more age.

Ageing a performer in his or her early twenties to old age will be difficult. There will be fewer clues to guide you to the way their face would age naturally, so wrinkles and other signs of age must be created. When ageing a middle-aged performer, lines and other signs of ageing can simply be accentuated and developed. In the case of younger performers it may be useful to look at photographs of older relatives whom they resemble, as visual patterns of the ageing process are often hereditary.

The make-up process

How you approach an ageing make-up design will depend on a number of factors. Remember the key issues of time, budget and suitability when planning for any job. As a general rule, the process of chiaroscuro (using light and shade painted on the skin, highlighting where skin needs to protrude and shading where skin needs to sink in) works well on the large stage but does not work in close-up. In this case, prosthetic appliances are often required to give a three-dimensional feel to the make-up. The most you can hope to age a performer for small

Images showing progressive ageing on a female:

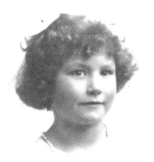

Childhood

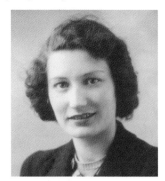

Twenties

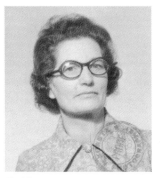

Forties

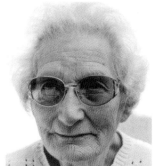

Old age

stage, television and film simply using chiaroscuro is by about 15 years. Beyond that other techniques such as old age stipple and prosthesis are required.

Skin tones and bases

Foundation is usually unnecessary as the natural blemishes and discolouration of the skin are more apparent in an ageing skin. Further colouration is often best applied in a stippling action, which also helps to break down the skin texture. The exception is when you wish to portray something particular to the character, for example a suggestion of illness.

* Grey skin tones suggest frailty in old age.
* Yellowy, green skin tones suggest illness in old age.
* Red skin tones suggest robust old age.

Ageing the hair

Bald caps can be used to create complete hair loss or can be used with toupees to suggest receding hair. Another way of creating the effect of a receding hairline is to lighten the front hairline, or more dramatically cut or shave the hair. For long shooting schedules some performers may prefer this option to spending lengthy periods of time in the make-up room day after day.

Men tend to 'grey' around the temples first. Adding grey here is a good technique for suggesting middle age on the male performer. Although women also grey with age, it is common for them to dye their hair to hide this. Whether a female performer wears grey hair or not will depend on her character. Wigs can be fitted to change the hair colour and style and are popular when ageing female performers.

The natural hair can also be greyed using temporary hair colours. There are many brands to choose from when buying off the shelf, and most are simply washed out. However, if you wish to create your own hair whitener, it is best to add a touch of yellow or silver to the mix to create a softer, more realistic colour.

Mixing colours for highlight and shade

Re-read the section on mixing highlights and shadows for skin tones in Chapter 5 'Developing the Artistic Eye' (page 69) to help you mix colours suitable for ageing. Remember to look at the natural shadows and highlights on the skin. As a general rule in most light skins, shadows are a greyed brown or browned grey and adding a reddened brown will give more emphasis and depth, whereas highlights are ivory with a hint of pink. Black skins have shadows that are dark blue and purple with black added for emphasis, and highlights are orange or yellow toned. However, the darker the skin tone, the less the lines and shadows will show and the use of highlight becomes the most useful tool.

Once you have mixed the highlight, the shader and a deepened version of the shader for lines of definition, check the colours by applying them to the performer's skin and squinting at them (this helps the eye to see the tonal value of the colours). The shader should look three tones darker than the skin tone, and the highlight three tones lighter. The deepest colour should look two to three shades darker than the shader. Once you are happy with the colours you are ready to proceed with the application.

KEY NOTE

There are simple rules to follow when creating this make-up:

* 'Lines' are really indentations in the skin that cause a shadow next to a highlight. Every line must have a highlight on each side of it to make the line look as though it is really indented in the skin.
* Use the performer's own lines and shadows for guidance.
* Folds have highlights on the raised side only.
* Progressive ageing must follow the same pattern of ageing.
* Once an ageing make-up has been applied and set, a straight or fashion make-up can be applied over the top.

STEP-BY-STEP **Ageing using light and shade**

The following procedures are suggested for the larger stage where the make-up will not be viewed in close-up. They are also an excellent exercise to help you understand the physical process of ageing on the skin and to practise the art of chiaroscuro. The procedures are a starting point in the art of ageing and once you become more accomplished, you will be able to adjust the make-up to suit the performer and character.

Equipment required

* Selection of brushes
* Selection of sponges including natural sea sponge
* Highlight colour suitable for the skin tone you are working on
* Shadow colour suitable for the skin tone you are working on
* Colour slightly darker than the shadow colour suitable for adding definition and lines
* Powder
* Spirit gum
* Grey, silver or white hair colour
* Rose or red colour
* Crimson lake (deep purpley-red) colour

The first stages of ageing

This make-up can be used in the following situations:

* to add maturity to a very young looking face
* to create characters in their late twenties and early thirties
* to add 'strength' to the face, particularly for men.

Use brushes or sponges to apply the make-up that are suitable for the area you are working on. Cream-based make-up is the ideal medium to use as it is easy to blend and control. The shadows, lines and highlights should fall into the natural pattern of the face so it is important to really study the model's face and apply make-up appropriately.

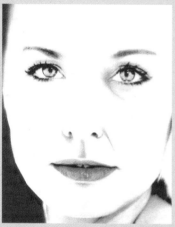

Face chart for first stages of age make-up

1 Cleanse, tone and moisturise lightly.
2 Place a small amount of shader in the natural shadow under the inner corner of the eye. Keep the shadow to the socket line, and do not make the shadow look too dark or you will make the performer look ill.
3 Add an area of highlight between the shadow and the eye.
4 Place a shadow in the hollow between the nose and the mouth.
5 Place a shadow under the centre of the lower lip.
6 Add a small highlight on the centre, fleshy part of the chin.
7 Place a gentle shadow in the naso-labial folds from the nostril to less than half way to the mouth. If the shadow is any longer you will make the face look too old. The shadows should exactly fit in the natural laughter lines when the model smiles.
8 Powder.

Progressive ageing

This make-up can be used in the following situations:

* to create characters in their early forties
* if the character ages during a play, you could add these details on top of the 'first stages of ageing' make-up.
1 Add highlights and shadows as for 'first stages of ageing' make-up above.

All design sheets for ageing make-up by Julia Conway

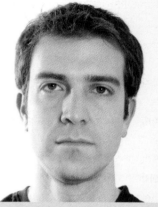
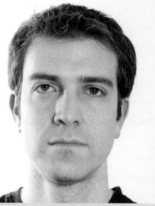

Model prior to ageing make-up being applied

Model after 'first stages of ageing' make-up has been applied

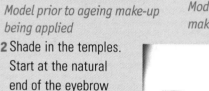

2 Shade in the temples. Start at the natural end of the eyebrow and continue up to the hairline in a fairly straight line, then blend down to the beginning of the cheekbone at the side of the eye.
3 Add chin shadows in the little hollow in the centre of the jaw line. Ask the performer to

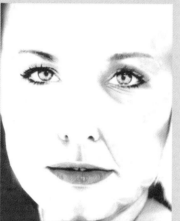

Face chart for progressive ageing

pull the chin into the neck. Where the skin creases, add small shadows either side of the chin. Chin shadows give the feeling that the skin on the jaw is loosening.
4 Add small shadows at the corners of the mouth.
5 Powder.
6 Strengthen the shadow under the outside corner of the eye.
7 You will now need to add more age lines using a fine brush. Trace a little of the deeper shading colour into a couple of lines under the eye. These lines will be coming from under the inner corner of the eye. You may see several, but use only two. Do not make them long – they should be no longer than the shadow under the eye. As you draw the line in, take a clean brush or cotton bud and fade the line a little. This will make it 'sink' into the skin and look real.

8 Shade the socket area of the eye.

9 Now go to the nasal fold. You have already put a shadow from the nose; now strengthen and lengthen it a little with the fine brush. Fade the line, then trace around the nostril shape.

10 Add shader under the cheekbone to *slightly* hollow the face.

11 Add highlights as follows.

* Highlight above the temple shadows on the outside of the forehead.

* Add highlights each side of the chin shadows.

* Highlight the outer portion of the brow bone down to the shaded socket to create the impression of a slight overhang.

* The lines under the eyes have highlights on both sides of them. These highlights are a little wider and longer than the lines. This is important. If they are the same width, the effect is one of stripes on the face.

* The mouth to nose lines have a highlight only on the cheek side. This highlight should be much wider than the line to give more depth.

* The shadow under the nose has a little highlight on each side of it.

* 'Bag' highlights are small highlights placed inside the socket you have shaded under the eyes to create the shape of the 'bag'. Also add a highlight on the cheekbone.

12 Re-powder to set the make-up.

Middle age

This make-up can be used in the following situations:

* to create characters in their late forties to late fifties

* if the character ages during a play, you could add these details on top of the progressive ageing or straight make-up.

1 Follow instructions for progressive ageing.

2 Powder.

3 Add forehead lines. Do not make them look like railway lines - break them up and avoid rows.

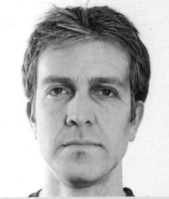

Second stages of ageing make-up

4 Ask the model to pull the eyebrows together. Using a fine brush, add frown lines.

5 Strengthen the nasal fold by lengthening the lines there.

6 Add more chin lines. Take the lines round to the outside of the jaw. Curve and blend them under the jaw line, otherwise they look painted and awkward.

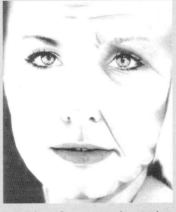

Face chart for progressive ageing

7 Add a fold above the eyelid by placing a finger over the end of the eyebrow and gently pushing the skin inwards and downwards. A fold usually appears from the inner end of the brow and goes down towards the outer corner of the eye. Draw the fold in with the darker shader and blend gently towards the nose.

8 Strengthen the shadows at the corner of the mouth.

9 Place highlights:

* each side of the additional chin lines where they curve upwards

* above and below each forehead line

* on each side of the frown lines

* at the corner of the mouth on the outside of the shadows

* on the brow bone to accentuate the eye fold.

Completed middle age make-up

10 If visible, the neck will also require ageing. Using the natural lines, proceed as for the forehead.

11 Powder the face and neck.

12 Partially grey the eyebrows, sideburns and temples on men (optional).

Old age

This is an extension of middle age. The older you make the face, the more you must think of the skull showing through the skin. Of course, if the character is a fat old person, this does not apply. If you have a round, fat face, don't attempt the 'skull effect'; it won't work. Instead, concentrate on the lines and corresponding highlights.

1 Add highlights, shadows and lines as for middle age make-up.

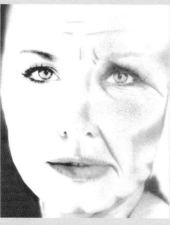
Face chart for old age

2 Powder.

3 To achieve a skull-like effect, the shading on the cheek must change shape. To get some idea of the effect, ask the performer to suck in the cheeks. Place the shader into the hollow the performer has made until you reach centre cheek. Then curve the shader towards the jaw. This is not a square shape, but a gentle curve. The highlight also follows the shape down.

4 Highlight the lips to take out the colour. Draw lines on the lips – you will see vertical lines on them. Take the lines on the top lips over the natural lip line. Highlight between the lines. Strengthen the shadows at the corners.

5 Now work on the neck.

 * **For thin *men:*** Highlight the Adam's apple and put a shadow on each side of it. Shade down the sides of the neck and above the collarbone. Stretch the neck and place shadows in the hollows on each side of the neck tendons. Highlight down the neck inside the shadows, on the tendons and on the collar bones.

 * **For thin *women:*** Ask the performer to put the chin out and pull the neck muscles up. You will now see a hollow. Put a shadow in the hollow and highlight on each side of it. Shade down the sides of the neck and above the collarbone; highlight above the collarbone.

6 Brush a little spirit gum through the eyebrows working in towards the nose. Brush the eyebrows towards the nose. This will give a sparse, untidy look. Lighten the hair.

7 Darken the eyelids and the area between the nose and the fold line on the brow bone with shader.

8 Extend the fold line downwards and highlight on top of the line.

9 Make the nose bonier and larger with shadows and highlights.

10 Powder.

11 Study the make-up so far and strengthen any highlights and shadows as appropriate.

12 Brush a highlight over the eyelashes to make them look sparse.

13 Add rose or redness around the rims of the eyes.

14 Take the fold of the eye down past the outer corner of the eye. Place a highlight above it and lengthen the highlight so that it is longer than the fold line.

15 Break down the skin texture by stippling on any skin discolouration, for example broken capillaries (lake crimson on a dry sea sponge), age spots, changes in skin tone, etc.

16 Powder again.

17 Add props, for example grey facial hair, glasses.

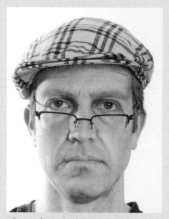
Completed old age make-up

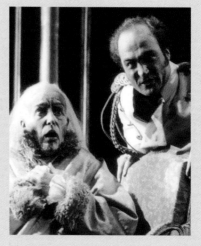

An example of an old age make-up for the large theatre. The performer was aged from the late twenties to look very, very old. A bald cap with hair inserted was applied and a simple chiaroscuro make-up was applied. The make-up is very effective from a distance but would look very crude close-up.

Ageing make-up for television and film

As discussed earlier, the application of highlight and shader to create an ageing effect is of limited use in television and film. Techniques such as applying old age stipple and prosthesis appliances are widely used to create effects that are three-dimensional and realistic close-up.

> **REMEMBER**
>
> Old age stipple should be applied in a calm, professional environment. Communication with the model is vital as he or she should keep the eyes closed when you are working near the eye area. If old age stipple gets into the eye, immediately carry out an eye bath. If irritation persists, seek medical attention.

> **KEY NOTE**
>
> Old age stipple is a latex-based product that is usually available in different skin tones. An allergy test should be carried out before use.
>
> This technique works best on models over thirty as there is more 'give' in their skin.
>
> Two people are required when using old age stipple: one to stretch, the other to apply the stipple, dry it and powder before the skin is released.
>
> The pattern of the wrinkles is determined by the direction of the stretch. If you stretch vertically, the wrinkles will be horizontal; if you stretch horizontally, the lines will be vertical.
>
> For subtle effects, the most common use of old age stipple is around the eyes and lips.

STEP-BY-STEP | **Applying old age stipple**

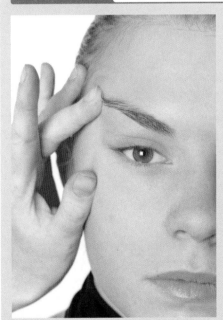 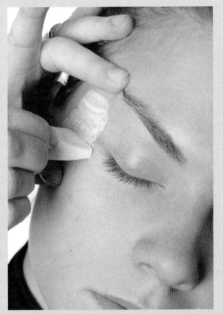 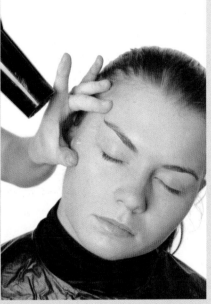

1 Stretch the skin (study your reference file and think about the way you want the lines to go).

2 Use an old, small, fine stipple sponge (a natural sea sponge is ideal for this) to apply the old age stipple. It is important to keep the layer thin. Do not let it touch the eyelashes and feather the old age stipple at the outer corners of the eyes. When applying to the lips the old age stipple should slightly overlap the lip line.

3 Keeping the skin stretched, dry with a hairdryer (cool setting).

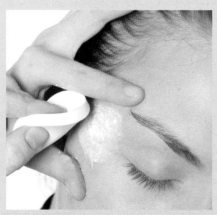 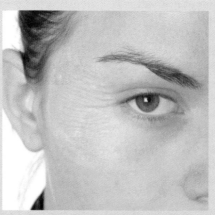 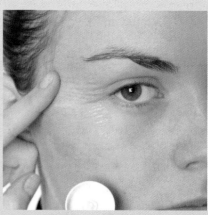

4 Keeping the skin stretched, powder generously and remove any excess.

5 Release the skin. It will form into wrinkles; these improve with time as they settle and become part of the model's face and natural expression. Repeat the process, adding as many layers as required. Keep the edges of the area thin. Stop before it begins to look false.

6 Apply lubricating jelly to take away any chalkiness. You can apply make-up over the top.

To remove the old age stipple use a little oil (Pro-clean) on a cotton bud. Gently lift the edges of the old age stipple. Do not pull the latex off in one piece; instead, gently stretch the skin as you wipe with the cotton wool. Take your time or you may damage the model's skin.

Evaluation

Make a list of the successful and unsuccessful aspects of your work. Think about how you could improve the finished result. Below is a troubleshooting table listing common problems.

Common problems	Troubleshooting
Make-up looks 'bitty' with raised areas and holes.	You need to work quickly when applying the old age stipple. Do not go back over areas whilst it is still damp as it will pick up the stipple underneath and make it look rough.
Make-up looks chalky and unrealistic.	Do not forget to apply lubricating jelly over the stipple. You may have applied too many layers, or your layers may be too thick.
Skin does not look very wrinkled.	Remember to hold the stretched skin until the stipple is dried and powdered.

Dramatic and fantasy effects can be created using old age stipple and layers of tissue all over the face. A layer of torn tissue is laid over the layer of stipple prior to drying. If you are applying latex to the whole face, work on small areas at a time, overlapping each one. The neck can be stretched vertically simply by holding the model's head backwards. Make-up can be applied as usual, but shading and highlighting are not usually necessary on top of the latex: the wrinkles are three-dimensional and create their own shadows.

STEP-BY-STEP Ageing for television and film

Once you have practised the technique of old age stippling and feel competent, move on to attempting the following ageing make-up for television and film.

Equipment required

* Selection of brushes and sponges
* Barrier cream
* Powder
* Old age stipple
* Selection of skin tone colours including a highlight and shader suitable for the skin tone you are working on
* Grey, silver or white hair colour

1 Apply barrier cream around the eyes and lips and powder well.
2 Apply old age stipple to the eyes and lips.
3 Emphasise folds with basic light and shade, using mainly highlights as shadows are picked up on screen. The make-up will get absorbed into the skin so make it a little stronger than you wish the final result to be. Do not go too theatrical; remember you can only age a performer approximately 15 years with this procedure.
4 Take out colour from the lips with highlight.
5 Stipple other colours on the skin tone to take out youthful, vibrant complexion, creating a mottled tonality. Avoid a repetitive pattern as the camera is sensitive to this. Keep it subtle.
6 Powder.
7 Lighten the eyebrows and lashes.

Ageing the hand

The hands can be aged using the same techniques as described earlier for the face. Study the real thing as well as photographs of aged hands and follow the diagrams below for details of where to apply highlight and shader. Mottled skin colouration and hyperpigmentation can also be added and veins can be accentuated.

Old age stipple can have excellent results when used on the back of the hands. Make-up can be applied before or after the application, but remember to make the make-up a little stronger than you require if you are applying it under the old age stipple. Follow the procedure below.

HANDS ON

Research films that contain excellent examples of ageing make-ups. The following are suggestions to get you started:
Charlize Theron in *Monster* (2004)
F Murray Abraham in *Amadeus* (1984)
Dustin Hoffman in *Little Big Man* (1970)

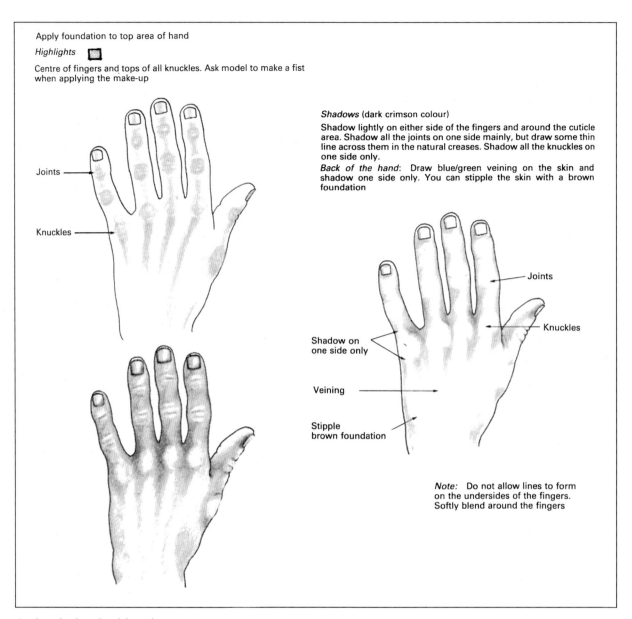

Apply foundation to top area of hand

Highlights

Centre of fingers and tops of all knuckles. Ask model to make a fist when applying the make-up

Joints

Knuckles

Shadows (dark crimson colour)

Shadow lightly on either side of the fingers and around the cuticle area. Shadow all the joints on one side mainly, but draw some thin line across them in the natural creases. Shadow all the knuckles on one side only.

Back of the hand: Draw blue/green veining on the skin and shadow one side only. You can stipple the skin with a brown foundation

Joints

Knuckles

Shadow on one side only

Veining

Stipple brown foundation

Note: Do not allow lines to form on the undersides of the fingers. Softly blend around the fingers

Ageing the hands with make-up

Fantasy ageing

Another technique you could try is to create an ageing make-up using fantasy colours. This works well when creating witches or wizards. Let your imagination go wild – try using complementary colours for highlighted and shaded areas for a really dramatic effect.

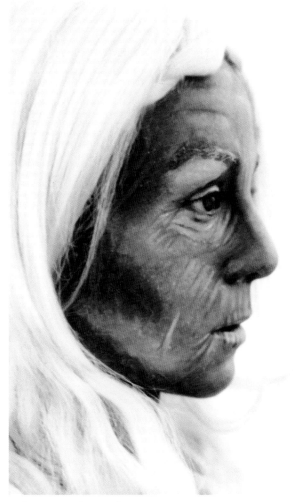

A fantasy ageing make-up

Gender changes

Why do men and women look different? The table below makes comparisons between the male and female skull and facial structures. It is important to remember there are variations and exceptions to these generalised observations.

Female	Male
Skull on average only two-thirds the size of the male's	Larger skull – on average one-third larger than the female's
Less prominent bone structure along the jaw and brow.	More pronounced bone structure along the jaw and brow
Smaller, narrower nose	Larger, longer and wider nose
Lips are fuller	Thinner lips
Smoother skin, less pronounced pores	Coarser skin texture
Downy, fine facial hair	Darker, coarse facial hair
Finer, higher eyebrows	Thicker, lower eyebrows
Eyes look more prominent	Eyes less prominent
Forehead more vertical	Forehead more angled
Thinner neck	Wider neck with pronounced Adam's apple

The make-up artist is rarely called upon to create a convincing gender change. Realistic changes are very difficult to achieve without the use of prosthetics and clever casting of the actor. More common is the suggestion of transgender, where a female is required to look masculine, or a male more feminine. Alternatively, gender change where limited realism is required, such as when the audience is supposed to be aware of the transformation, is also seen more frequently.

Examples are Robin Williams as Mrs Doubtfire, Dustin Hoffman as Tootsie or Gwyneth Paltrow in *Shakespeare in Love*.

When attempting to create a gender change for characterisation it is best to consider each point of application required to complete the process.

Female to male make-up application procedure

Make-up application	Technique
Foundation base	The skin needs to look coarser – omitting the use of foundation will help by maintaining an uneven skin texture. Additional skin texture can be added by stippling make-up on the skin's surface with a natural sea sponge or stipple sponge.
Contouring	To give the impression of a more masculine bone structure the following areas should be highlighted: jaw, lower frontal bone (above brows), bridge of the nose, outer edges of the nostrils, brow bone (below outer half of the eyebrow), sides of the neck and oesophagus (giving the impression of an Adam's apple).
Concealer	Blemishes can be removed, but the majority of shadows should be left to strengthen the facial features, for example shadows under the eyes and around the nose and mouth. Very deep, unattractive shadows with discolouration should be reduced.
Powder	As normal.
Eyebrows	Eyebrows should appear less groomed and thicker. This can be achieved be lightly brushing spirit gum through the hair and leaving it unkempt. Brushing slightly downwards can help them appear lower.
Eyes	No make-up required.
Lips	No make-up required. Blotted lip balm can be applied if lips are dry.
Hairstyle	A wig can be added as appropriate. Remember it is common for men to leave greyness in their hair showing. This can be added or incorporated in the wig for characters of a certain age.
Special effects	Facial hair can be added. Laying-on hair, lace facial pieces and application of stubble are all appropriate methods (see Chapter 10). Alternatively, for large theatre, make-up can be applied with a stipple sponge to create a five o'clock shadow.

Male to female make-up application procedure

Before this make-up is attempted, ensure the male model is clean-shaven.

Make-up application	Technique
Camouflage	Apply a 'beard cover' product to hide the five o'clock shadow. This is usually a camouflage-based product that provides excellent coverage. Apply a thin layer to the beard area and powder lightly.
Foundation base	Apply foundation to the whole of the face and neck, blending well. Ensure you use a foundation with excellent

	coverage – this means you will not be tempted to apply a thick, unnatural looking base. Do not try to change the natural skin tone with the base.
Contouring	To give the impression of a more feminine bone structure the following areas should be shaded: jawline, sides of the neck, sides and tip of the nose, temples, under the cheekbones. The tops of the cheekbones should be highlighted.
Concealer	Apply concealer in the usual places as for a beauty make-up, for example blemishes, shadows around the eyes, shadows around the nose, etc.
Powder	As normal.
Eyebrows	Permission should be gained from the model before making any semi-permanent changes to the eyebrows such as removing hair. Ideally, heavy brows should be plucked for definition and to make the eyebrows appear higher. Dark, coarse brow hair can be lightened for a softer appearance. Brows should be well groomed and the shape accentuated with colour.
Eyes	Appropriate eye make-up should be applied. The eyes should be brought forward and made to look larger.
Lashes	Lashes should be curled before mascara is applied. False lashes are useful for adding extra definition and femininity. Decide what effect you want before applying.
Lips	Use a lip liner for definition, outlining the natural shape of the lips but accentuating the Cupid's bow slightly. Avoid dark colours that will make the lips look thinner. A little gloss in the centre of the lower lip will act as a highlighter and make the lips look fuller. A highlight can also be added

	above the Cupid's bow for extra glamour and definition.
Hairstyle	A wig can be added as appropriate.
Special effects	If the hands are on show, body hair will need to be removed. False nails can be added and polish applied to complete the effect. The neck should remain hidden if possible as it is very difficult to hide the Adam's apple.

Ethnic changes

There are three accepted main groups of ethnicity in the human race:

* white
* Oriental–Asian
* black.

Within these three groups are a number of sub-groups, making human ethnicity a fascinating and complex subject area. For the sake of this chapter we will look at the main structural differences of the skull and face of the three main groups.

White

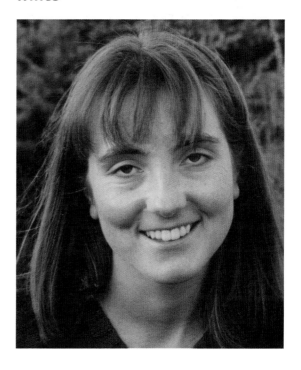

* The face shape is different variations of the classic oval.
* Skin tones vary with pink and yellow undertones.
* Eye pigment varies through blues, greens, greys and brown.
* Hair colour and texture vary.
* Eye sockets are defined.
* The nasal bone root is high.
* The nose is narrow and projects strongly.
* Lips are thinner than in other ethnic groups.

Oriental-Asian

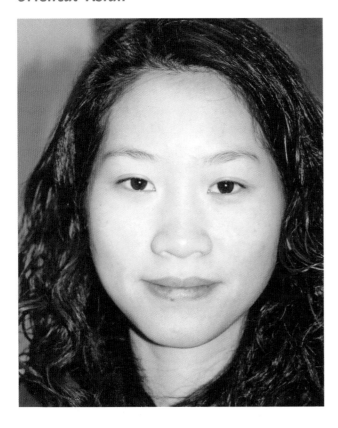

* The face tends to be rounder. Cheekbones flare outwards making the face appear flat.
* The skin has strong yellow undertones.
* Eye pigment is brown.
* Hair is black and very straight.
* Epicanthic eye folds obscure the eyelashes and give a tilted look. There is no deep eye socket.

* Eyelashes and eyebrows are short, sparse and straight. Hair appears to be tilted downwards.
* The nasal bone root is low and flat.
* The nose is medium broad.
* Lips are narrow in width and of medium thickness.

Black

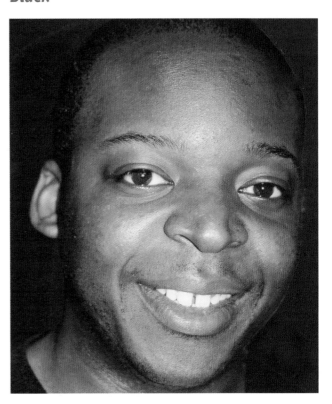

* The face has a strong chin with prominent cheekbones.
* The skin tone is yellowish brown to dark brown, often with red undertones.
* The eye pigment is brown.
* Hair is black, coarse and very curly.
* The eye sockets are defined and are sometimes hidden by a pronounced overhang from above the socket.
* Eyelashes and eyebrows are short and curly.
* The nose is broad.
* Lips are thick and everted with a deep indentation above the top lip.

White to Oriental–Asian make-up application procedure

Make-up application	Technique
Preparation of eyebrows	Block out the eyebrows, or part of the eyebrows, whichever you feel is more appropriate for your model.
Foundation base	Apply a base that has strong yellow undertones. Because you are changing the skin tone, it is critical to blend with precision and to take the base just past the costume line.
Concealer	Apply as normal.
Contouring	To make the white face appear more Oriental, highlight the following areas: the entire eyelid and eye socket from lash to brow, under the eye, the sides of the nose and across the top of the cheekbones, the temples. A shading should then be applied to the following areas: the bridge of the nose right to the tip, the angles of the jaw line to make it appear more rounded, the top of a high forehead, under the inner corner of the eye, under the outer corner of the eye.
Powder	As normal with a yellow-toned powder.
Eyes	Highlight the entire lid area. Apply kohl pencil in soft black or dark brown, extending the outer corner in a downward tilt. The inner corner should also be extended downwards (see diagram). Alternatively, prosthetics can be applied (see special effects below).
Eyebrows	If the natural hair has been left, brush downwards before adding colour (a soft black). The eyebrows can now be softly defined from the inner corner to the highest point. The outer portion should be kept very short.
Lashes	Black mascara can be added if the model is blonde or female, but lashes should be brushed downwards at the outer corner.
Lips	Lipstick can be added to a female model – a browny-maroon colour will give a natural look.
Hairstyle	A wig can be added – the hair should be straight and black in an appropriate style.
Special effects	Prosthetic Oriental eye pieces can be added – you can make your own (see Chapter 16, page 356) or buy them ready-made. Follow the instructions below.

Emphasising the oriental eye

Slanting brow

Highlight entire lid area

Extended shadow

Extended line

STEP-BY-STEP Applying prosthetic Oriental eye pieces

(It is assumed that you are familiar with the section on applying prosthetics in Chapter 10.)

Oriental eye pieces are designed to cover the socket line and create an epicanthic fold on a white person's eye. The pieces are applied at the start of the make-up process.

1 Ask the model to look straight ahead.
2 Hold the pieces to the eyes to check size and position.
3 Apply adhesive to the edges of the prosthetic piece (not the edge near the lashes).
4 Begin by placing the piece on the inner corner of the eye.

Pull the piece across the eyelid so the lower edge of the piece is in line with the lash line. When you are happy with the position, press it into place.

5 Seal the piece.
6 Apply make-up as described above.

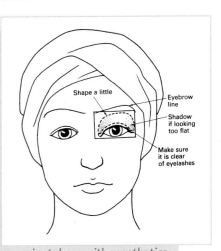

Shape a little

Eyebrow line

Shadow if looking too flat

Make sure it is clear of eyelashes

Creating an oriental eye with prosthetics

KEY NOTE

In 1990, English actor Jonathan Pryce was cast to play an Oriental Asian in the Broadway production of *Miss Saigon*. Pryce had previously performed the role on the London stage wearing heavy prosthetic eyelids until he was informed that some people might find this racially offensive. Members of the Asian-American artistic community complained about the show producer's refusal to allow them to compete for the role.

Dirtying down

Sometimes a script will require you to 'dirty down' a performer to create various characters. An excellent example of this is Baldrick from the British television series *Blackadder*.

'Dirtying down' refers to the process of making a performer look rather less than his or her best. It can be combined with casualty effects or used alone. Effects can be subtle or, as in the case of Baldrick, rather extreme.

Below are some examples of when dirtying down a performer may be appropriate.

* a character involved in an accident
* a character caught in extreme weather
* a homeless character or drug user
* a medieval peasant.

Medieval peasant make-up procedure

Make-up application	Technique
Foundation base	The skin needs to look weathered and textured. Fake tan (if the skin is not naturally tanned) will give the impression of working outdoors. Foundation should not be required, but texture can be added with a stipple sponge, for example dilated capillaries can be created using crimson red crème-make-up.
Contouring	No specific requirements.
Concealer	Concealer should be avoided. Let shadows and blemishes show as this will add to the finished effect.
Powder	As normal.
Eyebrows	Eyebrows should look untidy. Brush a little spirit gum through them to make them appear coarse and unruly.
Eyes and lashes	Eye make-up is not required.
Lips	Lips should look dry and uncared for.
Hairstyle	Backcomb a wig or natural hair into a messy, 'unstyled' style. A headscarf works well on a female model.
Special effects	The addition of skin disorders such as herpes simplex (cold sores) on the mouth, or pimples or boils on the skin using casualty effects works well, but avoid overdoing the effect. Ageing techniques can also be effective (peasants would have aged much more quickly than their wealthy counterparts). Coloured tooth enamel to create missing or discoloured teeth can also add to the effect.

Completed medieval peasant make-up

Examples of specific characterisations

STEP-BY-STEP **Geisha**

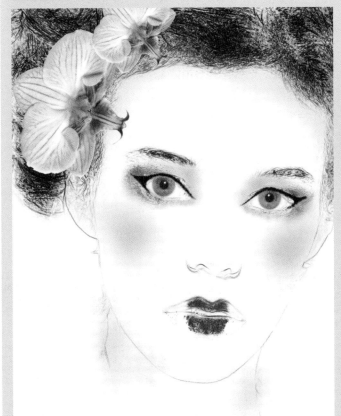

Design sheet for Geisha make-up by Julia Conway

1 Block out the eyebrows or part of the eyebrows as you see fit to achieve the final result (if required).

2 Apply prosthetic eye pieces (if required).

3 Draw a line around the face close to the hairline with a white pencil.

4 Fill in the face and continue down the neck (including the sides and back) to the costume line using a white base (you could add a touch a pink for softness or if pure white will cause problems with the lighting). Make neat and even. If they are on show, the hands will also need to be whitened.

5 Powder with transparent or white powder. Dust off excess.

6 Add soft black eyebrows, keeping them short and straight from the highest point outwards.

7 Line the top lid in black eyeliner accentuating the Oriental eye shape (keep the line thin).

8 Add a strong pink shader to the outer corner of the eye at the top and bottom.

9 Dust pale pink eye shadow just below the inner corner of the eyebrow and just below the inner corner of the eye. Blend to nothing.

10 Add black mascara but do not curl the lashes.

11 Very pale pink blush can be applied to the cheeks.

12 Draw small perfect lips in bright red (blue-toned, not orange).

13 Add a traditional Geisha wig or style natural black hair and decorate with flowers or another decoration.

Check out productions of the opera *Madame Butterfly* for interpretations of the Geisha make-up for stage.

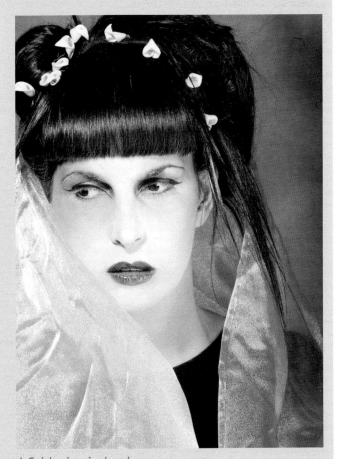

A Geisha-inspired make-up

STEP-BY-STEP Eighteenth-century make-up for stage (to be viewed from a distance)

Equipment required

* Cleanser, toner and moisturiser
* Selection of brushes and sponges
* Eyebrow plastic or wax
* Sealer
* Rose-coloured camouflage make-up (optional)
* Spatula to apply wax
* Off-white crème make-up base
* White powder

* White pan-cake make-up
* Blue eye shadow
* Eyebrow pencil in brown or black
* Dark blue eyeliner
* Brown or black mascara
* Red or bright pink blusher
* Red lipstick
* Black cake eyeliner

1 Cleanse the face and apply moisturiser or barrier cream (if required).

2 Block out the eyebrows with wax.

3 The base should be off white (white can cause problems with lighting). For a female character, add a touch of pink. For a male character, add a touch of beige. Apply a thin base with crème make-up all over the face, neck and chest (if exposed) using a damp latex wedge or sponge. Apply gently over the eyebrows using a brush. (You can use camouflage make-up to hide the eyebrows first: Apply pink (rose) camouflage, powder, match skin tone with camouflage, powder, apply off-white crème make-up. See the section on blocking out eyebrows in Chapter 10, page 212, for more detail.)

4 Powder generously with a white powder or talc.

5 Apply a very thin layer of white pan-cake make-up over the powdered crème base. This should give you an even finish.

6 Apply eye shadow. Blue is the best colour (you cannot tell the difference between blue and black from a distance, but blue seems to work better with the white base.) Apply it darker near the lashes and blend up fading to the brow bone.

7 Draw the eyebrows on – they should be long, thin, round and slightly higher than the natural brow (use the top of the wax or natural eyebrow as a guideline).

8 Apply dark-blue eye lines rather than black or brown ones to achieve more brightness in the eye area. Continue across the entire top lid, extending past the outer corner of the eye and fading to nothing at the ends. Apply lower eye lines just below the bottom lashes. Extend the lines past the outer corner, keeping them parallel to the top eye line. Apply mascara.

9 Apply red or bright pink blusher in a circle low down on the cheek.

10 Apply red lipstick in a bee-stung shape.

11 Add patches (beauty spots) in black (cake eyeliner is useful for this). Common shapes would be hearts, diamonds and circles.

Eighteenth-century make-up for television, film and stage

The table below describes the different approach necessary for the more subtle requirements of a television or film production and the more dramatic requirements of stage make-up. The television and film make-up is a restrained variation of a true eighteenth-century make-up. A contemporary audience would have difficulty relating to a heroine or hero wearing make-up that was historically accurate, as it would appear ugly and unsightly in the context of today.

Area of application	Theatre	Television and film
Base	Slightly off-white base	Foundation slightly paler than natural skin tone
Powder	White powder	Transparent (no colour)
Eyebrows	Eyebrows blocked out and redrawn so long, thin, rounded and raised	Eyebrows neatly groomed; filled in where appropriate
Eye make-up	Eye shadow (blue, dark at the lashes, fading up to the brow bone); theatrical eye lines and mascara	Neutral eye shadow applied to contour and flatter the eye shape; eye lines not necessary; mascara
Cheeks	Blusher – low and round in red or bright pink	Soft-red or pink-coloured blusher applied on the apple of the cheek
Lips	Red bee-stung shape	Red lipstick applied in natural shape
Other	Patches (beauty spots) – black and prominent in a heart, diamond or round shape	Patches (beauty spots) applied, but keep subtle

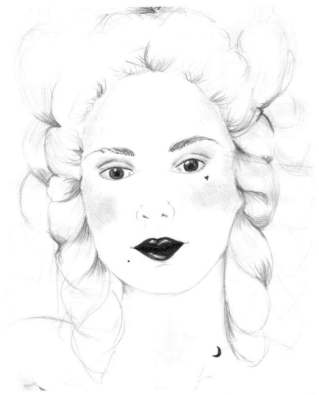

Eighteenth-century make-up design sheet by Fern Raymond

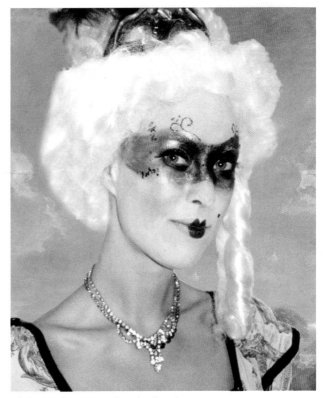

Eighteenth-century inspired make-up

Cleopatra

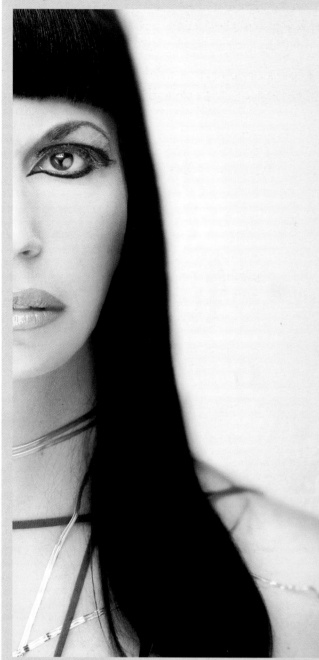

A Cleopatra-inspired make-up

1 For authenticity, the skin tone should be medium yellow brown to dark brown, so a change in skin colour may be necessary. Remember to blend the base well and take the colour to just below the costume line.

2 Apply concealer as required.

3 Contour the face to strongly define the features. Place highlight on the tops of the cheekbone and along the bridge of the nose. Place shading colour under the cheekbones, along the sides of the nose, from the tip carrying up towards the inner corner of the eyebrow and across to shade the area above the eye socket to the eyebrow.

4 Powder using a dark or orange-toned powder.

5 Darken the eyebrows to give them a strong shape that suits your model. Extend the outer edge, tapering as you go.

6 Apply eye shadow to the eyelids in peacock green or blue, extending the colour up into and just above the socket. Add a gold highlight in the centre of the lid above the lashes.

7 Apply black eye liner around the entire eye, extending it at the outer edge. Keep as close to the lash line as possible.

8 Add black mascara. You may curl the lashes first if you wish.

9 Apply lipstick – shades of orange-red, topaz or copper work well. Make sure you make full use of the lip area and make the lips look as full as possible. Add a gold highlight to the centre of the lower lip.

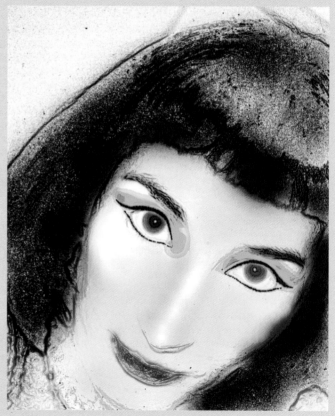

Design sheet for Cleopatra make-up by Julia Conway

STEP-BY-STEP Ballet and dance

Classical ballet make-up traditionally consists of pale skin tones and blue eye shadow for female performers, though dance in general tends to be less restrictive. Most dancers perform on stage, so the make-up is a variation of stage make-up, and is strong both in colour and application. Showgirl make-up is particularly striking and includes lots of lip gloss, heavy false lashes and sparkle.

1 Block out the eyebrows from the highest point outwards.
2 Apply a pale base all over the face, blending down to cover the neck and shoulders.
3 Powder generously. Dust off excess.
4 Fill in fairly dark eyebrows starting at the inner corners, extending outwards and upwards and tapering to a fine point.
5 Apply a light blue eye shadow across the entire eye area.
6 Define the socket with dark blue eye shadow, sweeping outwards at the outer corner.
7 Apply a pearlised highlighter to the brow bone.
8 Apply black liquid eyeliner across the entire top lid. Extend the eyeliner upwards past the outer corner of the eye to create a dramatic upswept line that tapers to a point.
9 Apply black liquid liner to the bottom lashes. Start approximately one-third in from the inner corner of the eye and extend the line under the lashes in a straight line and outwards, keeping parallel with the top liner.
10 Apply a highlighting colour between the eye lines on the outer corner of the eye.
11 Apply mascara and false lashes of your choice.

12 Apply strong blush to the cheekbones.
13 Apply a strong, bright-coloured lipstick.

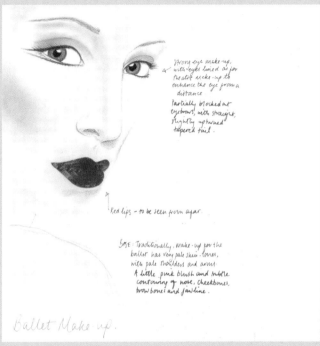

Design sheet for ballet make-up by Louisa Morgan

Knowledge Check

1 Give an example of an instinctive response to appearance.

2 Give an example of a learned response to appearance.

3 List four commonly accepted traits of the beautiful human face.

4 Discuss the use of stereotypes in the process of characterisation.

5 Why may it be important for the make-up artist to modify the realism of a characterisation?

6 List five considerations when ageing a performer.

7 Describe the procedure for using old age stipple.

8 When ageing a black performer should predominately highlight or shader be used?

9 List three characteristics of the black facial structure.

10 Discuss the differences between male and female facial structure.

CHAPTER 15

Looking back: the history of make-up and hairstyling

This is a huge subject area, which is impossible to cover in sufficient detail in a book of this nature. However, there are a number of books that specifically deal with the history of fashion and a reading list is included at the end of this chapter.

Instead, this chapter aims to give you an overview of the major trends in the development of hair and make-up design during the 20th century. Where it is relevant, references are listed that may be useful when sourcing visual material. These include fashion photographers, iconic figures and films set in each decade.

The information in this chapter should be regarded as a starting point to carrying out further research of your own. Research techniques are described in detail in Chapter 6.

Aim and objectives

Aim of this chapter: to provide you with the knowledge to enable you to research the history of make-up and hair design.

You should achieve the following **objectives:**

* Research the influential areas of art and design movements for each time period
* Research iconic figures of each time period
* Research images of hair and make-up for each time period using a variety of sources, for example books, films, internet, television, art
* Recreate make-up and hair designs for a number of time periods using techniques described in other chapters.

Roman Britain and Early Christian period

↓

Middle Ages (Medieval) (1200s to 1400s)

↓

Sixteenth century (1500s) *including*
Tudor period
Renaissance period
Henry VII's reign
Henry VIII's reign
Elizabeth I's reign

↓

Seventeenth century (1600s) *including*
Stuart period
Restoration period (late seventeenth century)

↓

Eighteenth century (1700s) *including*
Hanoverian period
French Revolution
Industrial Revolution

↓

Georgian / Regency period (early to mid
nineteenth century, 1811–37)

↓

Victorian age (mid to late nineteenth century,
1837–1901)

↓

Edwardian age (1901–14)

↓

Early twentieth century (1914–29), 1930s, 1940s,
1950s, 1960s, 1970s, 1980s, 1990s

Timeline of British history

KEY NOTE

The period from the accession of Queen Victoria to the outbreak of the First World War is often referred to as the Age of Empire because of Britain's expanding colonies around the world.

Recreating historical make-up and hairstyles for television and film

In most situations, recreating a historical make-up or hairstyle for a period production will require some adaptation. Many of the make-up and hair styles you will come across in your research may have been fashionable and considered desirable at the time, but to a contemporary audience they will appear unsightly, even absurd. It is therefore necessary to adapt the historically correct make-up into one that will appeal to the audience.

Interpretations of period make-ups will also be influenced by fashion trends that are around during the making of the production. A good example of this is the film *Cleopatra*, made in 1963 and starring Elizabeth Taylor. The portrayal of Cleopatra's make-up and hairstyles shows obvious influences of fashion trends that dominated the early 1960s and would have appealed to an audience of this era.

Make-up and hair designers have interpreted extreme periods of make-up in history, such as the eighteenth century or the 1920s, to appeal to their audience. Periods of history when make-up was not worn, such as the Victorian era, require the opposite approach. It would not be acceptable to send an actress or actor onto the set wearing no make-up at all. Make-up should therefore still be worn, but it should be applied in a minimal way that makes the performer appear completely natural. In these cases facial hair and hairstyles are often more useful in portraying a period look.

Occasionally a more historically accurate make-up may be applied to anti-hero characters with a view to gaining an unsympathetic response from the audience.

When designing the make-up for a period production it is important to remember the general principles of characterisation. Many of the fashion trends described in this chapter are applicable only to the wealthier members of society. The poorer classes may have worn much simpler costumes and hairstyles and may not have worn make-up at all. Likewise, the more mature members of society will not be wearing the most up-to-date fashions. It is therefore important to research each character thoroughly and to try to maintain a sense of individuality for each of the leading performers.

Extras can often be treated more generically.

In this chapter, we concentrate on the fashion and make-up trends of the 20th century. For more information about earlier historical periods, go to the Heinemann Make-Up Artistry website at www.heinemann.co.uk

Edwardian period (1901–14)

Art and design movements

* Fauvism (Matisse)
* Expressionism (Munch)
* Cubism (Picasso, Braque)
* Futurism (Carlo Carra).

Films set in the Edwardian period

* *Howard's End* (1992)
* *Titanic* (1997).

Iconic figures

* Camille Clifford
* Lillian Russell
* The 'Gibson Girls'

Trends in Edwardian hairstyling and make-up

Hairstyling

During the Edwardian period, women's hair was worn in a pompadour style consisting of waves backcombed and swept up over large pads of false hair to create fullness and width. The hairstyle was then decorated with a variety of finishes including combs, flowers and feathers. Women's hair played an important role in society status: when a young girl was considered ready for marriage, she would begin to wear her hair up. Long, loose hair was seen as a symbol of youth and innocence on young girls, yet on mature women, it was seen as a sign of promiscuity.

KEY NOTE

Elizabeth Arden opened her first salon in 1910 and went on to become head of the famous cosmetic chain.

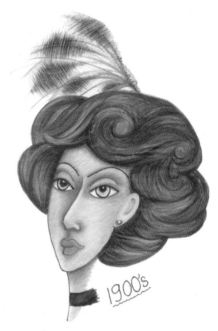

Design sheet for Edwardian era make-up by Kristin Tunley

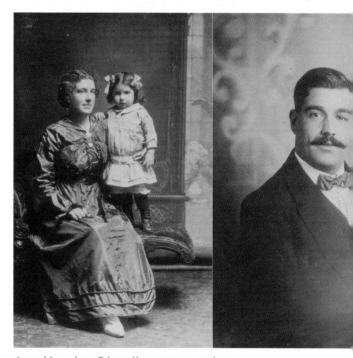

A working class Edwardian woman and man

Create an Edwardian hairstyle

Research pictures of Edwardian hairstyles. Choose one and 'break it down' so that you can recreate it accurately on a model using hairstyling techniques described in Chapter 12. Take a photograph of the finished hairstyle for your portfolio. Techniques you may need to use include:

* setting the hair in large rollers to create direction
* backcombing the hair
* using hair padding
* dressing the hair
* decorating the hair.

Make-up

Although make-up was slowly becoming more acceptable, the natural look was still fashionable. The emphasis on pale, matt complexions remained and cosmetics, such as liquid lighteners, were developed to enhance this effect. Rouge was returning to favour with the product 'Rouge de Théâtre' claiming this market. The popularity of face powder continued and products such as 'Papier Poudre' were used widely.

Early twentieth century, 1914–29

Art movements

* 1913–21 Constructivism
* 1916–22 Dadaism
* 1917–31 De Stijl
* 1919–33 Bauhaus
* Art Deco and Surrealism.

Fashion photographers

* Platt Lynes
* Cheney Johnston
* Madam d'Ora
* Man Ray.

Iconic figures

* Charlie Chaplin
* Clara Bow
* Louise Brooks
* Theda Bara
* Rudolph Valentino.

Films set in the 1920s

* *The Cotton Club* (1984)
* *The Great Gatsby* (2001)
* *Chicago* (2002).

Trends in hairstyling and make-up, 1914–29

Hairstyling

Following the popular androgynous look, young women cut off their hair into a short style.

* In the 1920s a short haircut called the 'bob' emerged.
* The bob of the early 1920s was abandoned for the shingle.
* In the late 1920s the Eton crop succeeded the shingle.
* Finger waves started to become popular.
* Fashionable men appeared clean-shaven at the beginning of the decade, and if moustaches were worn they were always clipped short. Men's hairstyles were worn short and close to the head, usually in a side parting.

KEY NOTE

During the First World War, an artistic elite dubbed the 'Bloomsbury set' revolutionised art, literature and dress. In keeping with their liberal views the fashions adopted by the set were exotic: rich fabrics, jewellery in elaborate metals, styles borrowed from the Far East, Byzantium and the European Middle Ages. Hair was soft and flattering, often worn in a loose Grecian bun or in loose, heavy waves. Pre-empting the shingle, hair was parted in the centre and swept into soft coils around the ears. The freedom of these Bohemian fashions paved the way for the 'roaring twenties'.

Area of application	Details
Base	Skin tones were still pale, though not whitened as in previous centuries.
Powder	Faces were thoroughly powdered; shiny noses were seen as vulgar.
Eyebrows	Eyebrows were plucked to become thin and round, but were kept long and were usually darkened.
Eye make-up	Eye make-up was soft and typically dark in colour – black, grey, blue, brown and plum was used. Colour was rubbed gently over the lid and blended into a delicate round shadow over the entire surface. Another faint line was drawn under the eyes and treated in the same way, but was even more shadowy and indistinct. Lashes were darkened.
Cheeks	Rouge became acceptable and positively fashionable in the mid- to late 1920s in natural shades of pink and peach. The desired effect was to give a natural flush to the face.
Lips	Lipstick followed the contour of the mouth, accentuating the curve of the upper lip but stopping short of the corners (bee-sting shape). Lipstick was bright and coral and pink in colour.
Other	Nail polish was created. Big cosmetic companies such as Yardley and Helena Rubenstein emerged. Eyelash curlers invented in 1923. Movie stars started to take on 'icon' status and began influencing fashion on the street; 'talkies' emerged at the end of the decade.

HANDS ON

Try to recreate a 1920s look on a model. Research pictures and photos from this decade, as these will be a valuable source of information.

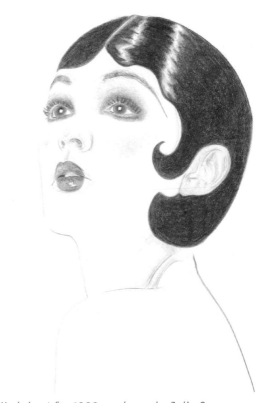

Worksheet for 1920s make-up by Julia Conway

Make-up

In the 1910s make-up was worn only by prostitutes, but by the late 1920s and early 1930s women's features were heavily made-up. From the late 1920s make-up was prepared using safe ingredients for the first time.

The 1930s

Art movements

* 1925–39 Art Deco influenced all aspects of design.

Fashion photographers

* P. Horst.

Iconic figures

* Greta Garbo
* Marlene Dietrich
* Clark Gable.

HANDS ON

Try to recreate a 1930s look on a model. Research pictures and photos from this decade, as these will be a valuable source of information.

Trends in 1930s hairstyling and make-up

Hairstyling

* Longer hair become fashionable again, worn close to the head.

Make-up

Area of application	Details
Base	More natural skin tones emerged for foundation.
Powder	The base was heavily powdered in natural shades.
Eyebrows	Eyebrows were long and narrow, but pencilled in for a more natural finish than the previous decade.
Eye make-up	Eye shadow was blended from the eyelids up to the eyebrows in subtle, smoky shades of blues, browns and dark greens. Lashes were heavily mascared.
Cheeks	Rouge or blusher was applied lower down under the cheekbones. Natural shades of pink were popular.
Lips	Lips were more natural in shape, with the mouth looking wider rather than smaller and the top lip taking on a more rounded appearance. Lipstick was still bright and was often in shades of red.
Other	Max Factor developed pan-cake, the first watered- soluble cake foundation. Plastic surgery emerged.

Sunbathing was now in fashion, and was reflected in more natural skin tones.
Nail varnish in both bright and dark colours was used.

* Finger waving, Marcelling and permanent waving were very fashionable.
* Bleached blonde hair was very popular.
* The men had short neat hairstyles and moustaches of different shapes, but no beards.

The 1940s

Art movements

* Abstract Expressionism.

Fashion photographers

* Cecil Beaton.

Iconic figures

* Lena Horne
* Veronica Lake
* Rita Hayworth
* Frank Sinatra
* Winston Churchill
* Vera Lynn.

Films set in the 1940s

* *Evita* (1997)
* *Tea With Mussolini* (1999).

Trends in 1940s hairstyling and make-up

Hairstyling

* Many women had shoulder-length to long hair dressed in a variety of pin-curled waves and rolls.
* Long hair had to be worn up and covered by women working in the factories so head scarves

tied on top became popular. Long hair was also pinned up away from the face and dressed in a 'victory roll'.

* Postiche hairpieces were used for styles requiring curls or chignons when dressing the hair.

* Men had short hair still, but cultivated waves in it using a comb and water.

* Men often wore moustaches.

* A photo of a wig dressed in a 1940s style can be seen in Chapter 13 (page 308).

Make-up

KEY NOTE

In the 1940s, because of rationing during the Second World War, less make-up was worn. The one readily available item was red lipstick, which continued to be produced as a morale booster for women. As a result, red lipstick has become a symbol of the 1940s.

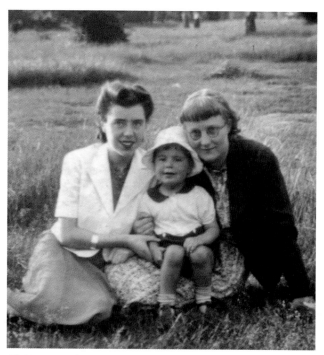

1940s portrait

Area of application	Details
Base	Foundation was more natural looking and sheerer in texture.
Powder	Powder was used less, but matt was still the preferred skin texture.
Eyebrows	Brows were natural and more angular, and darkened if required with pencil.
Eye make-up	Eye make-up was rarely used during the war period, but when available it could be found in shades of brown, bottle green and navy blue that were lighter than in previous decades. It was applied as a wash over the area, and lashes were darkened with mascara.
Cheeks	Cheeks had a natural-looking blush both in colour and placement.
Lips	Lips were red, and the top lip round in shape.

HANDS ON

Try to recreate a 1940s look on a model. Research pictures and photos from this decade, as these will be a valuable source of information.

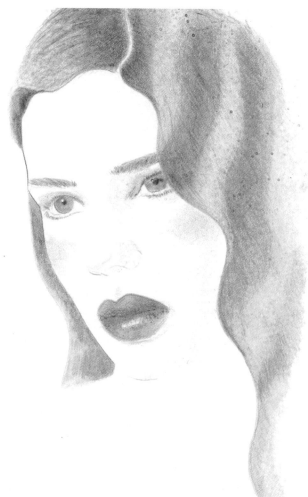

Design sheet for 1940s make-up by Julia Conway

The 1950s

Art movements

* Pop Art.

Fashion photographers

* Irving Penn
* Richard Avedon
* Clifford Coffin.

Iconic figures

* Marilyn Monroe
* Elizabeth Taylor
* Doris Day
* Brigitte Bardot
* Audrey Hepburn
* Grace Kelly
* Rock Hudson
* Cary Grant
* Elvis Presley
* James Dean.

Films set in the 1950s

* *Funny Face* (1957)
* *Grease* (1978)
* *LA Confidential* (1997)
* *The Talented Mr Ripley* (1999).

Trends in 1950s hairstyling and make-up

Hairstyling

* Elegant hairstyles were worn. Longer hair was often swept up in chignons and worn with short fringes.
* Hairstyles became shorter, fuller and curlier.
* Blonde was still a popular colour in US films and hairstyling fashions were strongly influenced by film stars.
* The men had shaven faces. Hair was worn short at the back and sides but left longer at the front and worn in a quiff or wave, like Elvis Presley. Crew cuts were also popular.

Make-up

Area of application	Details
Base	Skin tones varied from porcelain skin to sun-tanned complexions.
Powder	Complexions were still matt.
Eyebrows	Eyebrows were thick, shorter than in previous decades, arched, often darkened and precisely drawn.
Eye make-up	Colour became popular. Upper lids were shadowed up and out by blending browns in the socket line towards the brows. An obvious colour (often green or blue) was applied on the eyelids. Eyes were lined with pencil (thicker towards the outer corner) and extended at the outer corner as a small 'tick' in an upwards and outwards direction. Lashes were darkened and false eyelashes applied to the outer top corner.
Cheeks	Natural colours in pinks, peaches, etc. were brushed lightly over the cheekbone.
Lips	Lipstick gave lips a hard line in an array of colours. Liner was often used to outline the mouth.
Other	By the late 1950s many new make-ups contained 'guanine' which gave a shimmering lustre to the surface of the paints and powders. Fake tan for men, 'Man-Tan', was introduced onto the market. Pan-cake make-up was introduced and more than 10 million products were sold in 1953.

HANDS ON

Try to recreate a 1950s look on a model. Research pictures and photos from this decade, as these will be a valuable source of information.

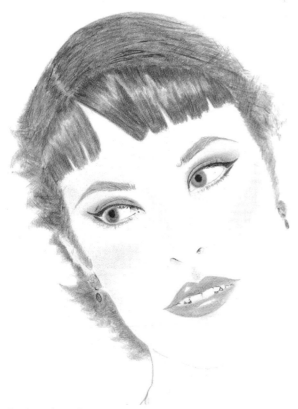

Design sheet for 1950's make-up by Julia Conway

The 1960s

Art movements

* Pop Art's popularity continued
* Op Art.

Fashion photographers

* David Bailey
* Hiro
* Snowdon
* Duffy
* Donovan.

Iconic figures

* Christine Keeler
* David Bailey
* Marianne Faithfull
* Jackie Kennedy
* Julie Christie

* Twiggy
* Mary Quant
* Jean Shrimpton
* Vidal Sassoon.

Films set in the 1960s

* *Alfie* (1966)
* *Austin Powers: International Man of Mystery* (1997)
* *The Doors* (1991)
* *Down with Love* (2003)
* *Catch Me if You Can* (2003).

Trends in 1960s hairstyling and make-up

Hairstyling

* The popularity of false hairpieces reached an all-time high in the 1960s.
* A style called the 'beehive' became popular, which was created by backcombing and padding the hair to create lots of height.
* Heavy fringes were popular, worn long and often covering the eyebrows.
* Twiggy made the short urchin cut popular.
* Straight, long hair was also popular accompanied by the heavy fringe.
* 'Hippies' wore their hair very long and deliberately unkempt-looking, often decorated with beads and flowers.
* Vidal Sassoon reinvented the bob.
* Men grew their hair long, and side burns, moustaches and beards were fashionable.

Make-up

Many looks came and went during the 1960s. The 'pale look' dominated the early sixties, but as the decade progressed, this was replaced by more and more adventurous make-up in colourful exotic designs. A face with child-like features was considered ideal, and make-up tried to create this with wide, heavily painted eyes and pale skin and lips.

Area of application	Details
Base	Pale to natural skin tones were lightly applied. Towards the end of the decade, young women would sometimes paint freckles onto their skin over the nose and cheeks. Complexions in the late 1960s were 'polished' and moist-looking with the aid of 'face gleamers'.
Powder	A light coating of powder created a natural, flattering texture.
Eyebrows	Eyebrows were neatly groomed, natural in colour and rounded in shape. Extra hairs were removed from the inner corners to create a wide-eyed effect.
Eye make-up	The upper lid was highlighted with a pale colour (white or aqua were good choices). The socket was shadowed with a darker shade, for example brown or charcoal grey, blended slightly upwards. A heavy black eye line extended over the corners of the eye, and a dash of white shadow in the corners created the look of a larger eye. The exotic look: during 1965 make-up became outrageous and bizarre, with inspiration coming from make-up artists such as Elizabeth Arden's Pablo.
Lashes	From the mid-1960s false lashes became hugely popular. As the decade progressed they got more and more wild and exotic.
Cheeks	Rouge was delicately brushed on the apple of the cheek to create a round, child-like face shape.
Lips	Lipsticks were predominantly pale in pinks, peaches and browns. The Cupid's bow was rounded off and the lips were gently curved to create a rose-bud shape.
Other	Fingernails were pale in 1964: tallow, ivory, tan, pearl and sometimes clear. Leg make-up became popular with the emergence of the mini-skirt. Face and body painting became very popular towards the end of the decade.

HANDS ON

Try to recreate a 1960s look on a model. Research pictures and photos from this decade, as these will be a valuable source of information.

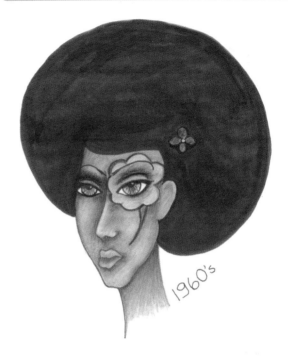

Design sheet for 1960s make-up by Kristin Tunley

The 1970s

Art movements

* Minimalism
* Conceptual Art.

Fashion photographers

* Guy Bourdin
* Helmut Newton.

Iconic figures

* Farrah Fawcett
* John Travolta in *Saturday Night Fever*
* Catherine Deneuve
* Woody Allen
* Joanna Lumley in *The New Avengers*
* Vivienne Westwood.

Films set in the 1970s

* *Saturday Night Fever* (1977)
* *Boogie Nights* (1997)
* *Shaft* (1971).

Trends in 1970s hairstyling and make-up

Hairstyling

* A wide range of styles were popular during this decade.

* Hair was still worn long and straight during the earlier 1970s.

* Perms became popular, particularly the stack perm. Crimping the hair was the alternative, less permanent option. Afro hair became huge.

* Red tints were applied to the hair with henna and highlights were first seen during this decade.

* Punks shaved parts of their hair and spiked the rest, creating a 'mohican', which they coloured with fluorescent dyes.

* The 'Charlie's Angels, Farrah Fawcett' hairstyle – big hair with lots of wave and huge flicks at the front – became highly popular in the late 1970s.

* Short hairstyles included the 'Purdey' cut, popularised by Joanna Lumley in The New Avengers.

* Layering the hair became fashionable. The 'Mullet' cut demonstrates this technique in its extreme.

* Men wore moustaches or sideboards and grew their hair long.

Make-up

Three specific looks dominated the 1970s:

* the disco craze, which led to the popularity of bright, iridescent colours

* the 'California Look' with golden suntans and polished make-up in tawny eye shades and glossy lips

* punk, representing the anarchic youth, with fluorescent-coloured hair standing on end and war paint applied to the face.

Area of application	Details
Base	Natural shades of foundation were used with the emphasis on contouring the face to show the bone structure. Pearlised highlighters were applied on the tops of the cheekbones. No base was used for punks as skin imperfections were part of the desired look.
Powder	Powder was used sparingly as the trend moved towards glossy, dewy textures.
Eyebrows	Eyebrows were thin and over-plucked, and medium to dark in colour.
Eye make-up	Eyes were usually heavily made up in a wide range of shimmery, frosted colours with a strongly highlighted brow bone. Popular colours included tawny shades; rose and plummy shades; earth tones – browns, greys and muted greens. For the evening, colours were frequently tinged with silver, copper or gold. Eye line was smudged for a softer look and lashes were darkened with mascara.
Cheeks	Soft shades of blusher popular at the beginning of the decade became increasingly stronger and brighter as the decade progressed.
Lips	Lips were outlined with pencils, filled in with matching colour and then covered with gloss. Colours were often dramatic: dark berry shades were popular.
Other	Safety pins, pierced faces and make-up applied in the style of war paint were all trademarks of the punk.

HANDS ON

Try to recreate a 1970s look on a model. Research pictures and photos from this decade, as these will be a valuable source of information.

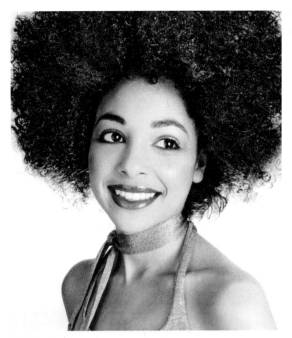

1970s make-up

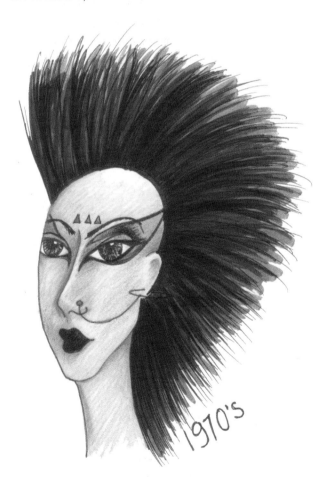

Design sheet for 1970s make-up by Kristin Tunley

The 1980s

Art movements

* Postmodernism
* Neue Wilde
* Figuration Libre.

Fashion photographers

* Patrick Demarchelier
* Herb Ritts
* Bruce Webber
* Steven Meisel.

Iconic figures

* Princess Diana
* Joan Collins (as Alexis Carrington in *Dynasty*)
* Margaret Thatcher
* Madonna
* Boy George
* George Michael.

Films set in the 1980s

* *Flashdance* (1983)
* *Desperately Seeking Susan* (1985)
* *The Wedding Singer* (1998).

Trends in 1980s hairstyling and make-up

Hairstyling

* Hair was big and often curly or backcombed and blow-dried into bouffanted hairstyles.
* Long hair was often dressed elaborately in braids, pleats and chignons decorated with large bows and slides.
* Also popular was hair that was short around the sides and back but left longer on top and either permed or gelled into spikes.
* The Gothics wore their hair black or bleached blonde with dark roots.

* Men's hair became short again, with 1950s hairstyles in fashion.

Make-up

Area of application	Details
Base	Natural-looking skin, often suntanned, was fashionable.
Powder	Matt skin was essential, so powder was applied.
Eyebrows	Influenced by Brooke Shields, eyebrows were left unplucked and very natural – the fuller the better.
Eye make-up	Three looks dominated the decade: * natural-looking eyebrows, soft colours and no hard lines around the eyes – grey, brown or olive green were popular colours * a dazzling array of colours: magenta, mauves and fuchsias, coppery reds, blues and oranges accented with blue, violet or green mascara; two or three colours including metallics might be used on the eyes, along with black or blue kohl eye liner applied on the inside rim of the eye * pale-faced gothic rockers with charcoal smudged eye sockets and bleached blonde or dyed black hair.
Lashes	Coloured mascara was popular.
Cheeks	Blushers ranging in colour from bronzed pink to soft apricot or coral, were applied across the cheekbone.
Lips	Lips might be in shades of pink, purple, bright red or red-orange. Sometimes lip liner was used in a slightly darker colour and left visible.
Other	In the mid-1980s the 'asymmetrical look' was in vogue. Various colours were applied to the eyelids, but not the same colours on both eyelids.

HANDS ON

Try to recreate a 1980s look on a model. Research pictures and photos from this decade, as these will be a valuable source of information.

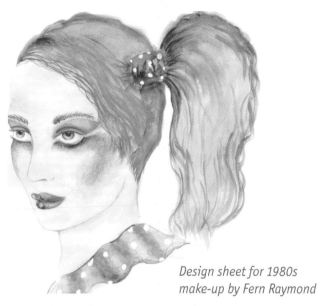

Design sheet for 1980s make-up by Fern Raymond

1990 to the present day

Individualism is the key word when describing the 1990s.

Art movements

* Installation Art
* Performance Art
* Digital Art.

Fashion photographers

* Corinne Day
* Nick Knight
* Elaine Constantine.

Iconic figures

* The Spice Girls
* Princess Diana
* Kate Moss
* David and Victoria Beckham
* Kylie Minogue
* Beyonce.

Trends in hairstyling and make-up, 1990 to the present day

Hairstyling

* The key to 1990s hair was simplicity. Hair was often worn long, flat and straight with a simple parting. It had to look healthy.

* Colouring techniques became increasingly advanced, with many brunettes choosing natural shades of red and mahogany. The severe bleached blonde look was out.

* Film star Meg Ryan influenced hairstyling by wearing a new short, choppy look with lots of texture and layers. The ideal look was feminine, but practical and easy to wear.

* Jennifer Aniston, from the popular series *Friends*, made the 'Rachel cut' very fashionable with its long layers.

* Men's hair was being worn shorter as the decade progressed. By the end of the 1990s, the hair was often shaved to a number 2 or 3. Facial hair was worn as 'goatie beards' (this look was epitomised by George Michael).

* The new millennium saw the popularity of hair extensions and a return to curlier hairstyles.

Make-up

On the whole, a natural, minimalist look based on neutral tones was fashionable for make-up and hair throughout the 1990s. Lips were stained in colours such as berry tones or soft reds that accentuated the natural lip tones. Matte was the key to the look.

However, during the latter part of the 1990s, perhaps in anticipation of the new millennium parties, sparkly, glittery and shiny make-up made a massive comeback. Matte was out; models on the catwalk announced the return of the glistening complexion with shimmering eye shadows, liquid blush that gave a flushed, stained look to the skin (often just placed on the apple of the cheek), and neutral lip colour smothered in gloss.

There was also an ethnic influence from the mid to late 1990s. Henna tattoos and mendhi designs painted on the hands and feet became a fashion accessory, introduced by the ever image-changing Madonna. Bindi jewels also became popular accessory items of the hip and trendy.

Area of application	Details
Base	Natural skin tones, with a very natural finish, were fashionable.
Powder	Powder and foundations were matt in the early to mid-1990s and dewy in the late 1990s, turning to positively shimmery for the new millennium.
Eyebrows	The popular look was for brows to look natural but groomed.
Eye make-up	Eye make-up was minimal throughout the 1990s, using soft neutral and earth shades. Matt in texture during the early to mid-1990s and shimmery in the late 1990s, a trend for stronger eye colour in metallics and glosses emerged in the new millennium.
Lashes	Natural colours were sometimes tipped with a colour. Aubergine-coloured mascara became a firm favourite with make-up artists.
Cheeks	Natural colours were placed on the apple of the cheek to give a flushed look. Liquid blush became popular during the latter part of the 1990s.
Lips	Large lips became fashionable. Mouths were made to look as large as possible. In the extreme, silicone or collagen injections gave a swollen look to the upper lip.
Other	Plastic surgery techniques continued to improve and society became obsessed with perfecting the appearance. The 'grunge' look with unmade-up faces and untidy hair became popular with young people in the early 1990s. Henna tattoos and bindis became a must-have fashion accessory in the late 1990s.

Try to recreate a 1990s look on a model. Research pictures and photos from this decade, as these will be a valuable source of information.

Reading list for further research

You may find the following sources useful when undertaking further research into the history of costume, make-up and hairstyling.

Fashion

Ewing, E. 1974. *History of 20th Century Fashion*. Batsford (looks at fashion and influences from the Edwardian era to 1970s)

Gernsheim, A. 1981. *Victorian and Edwardian Fashion: A Photographic Survey*. Dover (looks at changes in fashion as portrayed in photographs)

Kennett, F. 1983. *Collector's Book of 20th Century Fashion*. Granada (although aimed at collectors, this also looks at the social background and influences)

Laver, J. 1982. *Costume & Fashion: A Concise History*. Thames and Hudson (a comprehensive look at the development of costume and fashion from Egyptian to modern times)

Steeling, C. 2000. *Fashion: The Century of the Designer 1900–1999*. Konemann (considers designer fashion over the twentieth century, including the main influences)

Wilson, E. & Taylor, L. 1989. *Through the Looking Glass: A History of Dress from 1986*. BBC (outlines influences and fashionable trends from 1860 to 1990)

Make-up and hairstyling

Bryer, R. 2003. *The History of Hair*. Philip Wilson (a beautifully illustrated guide to the history of hairstyling)

Corson, R. 2001. *Fashions in Hair: The First Five Thousand Years*, 2nd edn. Peter Owen (the most comprehensive guide to the history of hairstyling – an invaluable resource for the make-up artist)

Corson, R. 2004. *Fashions in Make-up: From Ancient to Modern Times*, 3rd edn. Peter Owen (the most comprehensive guide to the history of make-up – an invaluable resource for the make-up artist)

Howell, P. & Erchak, G. M. 2004. *Hair: Untangling a Social History*. Frances Young Tang Teaching Museum

Mulvey, K. & Richards, M. 1998. *Decades of Beauty: The Changing Image of Women from 1890s to 1990s*. Octopus (an excellent guide to the history of costume, make-up and hairstyles that includes social and cultural influences)

Pacteau, F. 1994. *The Symptom of Beauty*. Reaktion Books (a psychoanalytic study of beauty)

Trasko, M. 1994. *Daring Do's: A History of Extraordinary Hair*. Flammarion

A large number of sites on the Internet cover the history of costume, make-up and hairstyling. Go to www.heinemann.co.uk/hotlinks and follow the links for some ideas.

Advanced techniques for the make-up artist

This chapter deals with techniques in which the make-up artist could become proficient after having mastered the basic skills required by industry. By developing and expanding their breadth of knowledge and application, make-up artists can increase their individual value to clients and ensure they are skilled for a wider variety of jobs and briefs.

Aim and objectives

Aim of this chapter: to provide you with the knowledge to enable you to:

* produce prosthetics to meet a design brief
* carry out cosmetic airbrushing.

You should achieve the following **objectives:**

* Produce a life cast safely
* Sculpt a prosthetic design
* Evaluate the different types of modelling materials available to the make-up artist
* Form a mould from a sculpture
* Cast the mould to form prosthetics
* Evaluate the different types of casting materials to make prosthetics
* Create a prosthetic using solid gelatine
* Use materials and perform procedures safely

* Discuss the purpose of multi-sections when creating overlapping prosthetic pieces
* Explain slush moulding and flat plate moulding
* List the requirements of a prosthetic portfolio
* List the advantages of airbrushing as an application technique
* Evaluate the specifications required of an airbrush and compressor for make-up application
* Evaluate the different types of products available for airbrushing
* Discuss the health and safety implications of airbrushing
* Discuss the importance and procedure of cleaning the airbrush
* Operate an independent double-action airbrush
* Control the airbrush to create a variety of marks
* Discuss masking techniques
* Create an airbrushed tattoo.

Producing prosthetics suitable for changing the appearance

The art of making prosthetics is wide-ranging and takes many years of experience to fully master. This section of the book will take you through the fundamental working procedures and will provide you with a foundation of knowledge that you can build on through experience and practice.

In order to make convincing prosthetics for make-up application it is important that you have an understanding of the anatomy of the head. This knowledge will enable you to produce prosthetic pieces that are realistic-looking and sit correctly on the natural contours of the face.

Refresh your knowledge of the anatomy of the head, neck and shoulders by re-reading the following sections in Chapter 4 'Anatomy and physiology for the make-up artist':

* Bones of the skull (page 46)
* Muscles of the head and neck (page 47).

Apart from knowing about structure and movement, it is also important to be aware of facial proportions. Again, refresh your knowledge by re-reading the following section on facial proportions in Chapter 5, 'Developing the artistic eye':

* Drawing the human head (page 80).

It is imperative that you have a complete understanding of all aspects of health and safety, which are discussed in Chapter 2, 'Health and safety', before embarking on the practical aspects of this chapter. Particular attention should be given to the sections regarding:

* legislation including Health and Safety at Work Act 1974, Personal Protective Equipment at Work Regulations 1992, Workplace (Health, Safety and Welfare) Regulations 1992
* insurance
* preparing the client.

Specific health and safety precautions relating to the production of prosthetics are discussed in this chapter.

Deciding to use prosthetics on a production means extra money, time and inconvenience for the performers. Therefore, it is a decision that should never be taken lightly. However, with the industry demanding nothing but near perfection from its make-up artists and the introduction of new technology, such as digital formats, a realistic-looking prosthesis is often the only viable option. Life casting (taking a three-dimensional, plaster impression of a model's features) is the first stage in the process of producing prosthetics.

Life casting

A life cast is a plaster copy of a model's face (or other body part) and is the basic building block for making prosthetics. It gives the make-up artist an accurate reproduction of the model's features and contours, ensuring the finished prosthetic piece fits the model it was designed for perfectly. It will involve you working confidently and accurately even under enormous pressure.

Life casting is straightforward and safe providing the make-up artist adopts professional working practices when carrying out the procedure.

The work area

It is preferable to have a separate area away from the main make-up studio for carrying out the procedures involved with making prosthetics. It is a wet and messy process, and because some of the materials are potentially harmful if breathed in, adequate ventilation is required.

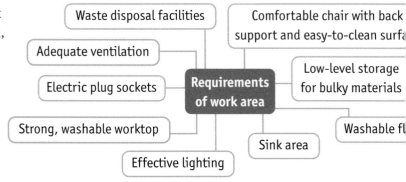

Before you begin the life casting session you should ensure all the materials you require are ready and set out in a logical way. You must never leave the model alone during a life casting session, so you will need to think about where to sit your model and then position your materials close to hand. The better you plan ahead, the more efficiently you will be able to work, ensuring the procedure is carried out smoothly and effectively. It is a good idea to make a checklist of all the materials you require and to prepare them before your model arrives.

Communicating with and caring for the life cast model

When the model arrives for a life casting session it is important that he or she feels comfortable and at ease. This can be achieved by the immediate work area and also by your manner towards the model. You must seem to be in control of the situation and confident of your own abilities if you are to instil confidence in the model. The life cast session may be the first time you meet the model and it is important to communicate well from the outset.

The model should be informed about each stage and its approximate timing – it may take up to 40 minutes to complete the life cast. The model should also be warned about the likely discomfort he or she may experience. Most models will have similar anxieties about the process.

helpless. Many of these anxieties will be alleviated by effective communication between the model and the make-up artist, both before and during the life casting procedure. The more you can prepare the model for the sensations he or she will experience, the less likely the model is to become distressed and panic during the procedure. Encourage your model to voice any concerns and try to alleviate these with clear explanations and reassurance. It is not enough to simply say 'don't worry about that'; you need to add a good reason why the model does not need to worry. For example, if a model is concerned about feeling trapped inside the cast, try to reassure the model by explaining *how* he or she can be released from the cast in the minimum time possible.

It is useful to work out a system of communication with your model that will enable your model to communicate whilst his or her head is covered in the alginate and plaster bandages. Try to keep it simple, for example a thumbs up for 'OK', a thumbs down for 'not OK' and a wave of both hands for 'get me out of here'. You should talk your model through each of the stages as you carry them out, and continually ask if everything is satisfactory for the model.

When you are ready to begin, the client should sit in a comfortable chair with a sturdy back and headrest (remove the headrest if you are carrying out a full head cast).

I may feel 'trapped' inside the cast

Will I panic?

Will I be cut off from my immediate surroundings?

Common concerns of a model undergoing a life cast

Will I have difficulty breathing?

Will I become claustrophobic?

Remember, the senses suddenly become diminished under the alginate and plaster bandages and the model may feel vulnerable and

KEY NOTE

In addition to the usual contra-indications (discussed in Chapter 2, page 29), specific contra-indications to life casting include:

* models who are known to suffer from claustrophobia
* models who have difficulty breathing through their nose (sessions with models who have a head cold should be postponed).

Sectional life casting

Before you begin, you will need to decide what part of the model you need to take a life cast of.

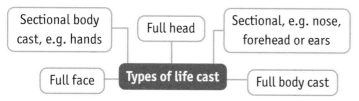

Sometimes, only a section of the face is required; this is very often the nose. Rather than taking a full facial cast, it is preferable to take an impression just of the required feature. This is cost-effective, less time consuming and more convenient for the model.

> **KEY NOTE**
>
> Having a life cast taken of your face or head is a unique experience. It is difficult to understand the sensations and emotions that may be felt by the model without having gone through the process yourself. If you intend to perform life casting on others, it is important that you experience the process for yourself.

Producing an original life cast

Equipment and materials

Below is a list of equipment you will need to produce a life cast:

* plastic sheet to cover model
* bald cap
* water-soluble marker pen
* petroleum jelly
* two containers for water (one for alginate, one for plaster bandages)
* alginate
* scissors
* plaster bandage (approx. three rolls)
* two flexible rubber bowls (one for alginate, one for plaster bandages)
* a blunt knife (such as a butter knife)
* duct tape (optional)
* denture adhesive (optional)
* small amount of modelling clay (optional)
* low-expansion plaster (approx 500 g for a facial cast and 1000 g for a full head cast)
* mixing equipment (electric hand mixer)
* plaster brush
* plaster tool
* plaster rasp
* glass or sand paper
* scrim (optional).

Alginate

Alginate is the material which is spread over the model's face to make a life cast. It is a powder derived from seaweed that becomes a paste when mixed with water and then sets into a solid, flexible material. Being temperature sensitive, the temperature of the water will determine how fast the alginate sets: the warmer the water, the faster it sets. The consistency of the paste is determined by how much water is added to the mix.

Many types of alginate are available. Dentists use a type that is very fast setting even when used with very cold water. However, this type would not give the make-up artist enough working time (i.e. the time between mixing the alginate into a workable paste and it setting into a solid, flexible material) to cover the model's face or body. Several manufacturers make 'prosthetic grade alginates' that provide a good working time even when used with tepid water, which is far more pleasant for the model.

When you are using a brand of alginate for the first time, it is important to experiment with it *prior* to the life casting session. Try mixing different proportions of alginate and water at varying temperatures and make a note of the effect on its working time. You should aim for a working time of between four and ten minutes, with a thickness of paste that can be applied to the face smoothly. Keep a record of your findings for future reference.

Plaster bandages

As alginate is flexible, you will need to reinforce it with plaster bandages to provide support so the alginate mould retains its shape. Plaster bandages are rolls of gauze saturated with 'plaster of Paris', which are dipped into warm water, squeezed out and applied to the alginate, setting hard in about ten minutes. They are available in different widths, usually varying between 7 cm and 15 cm. For a head cast, you should find three to four rolls sufficient.

Scrim (burlap)

A light, open-texture material usually made of cotton or flax, scrim is used to add strength to and reinforce the mould to prevent cracks from appearing. The scrim is cut into small squares, but the size will depend on the size of the mould – large moulds require larger squares.

Low-expansion plaster

As they set, all plasters expand to some degree. However, a low-expansion plaster is best as it expands less and is unlikely to crack. If you intend to use the life cast to produce hot foam latex prosthetics, the plaster will also need to be very hard to withstand the temperature of the oven. If you do not intend to make hot foam latex pieces, a softer, more porous plaster can be used.

> **REMEMBER**
>
> * Never wash plaster off in the sink because it will set in the drains and block them.
> * Never allow plaster to come into contact with eyes or skin.

Preparing the work area

Most of the materials you require for the life casting session can be prepared before the model arrives. The exception is the water for the alginate, which needs to be a specific temperature so should be prepared just before use. Begin by measuring out the alginate powder (approximately 400 g for a full head cast) and place it in one of the rubber bowls (the flexibility of the rubber makes for easy cleaning, as the material can be 'popped' out and the bowl wiped clean).

Next, cut the plaster bandages to the required lengths and lay them out in the order that they will be used:

* plenty of 15 cm strips for the forehead, eyes, mouth, chin and neck
* several 10 cm strips for the bridge of the nose
* several longer strips, approximately 20 cm in length, for around the back of the head if doing a full head cast, or around the perimeter of the cast if doing a sectional cast.
* a few small pieces, approximately 3 cm in length, to go around the nostrils.

Arrange the materials within easy reach of the immediate work area so you have plenty of everything you need to hand.

Preparing the model

The model's skin should be cleansed, toned and lightly moisturised.

Alginate is a messy material that will permanently stick to cloth so it is important to protect the model's clothes from inevitable splashes. The best way to do this is to wrap a piece of polythene around the model (a large bin liner with a hole cut out for the head could be used).

Ensure the model is comfortable with the back supported in an *upright position* so the features are not distorted. Alginate sticks to hair, so if you are carrying out a full head cast, you will need to apply a bald cap to the model (see Chapter 10, for this procedure). There is no need to use a custom-made cap; a cheap latex one bought from a supplier will suffice. Ensure there are no major wrinkles in the cap, but do not pull the cap so tight that it distorts the facial features. Once the bald cap has been fitted, take a water-soluble marker pen and draw the model's hairline onto the bald cap. The outline will transfer onto the alginate and then onto the plaster, acting as a guide to where the natural hairline falls. This is useful when sculpting a prosthetic that needs to stop here. A *thin* layer of petroleum jelly should then be applied to the bald cap (avoiding the marker pen) to aid removal of the cast later. For a facial cast, it is usually sufficient to clip the hair back from the face and apply petroleum jelly to the front hairline.

Other facial hair will also need to be protected from the alginate. This is achieved with a little petroleum jelly wiped over the eyebrows, eyelashes (using a cotton-tip) and any other areas of facial hair. You may have to use quite a thick layer over dense areas such as moustaches and beards.

The model should be asked to avoid smiling during the process, and to keep as 'blank' an expression as possible with the eyes closed. The model should also be warned that the alginate may feel cold on contact with the skin to avoid a 'shocked' expression forming on the mould.

Mixing the alginate

You should only begin to mix the alginate when you are ready to apply it to the model. Fill one of the containers with tepid water and pour the water onto the powdered alginate, mixing with your hand as you go. Working as quickly as possible, continue to add water until the alginate becomes thick and creamy in consistency. Refer to your own notes and records comparing alginate consistency, temperature and working times.

Applying the alginate

Working quickly, apply the alginate to the model starting on the forehead. Scoop a handful of alginate and use two fingers to spread it; allow the alginate to run down and add more alginate, letting it run down. Push the alginate upwards into the inner corners of the eyes and spread it over the eyelids. This is one of the areas referred to as **undercuts**, which require extra attention to avoid trapping air bubbles.

Continue to add the alginate, working down the sides of the face. Take care around the ears (another undercut area) and ensure that the alginate remains a good thickness (anything less than a centimetre is too thin). Thin areas may rip upon removal of the cast. Move onto the mouth, chin and neck, leaving the nose area until last. Push the alginate into the corners of the mouth and under the lower lip to get rid of any air bubbles (these are also undercut areas). The chin and neck area can be tricky because the alginate tends to fall from under the chin as you work. If this happens, simply spread the alginate back under the chin. The jaw line and chin are other areas of undercuts, so take time to ensure the alginate 'grabs' the contours beneath it, preventing air bubbles from forming.

If you are carrying out a full head cast, move to the back of the head. Begin at the top and work downwards in a similar manner.

The nose is the last area to be covered. Start at the bridge of the nose and work downwards. Clean your fingers of excess alginate and ask the model to take a deep breadth and hold it whilst you work around the nostrils. Work carefully but swiftly, ensuring alginate does not block the airways. The nostrils are another area of undercut so make sure you press the alginate into the crevices around the nostrils. When the area is covered, ask the model to blow hard through the nostrils to clear any excess alginate.

Throughout the application of alginate, communicate continuously with your model, checking they are happy with everything. Once you have finished, inspect the cast to make sure you have not missed any areas or created any thin spots. If you spot any problem areas, take steps to rectify them.

To complete this step, squares of damp scrim should be pressed into the wet alginate on the forehead and chin areas. This will ensure the plaster bandages, which are applied in the next step, adhere to the alginate and do not separate from it when removed from the model. If they were to become separated it would be difficult to replace the alginate mould in its original and correct position. This would cause distortion in the final life cast.

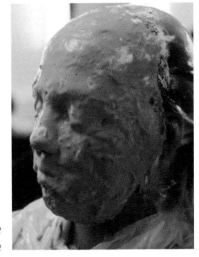

Applying the alginate

KEY NOTE

Removing the alginate in an emergency

The most important aspect of life casting is safety. If you find you have nearly finished the casting process, but your subject begins to show signs of distress or difficulty breathing, do not hesitate to destroy your work in favour of the model's safety and well being.

In an emergency, the alginate should be removed swiftly. Begin with the mouth and eyes as this should quickly alleviate any feelings of claustrophobia and panic on the part of the model. It is important that you remain calm and in control of any given situation. If the model continues to show signs of distress once the cast materials have been removed, a qualified first-aider should be called to provide assistance.

Casing the alginate with plaster bandages

Once you have completed the alginate cast, you need to add support and protection in the form of a casing made from the plaster bandages. You should already have a selection of plaster bandages, cut to various sizes, within easy reach. Fill the remaining bowl with warm to hot water (this will help the plaster to set quickly) and begin by dipping a 15 cm strip into the water. Squeeze out any excess water by holding the bandage at the top with one hand (over the bowl) and running the bandage between the index and middle finger of the other hand.

Starting at the forehead, place the bandage on the alginate and press firmly so it clings tightly to the contours of the alginate. Continue to work downwards, using the 10cm strips for the bridge of the nose. Take special care when placing the small 3cm strips between, under and around the nostrils. It is important to strengthen this area as it is particularly susceptible to damage and distortion. Remember to leave the nostril holes free to allow the model to breathe freely through the nose. The bandages should be placed so they overlap each other slightly. At least three layers of bandages are required to ensure the casing will hold its shape.

The casing is completed as follows.

* **For a facial or sectional cast:** When you have covered the alginate, go around the perimeter of the cast with a longer strip of bandage rolled up into the shape of a rope. This will give the cast extra strength and rigidity.

* **For a full head cast:** Complete the front half of the cast, making sure you go back no further than the ears and the top of the head. Wait for this to set and then apply a generous amount of petroleum jelly over the back edge of the plaster bandages. This is where the back half will overlap the front, allowing the casing to be separated at removal. Apply the back half just like the front, overlapping the front half of the casing where the petroleum jelly was applied. Take care to keep the back half away from any part of the front half that is not covered in petroleum jelly.

Allow the plaster to completely set (you should be able to press a finger against the plaster without leaving an indentation). This may take up to ten minutes. Do not forget to keep talking to your model, checking he or she is happy and giving regular updates on timing. The airways should be constantly monitored and kept clear.

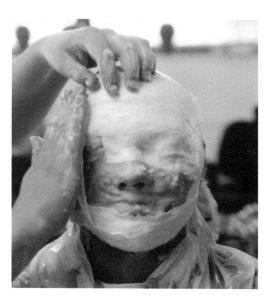

Applying plaster bandages

Removing the cast

When the plaster bandages are hard you can remove the cast from the model.

Facial or sectional cast

Begin by asking the model to bend forward whilst holding the front of the cast. Next, ask the model to wrinkle up his or her face to release the suction. Run your finger under the alginate and work your way around the cast. Lift the cast away without pulling at it, taking care to keep the alginate in place within the plaster bandage casing. If the alginate has come loose anywhere on the cast, you can use denture adhesive to stick it back in place. As alginate dries out, it shrinks causing distortion to the mould. It is therefore necessary to slow down the drying out process by placing moistened tissues or paper towels across the mould.

Full head cast

Draw a guideline across the two halves of the cast, to assist you when fitting them back together again. Lift off the back half of the plaster bandage casing and set it to one side. A slit now needs to be made in the back of the alginate mould so that it can be removed. Take a blunt knife in your working hand and slide your other hand between the alginate mould and the model's head. Even though the knife should be blunt, great care is still required to ensure you do not hurt your model. Continue to slice the mould in a single cut up towards the top of the head, working the back section loose as you go. Next, ask the model to hold the front of the cast and bend forward. Ask the model to wrinkle up his or her face to release the suction. Carefully work the mould off the model's head, taking care to keep the alginate in place within the front plaster bandage casing. Once the mould is clear of the head, the back of the plaster bandage casing is refitted over the alginate. Carefully adjust the alginate from the inside with your hand so that the cut is closed back together again. You should be able to see the transferred marker pen line outlining the natural hairline. Retrace the line to ensure it will be transferred onto the plaster cast during the next stage of the process. The two halves of the mould should now be secured together by wrapping more plaster bandages or duct tape around the neck area. Place moistened tissues or paper towels inside the mould until you are ready to cast it.

This alginate mould is referred to as the **negative** mould.

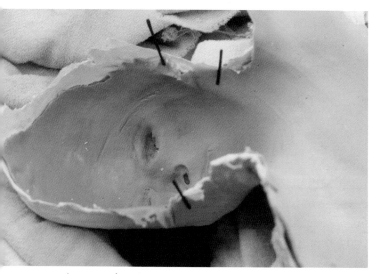

A removed cast

Inspect the mould. Minor imperfections such as a few small air bubbles are an inevitable part of the process, but any large distortions where the model's features are lost may mean you have to recast the model. Ensure you make notes recording the details of the session and evaluating the outcome for future reference.

Cleaning up the model

The model's skin should be restored to its original condition. A basic cleanse and tone should remove any residue left from the alginate. The skin can then be moisturised. If a full head cast was performed, the bald cap will need removing (see Chapter 10 for the procedure). Any contra-actions should be noted for future reference.

Alternative life casting materials

Life casting with silicone rather than alginate has been around for a while. However, it is still relatively unpopular with make-up artists, mainly because of the additional cost of the materials. The main drawback of alginate as a moulding medium is its weight: when applied to the skin it can sometimes drag the contours of the face (this is more evident when casting a mature skin). One advantage of silicone is that because less material is applied to the face (an application half a centimetre thick is sufficient), there is less distortion of the skin and features. Another advantage is that you can reuse a silicone mould time and time again as it does not shrink or distort, making it ideal for producing multiple casts. Silicone does not feel cold on application so it is more comfortable for the models and prevents 'goosing' of the skin, which can leave an impression on body life casts.

Preparation of the model is much the same as for traditional alginate life casting. The main difference is that silicone 'grabs' the skin a lot more than alginate. To counteract this, a rich moisturising cream should be applied over the skin and bald cap, and particular care should be taken with hairy or delicate areas such as around the eyes. Just as with alginate, scrim can be added to the silicone before it sets to add strength and aid adhesion of the plaster bandages. Because the application of silicone is thinner than alginate, there is less cushioning between the model's skin and the plaster bandage casing. Therefore extra care must be taken when removing the cast to ensure the model's skin is not bruised.

Casting the alginate mould

Now that you have a mould of the model's features you will need to produce a permanent plaster cast impression. This is referred to as the **positive** mould.

It is important you understand the difference between 'positive' and 'negative' moulds. Basically they are opposites of each other. When you perform a head life cast, the model's actual head is the **positive** and the alginate mould is its **negative** impression. When you make a permanent plaster cast from the alginate mould, you are creating another **positive**.

If you are to produce prosthetics of excellent quality that fit the model perfectly and have easy to conceal edges, the positive mould has to be first-rate.

You will need to support the mould as you work. A towel rolled into a sausage shape and placed inside a large container to create a 'nest' is a useful way to support facial and sectional casts. Place the cast, plaster bandage side down, so it is supported by the towel. On the underside, the nose should not touch the bottom of the container: once the cast is filled with plaster, the extra weight may push the cast down damaging the delicate nose area. Full head casts should be placed in a large bucket padded out with newspaper.

To begin with, it is necessary to plug the nostrils to prevent the plaster from leaking out of the mould. This can be achieved in several ways:

* with a small amount of modelling clay
* with a little alginate (mixed with warm water to set fast)
* with a single, small strip of plaster bandage.

Ensure the plugs do not protrude inside the cast. Whatever method you choose, work gently to avoid damaging this delicate area.

> **KEY NOTE**
>
> You should not inhale plaster dust as it is bad for your health. Always wear a facemask to protect yourself when working with plaster. If you are employed, your employer should provide you with adequate protection under the Personal Protective Equipment at Work Regulations 1992.

Scoop the required amount of plaster into the flexible, rubber mixing bowl (for large quantities of plaster you may need to use a large container). Then mix the plaster following the manufacturer's instructions. This usually involves sprinkling the plaster powder onto the surface of the water, a handful at a time, and allowing the water to soak up the powder before adding the next handful. Continue in this fashion until the powder is no longer being absorbed and begins to settle just above the level of the water. You can then begin to mix the powdered water with your hand, removing any clumps, until the consistency resembles a smooth, runny paste. When you are happy with the consistency, bang the container on a hard surface to encourage any air bubbles to rise to the surface. These can then be 'popped' by gently blowing on them.

The next step is to paint (using the plaster brush) an even coat of plaster onto the surface of the alginate mould, making sure you catch all the detail. This will help to prevent air bubbles from forming on the surface. This is referred to as the **splash coat**. As the plaster begins to set, build up this layer to an even thickness of about 1 cm. The remaining plaster in the mixing bowl should be fairly thick now and is suitable for applying to the cast as a finishing coat.

Continue to work the finishing coat until the plaster has almost completely set, smoothing the surface as much as possible and keeping the sides square. The cast should be approximately 2.5 cm thick all over and resemble the illustration on the right.

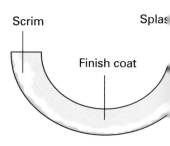

Layers of the plaster cast

Once the plaster cast has completely set, it can be removed from the mould. Turn the cast over so the plaster bandages are facing upwards. Peel off the bandages first, then peel off the alginate to reveal the life cast beneath. You should be able to see the transferred marker pen, indicating the natural hairline of the model. You can now dispose of the alginate mould and plaster bandage casing as they cannot be reused.

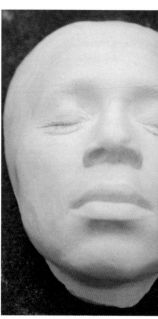

A positive life cast

> **KEY NOTE**
>
> **Strengthening the plaster life cast with scrim (burlap)**
>
> If you intend to create hot latex foam prosthetics from your life cast, then it is a good idea to add an additional layer of scrim between the splash coat and the finishing coat. This will hold your life cast together should a crack appear during the baking process. Take one of the squares of damp scrim that you prepared earlier and dip it into the plaster. Remove any excess plaster and place the scrim onto the splash coat, gently smoothing over the contours beneath to carefully remove any air bubbles. Cover the entire surface of the splash coat with one layer of scrim.

Correcting imperfections

Your life cast may have imperfections as a result of one or more of the following.

Imperfection	Cause	Action
The life cast is distorted.	The alginate shifted in the plaster bandage casing.	If the distortion is slight it may not be a problem. However, marked distortions will require you to repeat the life cast procedure.
The life cast is covered in raised spots.	Air bubbles have formed.	Remove the raised areas by filing them down with a plaster tool. Take care not to over file, as this will create indentations on the life cast.
The life cast is pitted in areas.	Air bubbles have formed.	These will need to be filled in with fresh plaster. Before you can add new plaster to the life cast, you will need to soak the cast in water (for about half and hour) so the new plaster will adhere properly. Mix up a small amount of plaster to fill in the holes. Finish by smoothing off with glass paper.

The underside of the life cast can be smoothed off with a plaster rasp. An even surface means the life cast will lie flat on a worktop and not wobble whilst you are working on it.

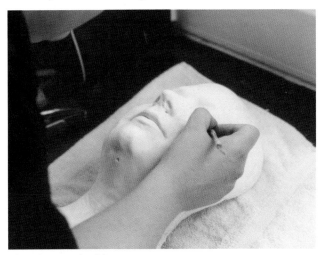

Cleaning up the life cast

Designing the prosthetic piece

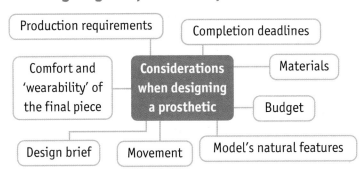

The design process of prosthetics will usually begin as a series of two-dimensional drawings that develop into a three-dimensional sculpture that is then cast into the final prosthetic piece.

Sculpting the prosthetic piece

The next stage in the production of prosthetics is to sculpt the prosthetic design onto the life cast, thereby altering the shape of the positive mould. You will need the following equipment:

* modelling material of your choice
* a selection of modelling tools
* Alcote (a dental mould release agent) or KY Lubricating Jelly.

Preparing the life cast for sculpting

The life cast should be covered with several thin coats of a material called **Alcote** (KY Lubricating Jelly can be used as an alternative). This creates a fine, invisible film over the surface that will allow you to remove the sculpted modelling material with ease later on by a process referred to as **floating off**.

Choosing the sculpting medium

Before you begin to sculpt your prosthetic piece, you will need to decide which medium you would prefer to work with.

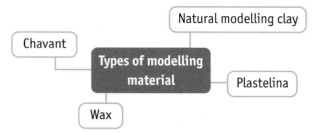

Each medium has advantages and disadvantages, but choice is down to individual preference.

* **Clay** is a natural material that maintains its working state by being kept continuously moist. It is very pliable and takes impressions of texture very well. The disadvantage is that it is constantly drying out and suffers shrinkage. When you are not working on the sculpture, it should be kept in a polythene bag with damp cloths. It is available in both firm and soft textures.

* **Plastelina** is a plastic modelling clay that will never harden, crust or deteriorate. It softens with the temperature of your hands. It tends to be less liable to accidental damage. This modelling medium is harder to work with but the advantage is that it does not require constant moisture. It is available in a variety of textures from soft to extra hard.

* **Wax** is sensitive to pressure and a good material for fine detail work: traditional recipes combined beeswax with turpentine, tallow or rosin in varying proportions for different degrees of hardness or malleability.

* **Chavant** is an oil-based versatile clay, which is non-drying. It shares many of the properties associated with plastelina and some of the modelling waxes.

Specialised sculpting tools are available for working with your chosen medium. These can be wooden, plastic or stainless steel and come in a variety of sizes and shapes. Do not forget your fingers – they are often the most useful tool of all.

Sculpting the design

Sculpting techniques vary enormously and there is no set technique, but you may wish to try the following to get you started.

1 Place the life cast on a solid surface so that you can work on it without it moving around.

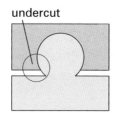
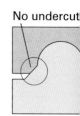

2 Begin by **blocking out** your design.
This refers to creating the basic structure and shape of your work. The clay can be rolled into strips and laid in place, forming the shape. Alternatively, pellets of clay can be built up into the desired shape. At this stage, it is important to check your work from all angles, and if necessary to check any important measurements you need to take account of. You should concentrate on the general shape rather than detail at this stage.

3 When your work is 'blocked out', the next step is to join the strips or pellets together, establishing the basic shape and form of the design. This is best done using a modelling tool.

4 At this stage you must check for **lock up**. This refers to areas of your sculpture getting caught when the mould section is being pulled apart from the sculpted life cast during the mould-casting stage of the procedure. These areas are called **under cuts** and must be eliminated by applying some modelling material to cover them. Check your sculpture carefully and try to imagine the mould section being pulled off: there must be no areas that could catch.

5 The edges of the sculpture (which in the final prosthetic will meet exposed skin) should be feathered out so they become very thin. This will ensure the edges of your prosthetic piece will become invisible when glued to the skin and covered in make-up.

6 Once you are happy with the shape of your sculpture and have checked that it meets with the design specification, you can begin to introduce texture to its surface. The most common way to apply texture is with textured pads. These are available in a variety of textures. You could also experiment with different textured surfaces, for example orange peel is excellent for creating the impression of skin texture.

Forming moulds from sculptures

Once you have completed the sculpture, you will need to produce its 'negative' mould (remember the sculpture is the positive element). Again, there are varying methods for creating moulds, one of which is suggested below.

Materials and equipment

To make the mould you will need to prepare the following materials:

* clay or other modelling medium
* low-expansion plaster
* plaster bandage
* petroleum jelly (or other release agent)
* plaster tools and brush
* key tool
* two flexible rubber mixing bowls
* clay board
* talc
* metal ruler
* acetone
* small bristle brush.

Creating the cutting edge

The first step to creating a mould is to create the **cutting edge**. This refers to applying a thickness of clay around the sculpture to create a cavity that will ensure the sculpture edges are kept thin. Roll out a piece of clay and cut several strips approximately 3 mm high and 6 mm wide. Place this strip to form a channel around the sculpture approximately half a centimetre from its edges. This channel acts as a drain for any overflow of casting material when the negative and positive sections are clamped together. The material which collects in the drain is referred to as the **flashing** on a prosthetic piece.

Using the key tool, you then put at least four **keys** (indentions) into the plaster – these will act as alignment keys, ensuring that the two halves of the mould (the positive and negative) fit together perfectly.

Building the retaining wall

The next step is to build a wall around the sculpture to create the mould height and shape. This is done with clay slabs. Dust the surface of the clay board with talc and roll out the clay to cover the board until it is approximately 1 cm thick. Use the metal ruler to even out the level of the clay. Cut a section from the clay, remembering to make it taller than the highest point of the sculpture (by about 3 cm), and place it in position approximately 2 cm away from the cutting edge. When the clay wall completely encases the sculpture, wrap a few strips of wet plaster bandage around the entire circumference to support the wall.

Sealing the sculpture

Once the clay walls have been built, you will need to seal all the surfaces within the wall (i.e. over the plaster, the sculpture and the inside of the walls) with a mould release. Petroleum jelly or soapy water work well, but there are a number of alternatives on the market. This mould release will ensure the easy separation of the negative and positive sections of the mould once the casting process has been completed.

Mixing the plaster and filling the mould

Mix the plaster as before (enough to fill the mould). Apply a splash coat using a plaster brush, making sure you cover all the detail on the surface and avoid forming air bubbles. Once this layer is complete, continue to pour the plaster over the sculpture, banging the work surface as you pour to release any trapped air. Continue until you reach the top of the clay walls. Disperse any air bubbles that form on the surface by blowing at them.

Once the plaster has completely set, remove the plaster bandages, then the clay wall. Providing you eliminated all the undercuts you should be able to separate the two halves of the mould fairly easily, using a modelling tool to prise them apart. If there is resistance you may wish to try soaking the mould in water for approximately twenty minutes before trying again.

Once the two sections of the mould are separated, remove the clay and clean the surface thoroughly with a little acetone on a small bristle brush. You can now tidy up the mould by smoothing off any rough edges and correcting any small imperfections.

The mould should now be allowed to dry out completely before you move onto the final stage of producing prosthetics. This may take a couple of days. You should now have a positive cast and a negative mould from which you can produce prosthetics in the casting material of your choice.

> **KEY NOTE**
>
> If you wish, scrim can be added on top of the splash coat to give the mould extra strength and durability.

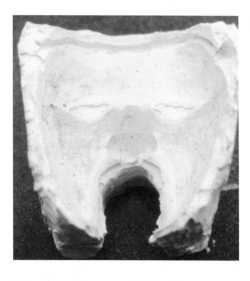

A prosthetic negative mould

Casting the mould to form prosthetics

This is the final stage in the production of prosthetics. The first step is to decide which type of material you are going to use to make your prosthetic from.

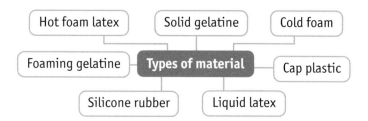

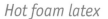

Cold foam

Cold foam is a polyurethane foam system. It is very soft, and is useful for small prosthetic pieces such as ears and noses. It is known as cold foam because it cures without having to bake or be heated. It expands right away; once you mix the parts you have between 45 and 90 seconds to work. Kits and components are available and should be used according to the manufacturer's instructions.

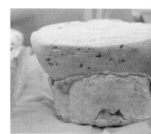

Cold foaming

Hot foam latex

Hot foam latex produces superior quality prosthetics with greater elasticity. However, it is more expensive and the process is much slower and harder to master. The fine cell structure makes for invisible blending of the edges into the face.

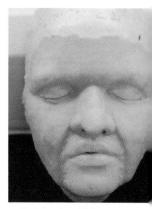

A finished cold foam piece

Most hot foam latex systems consist of four or five parts, which have to be precisely measured out before mixing and baking. The baking foam gives off by-products that will make the oven smell unpleasant so it is best to invest in a technical oven rather than use the one you cook in. The baking time depends on the thickness of the prosthetic piece, the thickness and type of mould, and the temperature of the oven.

The timings involved in the process (which is basically getting the foam to gel) can be difficult to get right, as the products are sensitive to room temperature and humidity: they are also affected by the amount and the speed of your mixing. It is therefore strongly advisable that you make notes and keep a record of your experiments with each new kit that you use. You will find these invaluable; they will prevent you from repeating mistakes and will ensure successes are not one offs!

The kits will contain:

* latex base
* foam agent
* cure agent
* gel agent
* releasing agent (usually soap based).

In addition, you will require an accurate set of scales, a stop watch, an electric mixer and bowl, and a foam injection gun (if unavailable, a spoon can be used instead).

Most kits work in the same way.

1 Begin by applying the mould release to each section of your mould, so the foam piece can be removed easily.

2 Measure out the ingredients precisely according to the manufacturer's instructions.

3 Mix the foam according to the manufacturer's instructions. You may have to adjust the mixing times if the mixer you are using is different from the one used in the instructions.

4 Once the foam is mixed, add the gel agent.

5 Working quickly, add the foam to the mould using an injection gun to reduce the risk of air bubbles forming. The gun gives you precise control over the placement of the foam, ensuring it fills all the detail of the mould. Once filled, the mould should be closed tightly (the tighter it is closed, the thinner the edges).

6 Once the foam has set, bake it in an oven (follow the manufacturer's guidelines, but be prepared for variations).

7 Take the mould out of the oven and allow it to cool before removing the prosthetic piece.

8 Trim the prosthetic and check for surface imperfections. Inspect the piece for large air bubbles trapped within the foam by holding it up to the light. If any are present, you may have to discard the piece and try again.

9 If you are happy with the piece, powder well.

REMEMBER

Some of the ingredients used to produce foam latex pieces can be very harmful. Please ensure you check the Safety Data Sheets supplied with the products and follow all recommended precautions.

Silicone rubber

Silicone rubbers can provide aesthetic qualities superior to those of foam latex or gelatine. They can capture the translucency and movement of human skin, creating realistic looking prosthetics in the most demanding of situations. Many types are available from many different manufacturers. The type most commonly used in mould making contains the **encapsulator** (a thin silicone membrane) and the **silicone gel**, weighed in the ratio 1:1, 2:1, etc. according to the manufacturer's instructions. Working and setting times vary depending on the brand of silicone. The silicone's softness and elasticity can be altered with the use of cosmetic grade silicone oils. Unlike gelatine, silicone will not melt under hot lights. Silicone can be cast in any kind of mould traditionally used for gelatine or foam latex.

KEY NOTE

* Do not use plaster with silicone unless it is primed and sealed first.
* Use plastelina as your modelling medium when casting or moulding with silicone as this will not rot it.

STEP-BY-STEP Producing prosthetics using solid gelatine

An old favourite, gelatine is cheap, easy to use and can be melted down and used again.

Ingredients
* 100 g sorbitol
* 20-30 g Gelatin 300 Bloom
* cosmetic grade pigments.
* 100 g glycerine
* 0.5 g zinc oxide (optional)

Remember that gelatine is a natural product and the quality can vary so slight alterations to the recipe might be needed.

1 Mix the dry products (gelatine, zinc and pigment) together. Assess the colour of the mix. If it is not correct, make adjustments to the pigments.

2 Mix the wet products (glycerine and sorbitol) together.

3 Mix the wet and dry mixes together and leave, preferably overnight.

4 Decant the mixture into a Pyrex jug and heat it gently in the microwave stirring every thirty seconds. The mixture should be ready after approximately two minutes. Do not allow the mixture to boil, because it will leave bubbles in your finished piece and destroy the gelatine fibres. The prepared mixture should be smooth.

5 Bang the jug onto the worktop to get rid of any bubbles that may have formed.

6 Pour the mixture carefully into the mould, letting it run down the side of the mould to reduce the chance of creating air bubbles. Fill the mould to about a quarter of its capacity.

7 Tilt the mould from side to side, coating the full surface and allowing any air bubbles to escape.

8 Gently press the positive cast into place.

9 Allow to cure.

10 Separate the sections, trying to keep the gelatine in the negative mould.

11 Remove the flashing, leaving a small edge, and powder the inside of your piece.

12 Removing your piece from the mould, powdering as you go.

KEY NOTE

If your moulds are large or complicated you can heat them to about 50-60 °C before putting the gelatine in. This will give you more working time before the gelatine starts to set.

KEY NOTE

When applying the gelatine piece to skin you must form a barrier between the gelatine and the skin or sweat will dissolve the piece. You could cover the back surface of the piece (avoiding the edges) with Pros-Aide. Dry and powder. Alternatively, an antiperspirant lotion can be applied to the skin on the areas where the prosthetic will sit.

Foaming sponge gelatine

A relatively new, alternative material to foam latex, foaming sponge gelatine is as easy to use but a fraction of the weight of solid gelatine. Foaming gelatine has chemical foamers that create a microcellular structure in the gelatine. This reduces the weight of the product by about 40 per cent, creating lightweight prosthetic appliances. Just as with solid gelatine, there are no hazardous ingredients or fumes. Kits are available that usually consist of two parts that are simply melted and mixed. They come with manufacturer's instructions.

KEY NOTE

Gelatine prosthetics should be stored in a polythene bag and kept in the refrigerator for longevity.

Below is a summary of the advantages and disadvantages of the different materials.

Material	Advantages	Disadvantages
Gelatine	Translucent Fast and easy to use Edges are easy to blend Completely safe (even edible) Can be melted down and re-used	Unstable – will melt under hot lights and when in contact with perspiration Does not move well Dries out Heavy Does not smell pleasant
Foaming gelatine	Translucent Fast and easy to use Edges are easy to blend Completely safe Lightweight Can be melted down and re-used	More delicate than solid gelatine (take care when removing from the mould) Dries out
Cold foam	Fast and easy to use	Only suitable for smaller pieces Can have crude edges Not suitable for close-up shots or fine casting
Hot foam latex	Light and flexible Adheres well to the skin Fine edges Stable – will not melt, etc. Durable	Ingredients are highly toxic and dangerous Expensive and time consuming Process is difficult to master and can be upset easily by variants in air temperature and humidity Timings have to be precise and will vary according to product batches Opaque finish
Silicone	Stable – will not melt, etc. Translucent Moves like skin Platinum silicone is safe as it does not give off by-products Waterproof Does not shrink Reusable	Expensive Heavy Process is difficult to master due to material sensitivity

REMEMBER

Always use medical or cosmetic grade materials and follow the manufacturer's instructions. If you are unsure of the potential hazards of a material, check the Safety Data Sheet.

Creating multi-sections for the application of overlapping prosthetics

Full-face prosthetic applications are best produced in sections for the following reasons:

* they are easier to apply
* they are more comfortable for the wearer
* they restrict movement less.

On application, these sections are overlapped so they merge with each other. When designing a full-face prosthetic piece, it is still preferable to work on a full-face cast to:

* allow you to see and judge the sculptured design in its entirety
* ensure symmetry and balance in the final prosthetic.

It is very important that you coat the surface of the face cast with Alcote or KY Lubrication Jelly before beginning to sculpt. Once you have finished sculpting the design, look at the sculpture to see how it would naturally divide into mould pieces. The most common way to divide a piece would be:

* the forehead
* the nose and upper lip
* each side of the face
* the jaw line and neck.

You will need to make sectional moulds and cast plaster positives for each of these areas.

Use a knife to cut through the modelling material so that it is divided into the desired sections. You must now 'float off' the sections. Immerse the face cast in water and leave it overnight (up to 24 hours). The water will dissolve the Alcote or KY Jelly, allowing the sculpted material to be easily lifted from the plaster cast. The sculpted sections can then be applied to the appropriate sectional cast and the edges feathered out to make them thin. This will ensure that when the sectional pieces are overlapped, they blend smoothly into one another.

It may not always be practical to feather out the edges of each section; perhaps the pieces are extra thick and thinning the edge to the level of the mould would not be appropriate. In this case, it is advisable to make additional casts as suggested for the following example.

Imagine you wanted to overlap a thick foam latex forehead piece, with a thick nose and upper lip piece. First cast a latex foam forehead piece on a sectional mould and then attach it to the original face cast and remould the whole thing. From the new mould produce a new face cast with the shape of the forehead section built onto it, from which you can then make subsequent sectional moulds. Attach the nose and upper lip sculpture to the latest sectional cast (which reflected the new forehead shape) and blend the edges. Then mould the new nose and upper lip shape and from that produce a prosthetic piece. When this prosthetic piece is applied it should have an undetectable join with the forehead piece.

> **KEY NOTE**
>
> Corresponding negative and positive sections should be identified with some sort of code for future reference. It would also be useful to note the name of the model and any other information that would help to identify the prosthetic piece in the future.

Slush moulding with liquid latex or cap plastic

Latex or cap plastic can be used in a process called 'slush moulding'. Paint a thin coat of either material over the surface of the mould (which has had a mould-release applied) to pick up all the detail, then pour a generous amount into the mould and 'slush' it around to cover the entire surface. Build up the thickness of the material in the middle of the piece but leave it thin at the sides and edges. Leave the cast to dry, preferably overnight. When it is dry, dust it with talc and carefully remove it from the mould.

Flat plate moulding

This kind of mould making does not require a life cast. It is used to produce simple prosthetics such as casualty effects, for example raised scars, eye bags, etc.

1 Take a plastic container, approximately 5 cm deep, and fill it with plaster to create the 'flat plate' on which you will work.

2 When the plaster has set, remove it from the container. Using the key tool, place 'keys' (indentions) into each edge of the plaster – these will act as alignment keys, ensuring that the two halves of the mould (the positive and the negative) fit together perfectly.

3 Seal the plaster with several thin coats of Alcote or KY Petroleum Jelly.

4 Sculpt the desired shape onto the sealed plaster using a modelling material of your choice. Make sure you keep the edges thin.

5 Create a low retaining wall using the clay, leaving a gap of approximately 1–2 cm around the edge of the sculpture and taking care not to cover the keys.

6 Cover the entire surface within the retaining wall with Vaseline or other mould-release agent.

7 Replace the flat plate into the original container and mix a fresh batch of plaster.

8 Paint a splash coat over the surface of the flat plate and sculpture and then pour the plaster to the top of the retaining wall. Allow the plaster to set.

9 Remove the mould from the container and clean away any clay using acetone on a bristle brush.

10 Allow the mould section to completely dry out, preferably overnight. Alternatively you could place it in the oven on a medium heat for approximately an hour and a half.

11 You are now ready to cast your mould – gelatine, liquid latex or cap plastic work well.

Colouring prosthetics

Prosthetics can be coloured during the production process by simply adding cosmetic grade pigments to the casting material. This is referred to as **intrinsic colouration**. It is usual to tint the piece a flesh colour and then to apply make-up on top. Cosmetic grade pigments, for example flocking, are available in a wide variety of skin and fantasy colours in wet or dry formats. 'Vein-like' material can also be purchased to add an ultra-realistic look to the piece.

Securing and applying make-up to prosthetic pieces

Please refer to Chapter 10, for this information.

Building a prosthetic portfolio

* Your portfolio should show a grasp of the basic skills behind prosthetic design: drawing and sculpting. If you are just starting out, nobody will expect you to have produced work involving the more expensive and technical procedures. However, do include some finished examples of prosthetics you have produced with make-up applied.

* Your portfolio should contain a variety of work. Even if your interest lies in a particular genre such as monsters, include examples of other work, for example ageing. Prospective clients will be looking for versatility.

* Do not include lots of different angles of a single piece.

* In your portfolio, quality is better than quantity.

* Take the best photographs that you can. Photographs should be in focus, shake-free and preferably taken with natural light rather than with a flash.

* Improve your skills and gain experience through practice and experimenting. Do not be afraid of failure, but do learn from your mistakes.

* There is a lot to be said for studying examples of the work of accomplished prosthetic artists.

* Keep a file for design inspiration. This may include images of interesting faces, figures, animals, plants, etc.

* Ensure your photographs do not feel 'amateurish'. Avoid photographing your friends wearing your monster prosthetics in 'monster poses'.

* Avoid recreating famous make-ups – you will be inviting clients to make comparisons with the real thing. Also, copying someone else's work shows little originality or creativity.

Cosmetic airbrushing

Airbrushing is considered to be a relatively new technique in make-up application. However, a rudimentary form was first used back in the 1920s as a way of applying body make-up to film extras quickly. Nowadays, with the development of sophisticated equipment and cosmetic grade pigments suitable for the airbrush, airbrushing has become an art form in itself. Most make-up artists will agree that although the airbrush is another valuable tool for applying make-up, it will never entirely take over from conventional brush work; each method has its place within the professional make-up artist's kit.

Airbrushing works by dispensing a large number of tiny droplets of pigment onto the skin (or prosthetic) via a pen-like tool. The colour product is pushed through this tool by air pressure supplied by a compressor. This produces a soft covering on the surface, which is built up in layers to achieve colour density. The technique is very hygienic because nothing other than the colour product touches the skin.

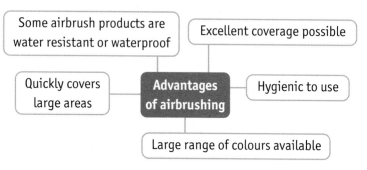

The airbrush lends itself to a variety of applications, in particular:

* camouflage and tattoo cover
* creating temporary tattoos
* applying foundation and contouring colours in beauty make-ups
* applying fine, almost invisible make-up for men
* applying colour to prosthetics
* body art and make-up
* applying fake tans.

Before you can begin to experiment with the art of airbrushing, you must familiarise yourself with the necessary equipment.

Airbrushing equipment

The airbrush

The airbrush is the tool that dispenses the pigment products onto a given surface. It is usually shaped like a pen and consists of several components:

* a 'cup' to hold the colour product
* an attachment for the lead to the air supply (compressor)
* a trigger to control the air flow and the flow of the product
* a nozzle, fitted with a cap, from which the product will be released
* the main body, housing a fine needle, which is controlled by the trigger.

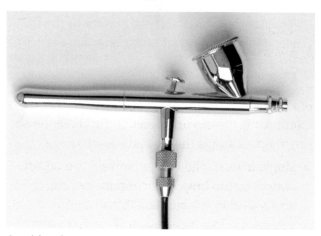

An airbrush

Although all airbrushes look similar, there are distinct differences in the ways they deliver the product to a surface. It is important to find an airbrush that meets the specific needs of the make-up artist. When choosing an airbrush you should give consideration to the following:

* the method of delivering (feeding) the colour product
* the trigger action
* the source of air supply
* the type of colour product to use.

The airbrush will need to have a container or 'cup' into which the chosen colour product can be poured. The position of this container will affect the method of delivery of the product through the airbrush and onto the skin. The three **colour feed methods** are as follows.

* **The side feed:** The container or cup is set to one side and raised above the airbrush. The colour product is siphoned from the container through the airbrush.

* **The suction feed:** The container is set beneath the airbrush. The colour product is suctioned from the container through the airbrush.

* **The gravity feed:** A cup is set directly on top of the airbrush. The colour product flows down from the cup and through the body of the airbrush.

Most make-up artists use a gravity feed airbrush. This is the best type for cosmetic work because:

* it is quicker
* it is more hygienic
* you can get closer to the face.

You will also need to consider the most appropriate type of **trigger action** for the airbrush. The trigger controls the air and colour action.

* **Single action:** The trigger works as an on/off switch, controlling the air supply and colour flow together. It is not possible to control the air and colour flow independently so the coverage has a coarser texture.

* **Fixed double action:** The trigger works as an on/off switch, but the air supply and colour flow can be operated independently of each other. However, the amount of air supply or colour flow cannot be adjusted; it is either on or off.

* **Independent double action:** The trigger works by controlling the pressure of air flow introduced through the airbrush and the amount of colour independently of each other. The air and colour supply can be varied.

The **independent double-action airbrush** is preferable for cosmetic work because you can control the air and colour supply separately with the trigger. The harder you depress the trigger, the more air will be expelled; the more you pull back on the trigger, the more colour will flow. This ensures the make-up artist has complete flexibility in the application of product onto the skin.

The air supply

The source of air supply is another important consideration for the make-up artist when choosing airbrushing equipment. Your choice will depend on budget and mobility. You must ensure it has a regulator fitted so you can control the air pressure. Commercially, airbrushes can be used up to pressures of 30 pounds per square inch (psi), but this is far too high for make-up application. Usually, a make-up artist will work at pressures of no more than 20 psi for the body and as low as 3 psi around delicate areas such as the eyes. Therefore, you need to be able to precisely control the air pressure entering the airbrush, via a regulator.

* **Canned or tanked air:** This is useful if you plan to use the airbrush infrequently or are working on location. Carbon dioxide types are suitable because they are noiseless, but you will need to purchase and fit an appropriate regulator. They serve well as a back-up, but generally compressors are a better option.

* **Tank compressors:** They have a reservoir tank containing compressed air, which is constantly ready to use. When the machine is switched on, a motor pressurises the tank of air (static pressure) and a regulator allows the pressure to be adjusted to the required level (working pressure). To adjust the working pressure, you will need to activate the air flow by pressing the trigger down on the airbrush and simultaneously turning the regulator. The compressor's motor does not run continuously, but activates when the reservoir tank pressure drops below the required level ensuring a steady, constant air flow. Larger compressors

are sometimes run on oil, but this type of compressor is meant to be kept stable and is not suitable for moving around. Battery powered compressors that are attached to a belt are useful for taking onto set for touch-ups. These work up to pressures of about 15 psi and last about an hour. The more expensive options offer the advantages of quieter operation and the capacity to handle several airbrushes at once. You must ensure your compressor has a moisture filter or trap integral to its design. If not, you will have to invest in an external one.

> **KEY NOTE**
>
> If you are not using a compressor, turn it off.

The air line

The airbrush is attached to the compressor by an air line. This is a thin, plastic tube with an attachment at either end. Most attachments are of the screw fit type and should only be tightened with the fingers. Some manufacturers can supply 'quick release' attachments that allow the airbrush to be attached and removed very quickly. This is useful when you are using more than one airbrush at a time, for example when alternating between colours.

Accessories

The following accessories are needed for airbrushing:

* airbrush holder to keep your airbrush stable when not in use, preventing spillage of the colour product
* flammable waste box to hold all waste flammable products, such as tissues soaked in alcohol-based cleaner, reducing hazardous fumes in the atmosphere
* soft brushes to clean the airbrush – do not use cotton buds
* dish or pot to soak airbrush parts when cleaning the airbrush (a 35 mm photo film canister works well)
* clean pot to dispense any spare products into without causing atmospheric hazards.

> **KEY NOTE**
>
> You may also wish to purchase some Teflon Tape, which is useful for trapping air leaks. Air-lube, available from airbrush suppliers, is used to lubricate the needle of the airbrush.

Airbrush colour products

Cosmetics designed for use with an airbrush are usually pigments suspended in a very thin liquid. They all need to be shaken vigorously to mix the pigments with the liquid suspension. Airbrush cosmetics are available in the following formulas.

Water-based	Similar to conventional liquid make-up, these products are cosmetic-approved pigments suspended in water. They have a similar longevity to conventional liquid make-up. Beauty make-ups are almost always applied with this type of product. They are removed from the skin with conventional cleansers.
Alcohol-based	These products are cosmetic-approved pigments suspended in alcohol (normally isopropyl alcohol). They are known within the industry as temporary airbrush inks, because they are used for creating fake tattoos. They normally last anything up to six days once sealed. They are available in a wide range of colours, including opalescent and metallic finishes. These products are removed with alcohol or oily cleansing creams.
Polymer-based	These products consist of cosmetic-approved pigments and polymer (a synthetic plastic) suspended in water- or alcohol-based formulas. Once the airbrushed product has dried, the polymer forms a 'film' on the surface that gives the make-up superb longevity. They are removed from the skin with alcohol or oily cleansing creams.

Silicone-based	The most recent formula to enter the market, these products consist of cosmetic-approved pigments suspended in a silicone base. Manufacturers claim the make-up not only has excellent longevity, but also retains a fresh 'just applied' look.
DHA (dihydroxy-acetone)-based	Used in 'sunless tanning' colour products, the active ingredient reacts with skin to produce a fake suntan.

KEY NOTE

Airbrushing conventional fluid foundations

Some conventional liquid foundations (Revlon Colour Stay Make-up is one example) may be used with an airbrush providing:

* they are diluted for airbrush work by adding Dow Corning 244 Cosmetic Grade Silicone Fluid
* the airbrushing is carried out at a slightly higher pressure than normal.

HANDS ON

Research airbrushing product ranges and suppliers.

Although you can overlay different types of products on the skin, you must never mix alcohol-based products with water-based products as this will clog your airbrush, sometimes beyond repair. Whenever you are switching from an alcohol-based product to a water-based product, always flush out the airbrush to remove any traces of the alcohol-based product from the airbrush with an alcohol cleanser, then flush through with a water-based cleanser before introducing water-based products to the airbrush – and vice versa.

Airbrush cleaning fluids

Cosmetic-approved cleaning fluids should be used through an airbrush. Most manufacturers of airbrush make-up include cleaning fluids as part of their product range. It is important to carefully follow the cleaning instructions provided, always

remembering to catch cleaner dispensed from the airbrush in a tissue or clean pot.

If you are in any doubt about how to handle a product safely, seek advice from the product manufacturer before use.

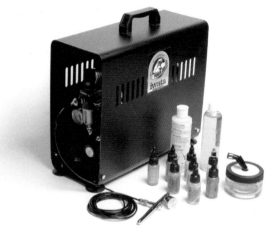

A selection of airbrushing colour products, clean pot, compressor and air lead

Cleaning the airbrush

Because of the mixture of air and colour product, the airbrush is prone to blockages. The airbrush should therefore be cleaned every time it is used as follows.

1 Run any remaining colour product through the airbrush.

2 Clean the cup out with a tissue.

3 Pour an appropriate cleaning fluid into the cup and run it through the airbrush. Using a higher psi than normal (up to 25 psi), 'jet wash' the airbrush to remove any stubborn dried product. Pull the trigger backwards and forwards as you do this to ensure the needle is thoroughly cleaned and lubricated.

4 Continue until the cleaning fluid runs clear from the airbrush.

5 Remove the cap from the airbrush nozzle and soak it in a pot of cleaning fluid to remove last traces of product.

6 Ensuring the needle is retracted, use a soft small brush to clean the nozzle of the airbrush.

7 Replace the cap.

A more thorough clean, involving disassembling the airbrush, should be carried out at regular intervals. When carrying out this type of clean, always ensure you follow the manufacturer's instructions. Take great care with the small and delicate parts, particularly the needle, which can be easily damaged.

> **REMEMBER**
>
> When running an alcohol-based cleaning fluid through the airbrush, it is important to protect the atmosphere from harmful fumes. Ensure you dispense the cleaning fluid into a 'clean pot' or use a tissue wrapped around the end of the airbrush (taking care not to block the outlet) to catch the cleaning fluid before it enters the atmosphere. The tissue should then be disposed of in a flammable waste box.

Basic airbrush techniques

The guidelines below are applicable when using an independent double-action airbrush.

1 Ensure the room is well ventilated.

2 Set your compressor to an appropriate psi (never exceed 10 psi for airbrushing the face).

3 Shake the colour product well and pour a very small amount into the cup on the airbrush.

4 Push the airbrush trigger down to begin the air flow through the nozzle. The harder you depress the trigger, the more air will be expelled.

5 Once you have achieved an adequate air supply through the nozzle, begin to pull back on the trigger to introduce the flow of colour product onto the skin (or paper if you are practising).

6 Always work at a 45° angle (downwards).

7 To stop the flow of product, continue to depress the trigger but move it forward, reducing the colour flow but still expelling air through the nozzle. This will remove the last trace of product from the airbrush and reduce the risk of blockages.

8 To discontinue the air flow, lift your finger off the trigger.

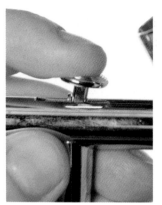 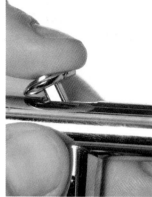

Depressing the trigger   *Pulling the trigger back*

Practise the action of stopping and starting the flow of air and colour through the airbrush. To prevent blockages, it is very important that:

* the flow of colour product is started after the flow of air

* the flow of colour product is stopped before the flow of air.

> **KEY NOTE**
>
> Learn to listen to your airbrush – you can usually hear any problems with the air or colour flow.

> **HANDS ON**
>
> **Controlling the airbrush**
>
> Learning to use an airbrush successfully takes time and practice. It is worth spending some time getting used to handling the airbrush using paper as your canvas before attempting to apply product to the skin.
>
> The following equipment is required:
> * sheets of A4 or A3 paper
> * masking tape
> * tissues
> * clean pot
> * flammable waste container
> * airbrush
> * compressor and air lead
> * airbrush colour products and cleaners.
>
> Using the masking tape, secure a sheet of paper onto a vertical surface. Using the airbrush as instructed above, carry out the following exercises. The exercises will improve your dexterity at handling the airbrush and

controlling the flow of air and colour to achieve the desired application on your canvas.
Create the following shapes with the airbrush.

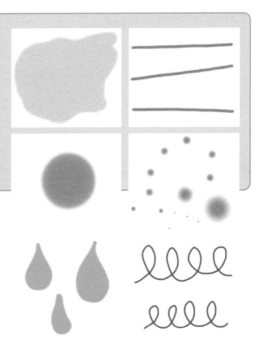

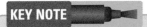 **KEY NOTE**

Make sure you close the top as soon as you have dispensed the colour product and wipe the top after use. You only need a few drops at a time. These products are expensive so do not waste them. Always remember to shake the bottle before use.

STEP-BY-STEP | **Applying an airbrushed beauty make-up to a female model**

This technique uses water-based colour products.

1 Prepare the model.
2 Apply a light water-based moisturiser.
3 Carry out corrective work using conventional brush techniques.
4 Powder these areas.
5 Set the compressor to between 4 and 10 psi. Keep it as low as possible – you can adjust it as required.
6 Begin by running airbrush cleaner through the airbrush to check the flow and remove any residue from previous use.
7 Mix foundation colour. You can do this in the airbrush cup or separate dish.
8 Spray colour into a tissue to check the colour tone and colour and air flow.
9 Protect the hairline with a tissue and ask the model to close her eyes.
10 Position your airbrush at a 45° angle (pointing slightly downwards) and about 5-8 cm from the face.
11 Begin by moving your hand in gentle sweeping movements.
12 Gradually begin the air flow by pressing the trigger down, then begin the colour flow by pulling the trigger back. Keep your hand moving.
13 Coat the skin evenly. When working around the ear, use an earplug or finger to protect the ear canal. Do not spray

colour up the nose (you will have to apply colour between the nostrils with a make-up brush afterwards). Reduce the psi to about 3 or 4 when working around the eyes. Remember that several thin coats give a far better application than one thick coat, so keep your hand moving at all times.

14 Mix a highlight colour and apply it to areas you wish to highlight. You may wish to add an even lighter highlighter to some areas to increase definition.
15 Mix a shading colour and apply it where you wish to add shadow to the bone structure.
16 Mix blusher colour and apply.
17 Use eyebrow templates and apply colour to eyebrows. Keep to about 3 psi. Alternatively, eyebrow colour can be applied using conventional techniques.
18 Apply mascara, eye make-up and lip colour using traditional procedures.
19 Run cleaner through the airbrush.
20 For longevity, water-based make up can be sealed. Various products can be used for this – Ben Nye Final Seal, Mehron Barrier Spray or Green Marble by Premier Products. Fill the cup with the chosen product and apply a thin layer to the face.
21 Flush out the airbrush with cleaner.

KEY NOTE

When changing colour, spray into a tissue until you see the colour change. This will prevent you making mistakes on the skin.

KEY NOTE

When contouring the model's face with airbrushed highlight and shadow, the same rules of positioning apply as when using conventional methods of application. However, a more diffused, subtle effect can usually be achieved with the airbrush.

STEP-BY-STEP **Applying a corrective airbrushed make-up on a male model**

This technique uses water-based colour products.

1 Skin must be clean-shaven
2 Prepare the model.
3 Apply a light water-based moisturiser.
4 Carry out traditional corrective work.
5 Powder these areas.
6 Set the compressor to between 4 and 10 psi. Keep it as low as possible – you can adjust it as required.
7 Run airbrush cleaner through the airbrush to check the flow and remove any residue from previous use.
8 If required, mix a colour to hide the five o'clock shadow (a product from Skin Illustrator called Coral Adjuster is excellent for this). Any colour correction is applied prior to the foundation colour.
9 Mix foundation colour. You can do this in the airbrush cup or a separate dish.
10 Spray colour into a tissue to check colour tone and colour and air flow.
11 Protect the hairline with a tissue and ask the model to close his eyes.
12 Position your airbrush at a 45° angle pointing slightly downwards and about 5-8 cm from the face.

13 Begin by moving your hand in gentle sweeping movements.
14 Gradually begin the air flow by pressing the trigger down. Then begin the colour flow by pulling the trigger back. Keep your hand moving. Coat the skin evenly. The result should be light and natural.
15 Mix a highlight colour to 'chisel' the features, for example to strengthen the jaw line and reduce a double chin. The cheekbone, temple and the area under the lower lip should be considered for camera work.
16 Mix a shading colour and apply.
17 Mix a blush colour and apply it to the centre of the cheek.
18 Fill in 'gappy' eyebrows, keeping to about 3 psi. Apply mascara if the eyelashes are blonde.
19 Fill in thinning hairlines.
20 Run cleaner through the airbrush.
21 For longevity, water-based make-up can be sealed. Various products can be used for this – Ben Nye Final Seal, Mehron Barrier Spray or Green Marble by Premier Products. Fill the cup with the chosen product and apply a thin layer to the face.
22 Run cleaner through the airbrush.

Masking techniques

Masking is the technique used to protect areas of the skin or model from being sprayed with the colour product.

To control the placement of colour

To protect the hairline

To protect the clothes

Reasons for masking

To blend colours

To apply tattoo designs

To shape the eyebrows

Materials for masking include tissues, templates and stencils. These can be used to create:

* hard masking, which involves holding the masking material directly onto the surface of the skin – this creates a hard, very precise outline and is used for creating tattoos

* soft masking, which involves holding the masking material above the surface of the skin to varying degrees – this creates a soft, graduated edge and is used when contouring the face and features.

A stencil is a mask with a shape cut out of it. The colour product is airbrushed over the stencil, leaving a positive impression of the shape on the surface of the skin. The skin surrounding the cut out shape is protected from the spray. Sometimes 'overspray' is created where the colour product reaches beyond the outline of the stencil. In such cases the excess product can be removed with the appropriate cleanser, although this may prove problematic if the colour has fallen on a previous layer of colour, rather than on bare skin.

Another common problem is known as 'creeping'. This is where the colour seeps behind the stencil, ruining the outline of the design. Holding the stencil firmly against the skin's surface should help to prevent this problem.

KEY NOTE

Stencils can be bought in, or if you need a specific design, you can make your own. Designs can be drawn or printed onto sheets of acetate. The shape is then cut out using a sharp scalpel knife on a cutting board. This should be done with great care to avoid injury.

Templates create negative impressions on the skin. The shape is cut out from the acetate and placed onto the skin. The colour product is them sprayed over the template and the surrounding skin. When the template is removed, a negative impression of the shape is left, free of colour.

Stencils and templates can be created from almost anything, provided it is safe for the material to come into contact with the skin. Wonderful effects can be achieved with a little imagination and experimentation; try using netting, lace, petals and feathers.

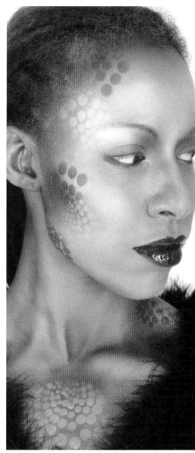
An airbrushed make-up

STEP-BY-STEP **Applying a fake tattoo using a stencil (using alcohol-based colour products)**

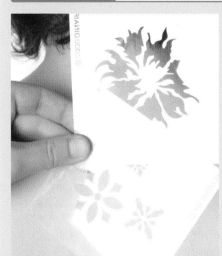

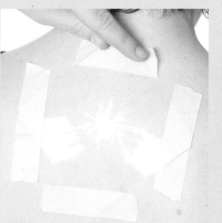

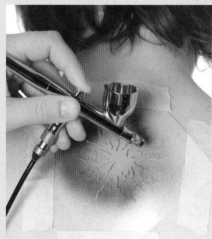

1 Choose a tattoo design. Ensure the model's clothes are protected. Before applying the colour product, clean the skin with an alcohol wipe.

2 Place the stencil on the skin ensuring it is tight to the surface. It can be fixed in place with a little masking tape.

3 Load the airbrush and apply the product colour as desired over the stencil, keeping your hand moving at all times.

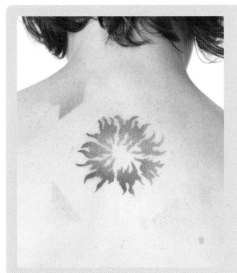

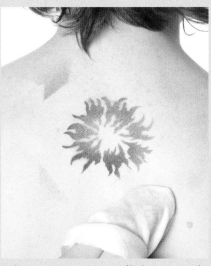

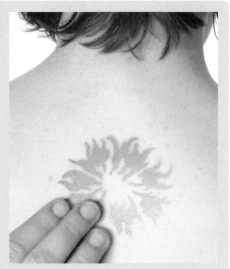

4 Allow the colour to dry and carefully remove the stencil.

5 Any overspray can easily be removed with an alcohol wipe.

6 Complete by airbrushing a sealing product over the tattoo to increase its longevity and maintain the vibrancy of the colours. Alternatively, to create an authentic-looking tattoo, dust with transparent setting powder and rub any excess powder off with clean fingers. This will give an authentic finish to the colours and restore the natural sheen to the skin.

KEY NOTE

For body art and self tan application, 20 psi is recommended. For extra strong fantasy colours, spray on white first and let it dry before applying colours.

Issues of health and safety

Although airbrushing is actually more hygienic than conventional methods of make-up application because the skin is not touched by anything other than the product and air, the technique does present other health and safety issues. Inevitably, because the products are being sprayed onto the skin, particles will enter the immediate atmosphere. Where the products contain ingredients that may be harmful if expelled in large doses, precautions need to be taken to protect both the model and yourself.

* You should ensue the work area has adequate ventilation. Avoid working in small, enclosed spaces.

* If you are airbrushing frequently or suffer from respiratory complaints, you should wear appropriate personal protective equipment, for example a face mask.

* Many of the cleaning products are not designed for skin contact. Take care and wear gloves for protection.

Because alcohol products are volatile and may enter the atmosphere, it is essential that adequate fire precautions are taken:

* no smoking should be allowed in the vicinity

* no unshielded electrical equipment, for example hairdryers, should be used in the same area

* fire extinguishers should be available.

Other precautions include the following.

* Do not eat in an area where airbrushing is being carried out – particles may drop onto the food.

* Check for contra-indications and known allergies. If contra-actions occur, discontinue

use and remove the product. If irritation continues, seek medical advice.

* Ensure your compressor regulator is working correctly and is set to the correct pressure. Always work at minimum psi necessary to achieve results. Never exceed 10 psi on the face and 3 to 4 psi around the eyes. If this pressure limit is exceeded, air may be forced into the dermal layer of the skin causing severe bruising, or in rare cases even death from embolisms. If the colour product bounces from the skin during application, the air pressure is too high and should be reduced.

* Never spray paint into the eyes, ears, nose or mouth. At no time should compressed air or colour product be sprayed directly into the eyes, nor should the angle or pressure of the airbrush force open the closed eye.

* Do not spray red around the eyes as this stains badly.

* When airbrushing, never remove the cap from the airbrush to expose the internal needle. This is dangerous as it may pierce the model's skin.

> **KEY NOTE**
>
> **Contra-indications to airbrushing**
>
> In addition to the usual contra-indications for make-up application, airbrushing should be avoided around anyone who is trying to conceive, is pregnant or is breastfeeding.

Troubleshooting

Colour splatter

* There is a problem with the moisture trap in the compressor. Water condensation accumulates inside the moisture trap and air storage tank. Follow the manufacturer's instructions to drain the excess moisture.

* Dried colour product is left in the nozzle or on the tip of the needle. Remove the nozzle or tip of the needle and carefully clean it with appropriate cleaner on a soft brush.

Blow-back (when the product in the cup 'bubbles')

* The airbrush is totally blocked. A complete clean may be necessary. Always stop the colour flow before the air flow to prevent blocking in the future.

* Colour is clogged in the base of the cup.

* The nozzle cap is loose.

* The nozzle is damaged.

Colour is blobby, sluggish or skipping

* The airbrush needs cleaning.

* The pigment is not mixed or diluted enough. Shake the product bottle vigorously. If using conventional cosmetic, dilute it further.

* The air pressure is too high.

* The nozzle is partially blocked.

* Dried paint is left on the tip of the needle.

* The airbrush may be leaking air.

* If you are using a tank of air, it may be running out.

Double line

* The airbrush is dirty.

* The needle is bent.

* The nozzle or cap is dirty.

* Dried paint is left on the tip of the needle.

Splattering

* The airbrush is dirty.

* The colour product is too thick.

* The air pressure is too low.

* Dried paint is left on the tip of the needle.

No air or colour

* Check the compressor is working and connected to the airbrush correctly.

* The air pressure is not correct.

* The nozzle is clogged or damaged.

* The nozzle cap is loose.

* The needle is loose or damaged.

* The paint is too thick.
* If you are using a tank of air, it may be running out.

The trigger sticks or does not move smoothly

* Use Super Lube to lubricate the trigger.
* A part may be broken or bent.

Knowledge Check

1 List the requirements of a prosthetics work area.

2 Suggest a communication system between the model and make-up artist when carrying out a facial life cast.

3 What health and safety precautions should be taken when working with plaster?

4 How should the model be prepared for a full head life cast?

5 What are the advantages of casting prosthetics in foaming gelatine?

6 What are the specific contra-indications to life casting?

7 What are alcohol-based airbrush products also known as?

8 Describe how an airbrush should be cleaned after each use.

9 What are the specific contra-indications to airbrushing?

10 Explain the difference between hard and soft masking.

CHAPTER 17

SECTION 4:

Business skills

As a make-up artist you may find yourself working within a large organisation, such as a theatre or make-up retailer, or you may become freelance, working on a self-employed basis. In either situation it is critical that you develop skills outside of those that relate purely to the design and application of make-up.

Aim and objectives

Aim of this chapter: to provide you with the knowledge to enable you to:

* implement marketing strategies
* contribute to the financial effectiveness of a business
* agree contracts for hair and make-up work.

You should achieve the following **objectives:**

* Break marketing strategies down into objectives and actions
* Evaluate appropriate timescales for action plans
* Acquire resources required to implement action plans
* Identify uncertainties and potential problems of proposed marketing strategies
* Identify and organise other people involved in implementing action plans
* Monitor action plan activities and evaluate their progress
* Identify new opportunities and potential threats to the action plan
* Evaluate ways in which you can improve your productivity at work

Note: Go to the Make-up Artistry website at www.heinemann.co.uk for more information about:

* Legislation (Working Time Directive 1998) and consumer protection legislation.
* The effective use and monitoring of resources including stock, human resources and time.

* Discuss legislation relating to the use of resources
* Discuss considerations for the employer relating to the acquisition of resources
* Identify methods for monitoring stock levels and ordering additional supplies
* Discuss appropriate procedures for checking stock
* List ways in which waste of stock can be avoided
* Evaluate the importance of security and insurance in relation to stock
* Identify the importance of monitoring the performance of resources.
* Select and co-ordinate a design team
* Meet productivity and development targets
* Negotiate and agree contracts for hair and make-up work.

Improve your sales and marketing

As a make-up artist you may find yourself working within a large organisation, such as a theatre or make-up retailer, or you may become freelance and work on a self-employed basis. In either situation it is critical that you develop skills in addition to those that relate purely to the design and application of make-up. In a commercial environment you need to be able to plan and analyse your actions to improve sales and marketing, deal with other members of a team and generate a consistent workload, particularly if you are self-employed with a single source of income. These and other 'business' skills will provide you with a solid basis on which you can develop a career path and gain opportunities to work in your chosen field.

Developing a marketing action plan

In your role as a make-up artist, you will be required to perform a variety of tasks and your success will be founded on careful planning of each aspect of the tasks. When working freelance you must be capable of generating work, and this will inevitably involve the 'marketing' of yourself as a make-up artist. Successful marketing requires a methodical approach and the establishment of an action plan at the outset. Once your plan is in place, which might consist of a list of objectives and actions, you should measure and evaluate your progress.

List your objectives
↓
List actions to achieve each objective
↓
Assign a timescale to each objective
↓
Evaluate your progress
↓
Identify where further action is needed

Action plan objective	Action	Evaluation of progress
Ensure local photographers know about you	Network and make contact (see below)	Contacted six photographers. Heard from two, visited one with portfolio. Good feedback.

Example of breaking activities down into objectives and actions

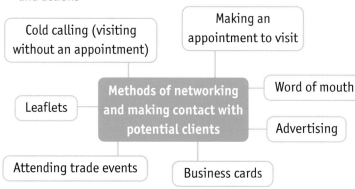

Methods of networking and making contact with potential clients:
- Cold calling (visiting without an appointment)
- Making an appointment to visit
- Word of mouth
- Advertising
- Business cards
- Attending trade events
- Leaflets

Appropriate timescales for your action plan

Once the objectives are set, you should assign timescales to each item. This way you can evaluate progress and identify where further action is needed. For example, you could start by identifying and contacting the photographers or television and theatre companies you would most like to work with. But set a deadline. If the work is not coming in within a defined period, move on to other contacts.

The resources you might need to put your plan into action

Your marketing strategy will require a variety of resources. You will probably need a business card, which will have to be designed and printed. Some high street printing shops will provide a design service, but make sure you see what the final product will look like before you agree to the printing going ahead. Your card or leaflet could include examples of your work, which will make them more eye-catching and provide a conversation point when you finally make contact with your target. You could use the same design format for all your business correspondence including invoices, receipts, etc.

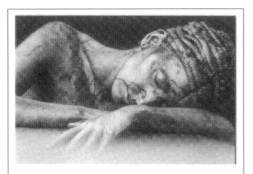

Example of a business card

HANDS ON

Design a business card for yourself. It is not a good idea to put both your phone number and address on the card, in case it ends up in the hands of someone unscrupulous. However, a phone number, email address and website details (if applicable) are all useful information for potential clients. Remember, clients will receive many business cards, so try to make yours stand out.

KEY NOTE

Although it is usually more economical to place a larger order with printing firms, remember that personal details such as telephone numbers and prices may change over time, leaving you with out-of-date marketing material.

To develop your portfolio you may need to locate studios, models and stylists, and gain the services of a photographer. You should plan your budget for

such activities carefully and try to come to an agreement that benefits not just yourself but also the photographer, stylist and model. Test shoots are an excellent example of how resources can be shared for the mutual benefit all parties involved.

Once you have identified the resources you need it is important that you monitor their use and results. For example, you might spend a lot of money on a leaflet and so you need to know that it was well spent. Check how many responses the leaflet generated, how many jobs resulted, what income they brought in and whether it was more than the initial outlay.

You will have to speculate to gain work opportunities, but make sure you get the balance right. An advert in a bridal magazine, for example, will be very expensive but might be worthwhile as it is a sure way of reaching your target audience.

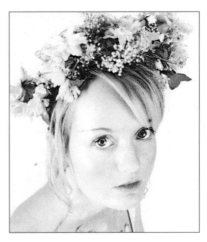

Bridal Make-up

North-West based professional make-up artist offers a make-up and hair design service to transform you on your wedding day.

Bride, bridesmaids and mother of the bride can all be transformed at the location of your choice. For full details, consultation and to view portfolio of work, please contact Amanda Smith on 07950 823 *** or visit www.bridalmakeup****.co.uk

Example of an advert. Make-up artist: Gillian Curd

Sometimes you need to speculate with your time, not just your money. In the early days of your career expect to do lots of test shoots, but don't always expect to earn from these. However, non-fee-earning jobs must be worth your time in other ways, for example you could gain quality images for your portfolio or meet valuable new contacts. Working hard and enthusiastically in the beginning will pay dividends in the long run.

Identifying uncertainties and potential problems in the action plan

One key to success in achieving your aims is to anticipate potential problems. When developing your marketing plans you should always consider what might go wrong, or what is out of your control. Marketing is a fundamentally uncertain process as you cannot predict how your approaches will be received. Your success will also depend on global issues.

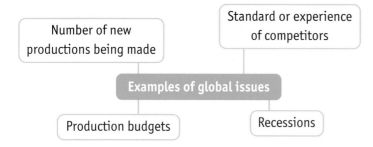

It is important that you spread your marketing over a broad range of targets. In this way you can avoid wasting lengthy periods of time waiting for responses from one type of contact, which may all prove to be unsuccessful.

Involving other people in implementing your action plans

Your action plan for a particular objective will undoubtedly involve other people. You must therefore ensure that you identify these people at the outset and that you establish a set pattern of communicating with them. As a freelance make-up artist, you may have sought financial backing from a bank, or perhaps obtained a career development loan. The progress of your career, and how you obtain work, will therefore be of interest to other people. You should ensure that you are aware of what requirements your backers will impose on you in terms of reporting your finances and, most importantly, you should keep detailed records of the work you do. Agencies will want to see that you are networking, meeting with contacts they have provided and attending interviews they have arranged.

Methods of monitoring marketing activities

There are various ways in which you can monitor the progress of marketing activities. The method you choose will depend on the activity itself and the context in which you are working. For example, when working within a large studio environment, you will become very familiar with the need for meetings, briefings and report writing. The larger the organisation, the more formal the approach will be. An environment such as a television studio will have a set strategy that includes when meetings are required, how reports should be written and who needs to know what and when. In terms of marketing, it is likely that a group of key personnel will be formed to address a particular aspect of a marketing strategy and will meet at regular intervals to discuss progress. Individuals within the group will be given specific responsibilities and will have to report to the meeting, either verbally or in writing.

In any working environment, the best way to monitor the progress of your marketing is to speak to the people you are trying to reach. Once you have made your first approach, i.e. a business card, a phone call etc., allow some time to elapse and then contact the target. Ask how your approach has been received and request a meeting. Always be polite – nobody likes a pushy salesperson. Once you receive feedback, keep notes and then evaluate your progress against your action plan, checking the time you have allowed yourself to achieve a positive result. If the response is poor, move on to other ideas; you can always contact people again in the future.

New opportunities and threats to your action plan

Marketing is a fluid process. The opportunities and methods of marketing which are open to you will be changing constantly. A good example of this is the increasing use of electronic communication in advertising. An undoubtedly efficient and cheap way of contacting lots of people is to email your approaches, though the success of this method might be questionable – we all know how easy it is to delete a message from someone trying to sell us something. A website address that displays your portfolio, CV and contact details is a popular method of self-promotion with make-up artists. The key to success is to be selective about your approaches and to choose the most appropriate means.

Sometimes, opportunities arise unexpectedly. A client may telephone out of the blue, a competitor may fail to turn up for a job, a contact may recommend you without your knowledge. However, your best chance of obtaining work is through networking and ensuring you are the best person for the job. You should be trained:

* complete relevant courses of study

* continue to train throughout your career (Continued Professional Development – CPD)

* investigate new products and their use.

You should be able to:

* practise and improve on the skills you have learned

* be positive, enthusiastic and pleasant to work with

* be reliable

You should be informed:

* join a union such as BECTU

* subscribe to a trade magazine

* keep up to date with trends

* talk to as many people within the industry as you can.

KEY NOTE

Remember, you are only as good as your last job and a poor reputation is very hard to shake off.

Even if you have done all of the above, some factors will affect your career which are out of your control. New competitors may arrive on the scene, a studio may close down, a photographer may change from fashion to commercial, your assistant might leave. Always try to keep your options open. Try to build a broad range of contacts and only specialise when you are sure you have found the role that suits you best and will provide as secure an income as possible.

Meeting productivity and development targets

This section looks at:

* productivity – your effectiveness in the workplace

* development targets – ways in which you can improve your skills to increase your effectiveness.

Productivity

Whether working freelance or within a studio or production environment, your productivity generates income. Put simply, the more work you do of a good standard, the more income you generate. In an 'arts' environment, however, it is not always easy to measure productivity. The best measure for your employer will be whether you perform the tasks assigned to you to the satisfaction of the client and to the agreed deadline.

To ensure you are successful, it is important that you understand what is expected of you. Always make sure your employer explains the extent of your role at the outset and be clear you know what timescales have been allowed. When carrying out an element of work, such as designing a make-up application, monitor your own progress and make sure you notify your line manager early if you think you may miss the deadline. This will give you the opportunity to rectify the problem. However, be mindful that more time or more help will mean less income in the eyes of your employer. On the other hand, if you finish work ahead of schedule, tell someone!

To understand how your productivity is perceived, ask for feedback if it is not automatically offered. Larger organisations should have formal procedures for this. This feedback will help you identify areas for improvement and you will be able to discuss where you see opportunities, both in new trends and in your future development.

Development targets for personal learning and improvement

In the make-up industry, where techniques and materials are continually being updated and improved, it is vital you stay in touch with developments. In addition, with more and more talented, well-trained make-up artists entering the profession you need to stay ahead of the game by updating technical skills with professional training, otherwise known as Continued Professional Development (CPD).

The most important aspect of CPD is that it should be a part of your career at all times. Rather than try to rectify deficiencies in your skills when it is too late, you should have an action plan that you agree with your employer if necessary. Your plan should set out which areas of make-up artistry you wish to explore further, where you consider yourself weak and which innovations you feel are important to you. You should set a regular timescale for reviewing your improvement targets and take action if the targets are not being met. You should also keep records of your CPD activities, which might include formal training, individual research and reading, attending seminars, etc.

Development targets set by your employer should be agreed, rather than imposed on you. If you feel any targets are unreasonable, you should negotiate changes and document what is agreed. There may be aspects of make-up that your employer wishes to expand into, or you may be able to suggest areas that might be of interest. Try to consider CPD as a positive aspect of your working life and be excited by new opportunities and challenges.

Agreeing contracts

Whether you are in the position of employing a make-up artist or assistant, or you are being employed by others, it is critical that the scope of work, responsibilities, time, costs and how the employment may be terminated are agreed at the outset. These factors should be enshrined in a formal contract, which must be agreed and signed by both parties. A contract protects the interests of both sides and will be the most important document if things go wrong. It is important that you know how contracts are formed and understand the implications of signing.

The scope of services

Before agreeing to accept a job, or to employ others, the first step is to establish what is required. When deciding to employ another person or company, you must be confident in their capability to complete the task. Be very clear about your requirements and document them. Ask for confirmation that the other party:

* has experience of each aspect
* has the equipment required (or has allowed for its hire)
* can provide documentary evidence of training or intention to gain training through CPD
* can provide references from satisfied clients or employers
* can provide evidence of professional indemnity insurance.

If, on the other hand, you are the one being employed, you must ask the client or employer to confirm in writing the services required of you. If you are told verbally, confirm the conversation in writing. Before agreeing to do the work you must also go through the above checklist, assessing your own capabilities in an objective manner.

In legal terms, you will be expected to carry out your duties with 'the reasonable skill and care expected of a competent make-up artist'. This means that the law requires you to do the work not as the best make-up artist in the world, but as someone capable of completing the work satisfactorily and safely. You must therefore never be tempted to agree to a job that you know you cannot complete. If you do you will run into trouble during the work, will probably lose the client and may even be sued for breach of contract!

When considering the job, the type of production will have a major influence on your assessment of your ability to complete the work in terms of skill and time. The following table highlights some of the questions you should ask yourself.

Theatre	Can I do hair and postiche work? Can I work unsocial hours? Can I commit to a long production run? Can I work under pressure?
Television and film	Can I deal with continuity issues? Can I deal with close-up work? Can I work long hours? Can I travel? Can I accept short contracts?
Fashion and photographic	Can I accept very short contracts, i.e. one day? Can I travel? Do I have a suitably up-to-date kit (latest products and colours) Can I work quickly?

Negotiating and accepting contracts

Your reasons for accepting or declining a make-up job can vary. Possible factors are the following.

* **Money:** Will you get paid a sufficient amount to make the job worthwhile? Will the fee cover your expenses such as equipment, materials, travel, insurance and other overheads?

* **Time:** Are you available for the full duration of the contract? Do you think the time allowed is sufficient to complete the work to acceptable levels of quality and safety?

* **Publicity:** Is the job something you want to be associated with? Does the opportunity outweigh the low fee? Will the job further or hinder your career?

* **Experience:** Is the job something that interests you? Is it a new area that you want to get into (be sure you are capable)? Will the work make you a better artist?

* **Other people:** Have you worked with other members of the team before and if so, was the team successful? Have other members of the team been recommended? Do you need to interview other people and if so, does their portfolio demonstrate a compatible approach to the production?

Negotiations

Once you have assessed the above factors and decided the production is of interest, you must negotiate your appointment. This will require your communication skills to be at their very best. Always be pleasant and tactful during negotiations, but don't be a 'pushover'. You should know what you want and what you can concede. For example, know what your costs are so that you can set a minimum fee in your own mind. If you have worked with the employer or client before, use the previous agreement as a basis. If you did a good job, try to improve the current agreement on the strength of this. You should also be aware of where your position is weak, for example are there a number of other make-up artists capable of doing the work and for less money? Be honest about your abilities and emphasise where you have a special expertise. This will help give an impression of your 'worth'.

If the negotiations go badly or you decide you are unavailable, you must relay this information carefully. Be courteous and apologetic and give clear reasons why you have declined the offer, for example the work might clash with another commitment. Never just say 'it wasn't worth doing'! Say that you would like to be considered for future opportunities and suggest a colleague who may wish to take the job instead.

Acceptance

If you decide to accept the work, you must then agree the content of the contract, known as the 'terms and conditions'. You should always make sure the agreement you have reached, verbally or otherwise, is confirmed within the contract. Ensure that both parties are left in no doubt as to the type of job being undertaken and what is required of the make-up artist. Be very specific on timescales and agree detailed programmes if possible. If there are key dates, make sure they are recorded and agree what will happen if dates are missed, i.e. extensions of time allowed, reductions in fee, etc. Always set an end date to the agreement.

As part of the negotiations will undoubtedly have included the subject of money, it is now time to record what was agreed. It is worthwhile stating not just the total cost of the work but also how this was calculated and how any extra costs are dealt with. The fee calculation should make reference to:

* whether the fee is an all-inclusive lump sum to be paid at the end of the job

* whether the fee is a percentage of the total production cost – if the production gets a bigger budget you may get a bigger fee for the extra work involved

* whether the fee is time charged and based on an agreed hourly rate

* whether there will be extra money if there are changes to the brief or timescales

* whether payment is to be staged and what the intervals will be

* how long after the date of the invoice payment will be made (this can be up to 60 days).

The contract

When one thinks of a contract, the image of a hefty legal document springs to mind. In fact, contracts can range from lengthy documents to just a single page. The extent of the document will depend on the size and value of the work being agreed upon. A single day's work for a relatively small sum of money will not require a weighty set of terms and conditions. Conversely, a production worth several thousand pounds should not be agreed on the back of an envelope!

The effectiveness of the contract will stem from whether it states the important issues that have been agreed during negotiations, namely the 'terms'. It is advisable that these include the following.

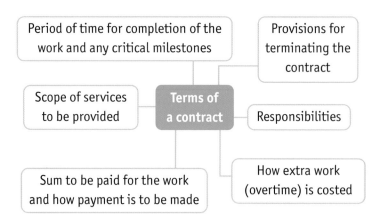

Whilst a simple exchange of letters, including confirmation of the above, should be sufficient for many jobs, you may well be asked to sign a more comprehensive document. This will be the case particularly when working for a large organisation that is likely to use a standard contract drawn up by solicitors. Whilst this might seem daunting, you should welcome the document as it should leave no room for doubt about what is expected of both parties. If you are asked to provide a contract by an inexperienced client, try to obtain a standard form that has been approved by the industry. Standard contract forms should be available from unions, insurers, etc.

Once you have checked that the contract correctly states the terms listed above, you should check the 'small print', known as the 'conditions'. You may find that some contracts are easy to understand. However, if you are ever in any doubt as to the meaning of any conditions, *do not sign the contract* until their meaning has been fully explained to you, preferably through consultation with a solicitor. You should be aware that once you have signed a contract you are deemed to have agreed with its content. 'Not understanding' what you have signed will not be a good defence if things go wrong and you find yourself in legal difficulties.

It is important that the contract conditions do not contravene the laws that affect the work of a make-up artist. These include:

* health and safety legislation
* employment law
* working time directives
* workplace regulations.

If you do discover that the contract contains conditions that you cannot or must not agree to, you should mark this clearly on the document (known as 'red-lining') and raise the issue with the other party. You should sign your name against the change and ensure that the other party does the same. Never amend a standard contract form without gaining legal advice as you might be changing the meaning of other clauses without realising it.

Once you are confident that the terms and conditions are satisfactory, you should confirm your acceptance. This is normally done by signing and dating two copies of the contract then sending them both to the other party, who will sign both copies and send one copy back to you for your records. Make sure that both copies are identical and that any amendments are recorded and signed on both.

The signed contract, once back in your possession, is a very important document. It protects you should things go wrong during the production as it confirms the obligations of the other party, to which they have agreed. Therefore, it is very important that your copy of the contract is kept safe. Keep the contract where you can find it but in a location where it will not get damaged or thrown away by mistake. Ideally, it should be held in a locked filing cabinet. Remember, the bigger the production, the bigger the value and the more important the contract.

Knowledge Check

1. List some methods of reaching your target audience when marketing yourself to potential clients.

2. Explain how to acquire resources to implement action plans.

3. Identify the global issues that may affect the success of marketing strategies.

4. How can you improve your chances of obtaining work?

5. Explain how you could contribute to the financial effectiveness of a production, photo shoot or retail outlet

6. Discuss the four main areas of impact that the Working Time Directive 1998 has had on employment law.

7. Discuss methods of monitoring stock levels.

8. List the ways in which waste of stock can be avoided.

9. What does CPD stand for?

10. List ways in which you could contribute to your CPD.

Index for Make-up Artistry

The following bonus information can be found on the
Make-Up Artistry website at **www.heinemann.co.uk**:

✳ Qualification mapping tables
✳ Working in the theatre
✳ Working in film and television
✳ First Aid
✳ Colour psychology
✳ The history of fashion and make-up before the
    20th century
✳ More business for make-up artists

Photo acknowledgements
All photographs by Gareth Boden or Julia Conway
except:
ADF Management: pages 179, 181
Conde Nast: page 6
Corbis: pages 2, 3, 245, 246
Amanda Duxbury: pages 229, 233, 255
Samantha Higgins: page 233
Sandi Hodgkinson: page 184
Kobal: page 76
Pilal Lannon: pages 78, 232
Louisa Morgan: pages 229, 231, 233
Gerald Murray: pages 96, 224, 324
Joanne Price: page 329
Shu Uemura and Kiehls: page 164
Mark Tasker: cover; pages 112, 297, 335, 338
A J Wilkinson: pages 294, 295, 297, 381, 351